EXAMINATION REVIEW FOR

MEDICAL TECHNOLOGY

Edited by

NEVILLE J. BRYANT, A.R.T., F.A.C.B.S.

Serological Services Ltd,
Toronto, Ontario, Canada

W. B. SAUNDERS COMPANY

Philadelphia • London • Toronto • Mexico City • Rio de Janeiro • Sydney • Tokyo

Tony Travis

W. B. Saunders Company: West Washington Square
Philadelphia, PA 19105

1 St. Anne's Road
Eastbourne, East Sussex BN21 3UN, England

1 Goldthorne Avenue
Toronto, Ontario M8Z 5T9, Canada

Apartado 26370—Cedro 512
Mexico 4, D.F., Mexico

Rua Coronel Cabrita, 8
Sao Cristovao Caixa Postal 21176
Rio de Janeiro, Brazil

9 Waltham Steet
Artarmon, N.S.W. 2064, Australia

Ichibancho, Central Bldg., 22-1 Ichibancho
Chiyoda-Ku Tokyo 102, Japan

Library of Congress Cataloging in Publication Data

Bryant, Neville J.

Examination review for medical technology.

1. Medical technology—Examinations, questions, etc.
I. Title.   [DNLM; 1. Technology, Medical—Examination
questions. QY 18 B915e]

RB37.B83 1983   616.07′5′076   83-43013

ISBN 0-7216-2165-1 (pbk.)

Examination Review for Medical Technology   ISBN 0–7216–2165–1

Last digit is the print number: 9   8   7   6   5   4   3   2

CONTRIBUTORS

PETER K. HUGGARD, A.R.T.,A.N.Z.I.M.L.T.
Chief Technologist
Division of Clinical Chemistry
The Hospital for Sick Children
Toronto, Ontario, Canada

J. BARRY ATKINSON, A.R.T.,F.I.M.L.T.
Chief Technologist
Hematology – Oncology
The Hospital for Sick Children
Toronto, Ontario, Canada

SHARON LAYNE, M.Sc.
Chief Technologist
Microbiology
Toronto Western Hospital
Toronto, Ontario, Canada

NEVILLE J. BRYANT, A.R.T.,F.A.C.B.S.
Technical Director
Serological Services Ltd.
Toronto, Ontario, Canada

GEORGE L. MUNROE, F.I.M.L.S.
Chief Technologist
Laboratory and Nuclear Medicine
York Finch General Hospital
Toronto, Ontario, Canada

ACKNOWLEDGMENTS

Special thanks are due to many friends and colleagues who in one way or another contributed to the preparation of this book. In particular, I would like to thank Mrs Patricia O'Brien, who typed the entire manuscript, and who was always patient and enthusiastic in the task.

Thanks are also due to my staff at Serological Services who helped so much with the final preparation of the manuscript, and to Baxter Venable of W. B. Saunders who is a constant source of encouragement and support.

Neville Bryant

PREFACE

The purpose of this book is to act as a study companion
for students of Medical Technology - to provide appropriate examination questions and explanatory answers
so that the student can test his/her knowledge of the
various subjects. The book covers the five essential
areas of study - Chemistry, Microbiology, Hematology,
Immunohematology and Histopathology.

It should be stressed that this book does not preclude the
study of other texts related to Medical Technology. A
list of references has therefore been provided with each
section so that the student may find explanations of the
sections that he/she finds difficult or confusing.

The purpose of this book, can be more correctly
stated, therefore, as a means to identify areas of difficulty, so that the student may be guided in his/her knowledge and directed towards those aspects of the subject
that require additional effort.

Neville J Bryant

CONTENTS

CLINICAL CHEMISTRY

PETER K. HUGGARD
A.R.T.,A.N.Z.I.M.L.T
Chief Technologist
Division of Clinical Chemistry
THE HOSPITAL FOR SICK CHILDREN
TORONTO, ONTARIO, CANADA

The following values have been used in calculations in the text.

Molecular weight

Glucose	180
Bilirubin	585
Creatinine	113
Calcium	40
Phosphorus	31
Uric Acid	168
Cholesterol	387

Atomic weight

Barium	137.3
Chlorine	35.5
Hydrogen	1
Oxygen	16
Sodium	23
Sulphur	32

QUESTIONS

SECTION A: MULTIPLE CHOICE

Select the phrase, sentence or symbol which completes the statement or answers the question. More than one answer may be correct in each case.

1. Alkalosis can result from:
   (a) hyperventilation
   (b) acute vomiting
   (c) hypoventilation
   (d) (a) and (b) are correct

2. Factors governing the rate of enzyme reactions are:
   (a) hydrogen ion concentration
   (b) temperature
   (c) substrate concentration
   (d) cofactors
   (e) all of the above

3. A cerebrospinal fluid sample (CSF) obtained from the lumbar region of the spine was analyzed and the following results obtained. Indicate the abnormal result.

   (a) Glucose 70 mg/dl
   (b) Protein 65 mg/dl
   (c) Appearance: clear and colorless
   (d) Total cell count: 1 WBC/mm^3

4. If a patient has been on a diet containing 60 - 150 g of fat/day, the normal fat excretion in a 3-day stool sample is:
   (a) $<$ 15 g/day
   (b) $>$ 20 g/day
   (c) $<$ 6 g/day
   (d) none of the above

5. The Leiberman-Burchardt cholesterol reaction is one which is based on:
   (a) an enzymatic reaction with glycerol
   (b) a reaction with sulphuric acid and acetic anhydride
   (c) a reaction with alcoholic potassium hydroxide (KOH)
   (d) separation by gas chromatography

1

6. Mature fetal lungs have a lecithin-sphingomyelin (L/S) ratio in amniotic fluid of:
   (a) > 5.0
   (b) 1.0 - 1.5
   (c) < 1.0
   (d) > 2.0

7. A lack of the enzyme phytanate alpha-oxidase and subsequent build-up of phytanic acid is seen in:
   (a) Tay-Sachs disease
   (b) Gaucher's disease
   (c) Fabry's disease
   (d) Refsum's disease

8. A typical phospholipid found in human serum is:
   (a) lysophosphatidyl choline
   (b) phosphatidyl ethanola-mine
   (c) sphingomyelin
   (d) all of the above

9. Which of the following are characteristic of IgG in serum?
   (a) It has a concentration 600 - 1800 mg/dl
   (b) It shows major anti-bacterial activity
   (c) It has a Svedberg co-efficient of 19S
   (d) It has a half-life of 23 days

10. A serum bilirubin concentration of 16.0 mg/dl expressed in System International (S.I.) units is:
    (a) 274 mol/l
    (b) 278 mol/l
    (c) 176 mol/l
    (d) 400 mol/l

11. The following results were obtained on a patient:

    Serum creatinine 1.8 mg/dl

    Urine creatinine 60 mg/dl
    24 hour urine volume 900 ml

    The creatinine clearance on this patient is:
    (a) 100 ml/min
    (b) 53 ml/min
    (c) 500 ml/min
    (d) 21 ml/min

12. A bilirubin solution gave an absorbance of 0.468 when measured in a 1 cm light path curette at 450 nm. The concentration of the bilirubin solution was 4.53 mg/l. What is the molar extinction coefficient?
    (a) 30300
    (b) 6.05×10^3
    (c) 12100
    (d) 60500

13. One Torr is equal in pressure to:
    (a) 1 atmosphere at sea level
    (b) 760 atmospheres at sea level
    (c) 1/760 of an atmosphere at sea level
    (d) none of the above

14. The pk value of the hydrogen ion concentration in normal blood at 37°C is:
    (a) 1.9
    (b) 3.0
    (c) 6.0
    (d) 6.10

15. Oxygen moves into the blood from the lungs by the action of:
    (a) hemoglobin affinity
    (b) osmosis
    (c) passive diffusion
    (d) active diffusion

16. What would be the likely blood

ethanol concentration in a
patient who did not have increased tolerance to ethanol,
and exhibited the symptoms
of euphoria, loss of inhibitions and prolonged reaction
times?
   (a)   200 - 300 mg/dl
   (b)   100 - 150 mg/dl
   (c)   Above 400 mg/dl
   (d)   20 - 50 mg/dl

17. An electrophoretic separation
     and integration of serum pro-
     teins on a patient show that
     the globulins comprise 71 per
     cent of the total proteins.
     If the total serum protein
     is 6.7 g/dl, what is the con-
     centration of albumin?
        (a)   3.4 g/dl
        (b)   1.9 g/dl
        (c)   4.8 g/dl
        (d)   None of the above

18. The final color formed by the
     copper reduction method for
     urine sugar is:
        (a)   blue
        (b)   orange-red
        (c)   brown
        (d)   none of the above

19. When making a microscopic
     examination of feces, which
     of the following may be
     found in a normal sample?
        (a)   A few epithelial cells
        (b)   Occasional white blood
              cells
        (c)   Neutral fat globules
        (d)   All of the above

20. A 1 hour basal acid level of
     $>$ 20 mEq in a gastric aspir-
     ation usually indicates:
        (a)   a normal result
        (b)   gastric ulcer
        (c)   duodenal ulcer
        (d)   Zollinger-Ellison syn-
              drome

21. The protein concentration
     of a transudate is:
        (a) $>$ 50 g/l
        (b) $<$ 1.0 g/dl
        (c) $<$ 30 g/l
        (d)   6 - 8 g/dl

22. In cystic fibrosis the
     sweat chloride concentra-
     tion is:
        (a)   usually $>$ 70 mEq/l
        (b)   40 - 60 mEq/l
        (c) $>$ 120 mEq/l
        (d)   equal to the plasma
              chloride concentra-
              tion

23. Which of the following
     tests on amniotic fluid
     may be used to assess fetal
     lung maturity?
        (a)   "Shake" or "Foam"
              test
        (b)   Nile-blue stain of
              fetal squamous cells
        (c)   Creatinine concentra-
              tion
        (d)   All of the above

24. Which of the following
     sets of results correspond
     to normal findings in syno-
     vial fluid?
        (a)   Clear and straw-
              colored, fibrin clot
              usually absent, mucin
              clot good
        (b)   Clear and colorless,
              fibrin clot absent,
              mucin clot good
        (c)   Turbid yellow, fibrin
              clot present, mucin
              clot fair to poor
        (d)   Xanthochromic, fibrin
              clot usually absent,
              mucin clot variable

25. Seminal fluid analysis in
     a normal male will usually
     show the following results:
        (a)   volume 5 ml, sperm

count 10^6 sperm/ml
(b) volume 1.5 ml, 8 x 10^7 sperm/ml
(c) 9 x 10^7 sperm/ml, volume 4 ml
(d) 70 per cent of sperm motile, 60 per cent of normal morphology

26. Normal alkaline urine may contain which of the following crystals?
    (a) Ammonium biurate
    (b) Triple phosphate
    (c) Amorphous phosphates
    (d) Calcium oxalate

27. Which of the following is a definition of specific gravity?
    (a) A measure of the number of solute particles per unit of solvent
    (b) The ratio of the weight of a given volume of solution to an equal volume of water at a specified temperature
    (c) The ratio of the velocity of light in air to the velocity of light in solution

28. A molal solution:
    (a) contains 1 mole of the solute in 1000 g of solvent
    (b) contains 1 gram-equivalent weight of the solute in 1 liter of solution
    (c) contains 1 mole of the solute in 1000 ml of solvent
    (d) none of the above

29. Twenty-five grams of $BaCl_2 \cdot 2H_2O$ is equivalent to what weight of $BaCl_2$?
    (a) 29.32 g
    (b) 1.17 g

(c) 21.32 g
(d) 0.853 g

Atomic Weights:
Ba   137.3
Cl   35.5
H   1
O   16

30. The standard error of a population of values can be calculated by the formula:
    (a) $S\sqrt{N}$
    (b) $\dfrac{\sqrt{N}}{S}$
    (c) $\dfrac{S}{\bar{x}}$
    (d) $\dfrac{S}{\sqrt{N}}$

31. The relative centrifugal force for a centrifuge with a rotating radius of 12 cm and a starting speed of 8000 r.p.m. is:
    (a) 103034
    (b) 0.0119
    (c) 8586
    (d) none of the above

32. In a series of numbers, the mode is:
    (a) equal to the middle value
    (b) equal to the sum of the values divided by the number of values
    (c) equal to the most frequently occurring value
    (d) equal to the standard deviation of the series divided by the mean

33. An ideal analytical procedure should be:
    (a) accurate
    (b) precise
    (c) sensitive
    (d) specific

34. Which of the following vitamins are fat soluble?
    (a) A
    (b) K
    (c) E
    (d) C

35. Which of the following chemicals have been used as substrates in alkaline phosphatase assays?
    (a) p-nitrophenylphosphate
    (b) β-glycerophosphate
    (c) Phenylphosphate
    (d) Phenolphthalein monophosphate

36. Serum contains an enzyme which migrates electrophorectically as an alpha$_2$-globulin, is a metalloprotein, and catalyzes the oxidation of p-phenylenediamine by oxygen to a purple-colored compound. What is the enzyme?
    (a) Cholinesterase
    (b) Transferrin
    (c) Ferritin
    (d) Ceruloplasmin

37. Which lactate dehydrogenase isoenzyme is the predominant one in lung tissue?
    (a) LD_1
    (b) LD_1 and LD_2
    (c) LD_5
    (d) LD_3

38. Which of the following biochemical abnormalities are seen in Wilson's disease?
    (a) Increased cystine and lysine in urine
    (b) Decreased cystathionine synthetase in liver
    (c) Disorder in copper metabolism
    (d) Increased serum CK

39. Aspartate aminotransferase (AST) catalyzes the reaction between L-aspartate and alpha-oxoglutarate to form:
    (a) L-alanine, alpha-oxoglutarate
    (b) pyruvate, L-glutamate
    (c) oxalacetate, L-glutamate
    (d) pyruvate, oxaloacetate

40. Free bilirubin in the serum is attached to:
    (a) alpha$_2$-globulin
    (b) beta-globulin
    (c) albumin
    (d) gamma-globulin

41. Which of the following criteria must be met to make a diagnosis of cystic fibrosis?
    (a) Characteristic lung pathology
    (b) Pancreatic insufficiency
    (c) Increased sweat electrolytes
    (d) Family history

42. Which components can be used as voltage sources in instruments?
    (a) Photocell
    (b) Thermocouple
    (c) Quartz crystal
    (d) All of the above

43. A micron is:
    (a) 10^{-6} m
    (b) 10^{-6} cm
    (c) 10^8 m
    (d) none of the above

44. An Allen correction is:
    (a) an adjustment made to correct Na measurements made by a specific ion electrode to flame results
    (b) a special hexagonal wrench
    (c) the allowance for body surface area in clearance calculations

(d) a correction for interfering substances in
spectrophotometric
measurements

45. Narrow bandpass filters are
desirable in flame photometry
because:
(a) they stop interfering
substances affecting
the results
(b) they are cheap to manufacture
(c) they isolate emission
energy at a given wave-
length
(d) they are not affected
by the heat of the flame

46. The rate of migration in an
electrophoretic system depends
on the:
(a) net charge on the molecule and strength of
the electric field
(b) the size and shape of
the molecule
(c) the nature of the sup-
porting medium
(d) temperature of operation

47. When a solute is dissolved in
a solvent which of the following occur?
(a) The osmotic pressure is
increased
(b) The vapor pressure of
the solution is lowered
below that of the pure
solvent
(c) The boiling point of
the solution is raised
above that of the pure
solvent
(d) The freezing point of
the solution is lowered
below that of the pure
solvent

48. Which of the following detec-

tors have successfully been
used on a gas chromatograph?
(a) Thermal conductivity
detector
(b) Flame ionization
detector
(c) Electron capture
detector
(d) All of the above

49. Mass number is represented
by the letter:
(a) H
(b) N
(c) A
(d) Z

50. Which of the following cause
an increase in blood glucose?
(a) Growth hormone
(b) Epinephrine
(c) Insulin
(d) Thyroxine

51. Which of the following is
the formula for glyceraldehyde?
(a) - CHOH - COH
(b)
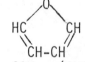
(c) $COH - (CHOH)_4 - CH_2OH$
(d) $COH - CHOH - CH_2OH$

52. Which of the following is
the formula for cysteine?
(a)
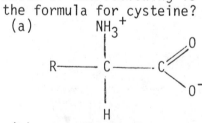
(b) CH_3CHNH_2COOH
(c) $S - CH_2CHNH_2COOH$
       |
       $S - CH_2CHNH_2COOH$
(d) $HSCH_2CHNH_2COOH$

53. Which of the following numerical
prefixes describes the term

femto?
(a) 10^{12}
(b) 10^{-12}
(c) 10^{-9}
(d) 10^{-15}

54. Which of the following is a site of action of prolactin?
(a) Mammary gland
(b) Liver
(c) Symphysis pubis
(d) Thyroid

55. The suffix for a saturated hydrocarbon is:
(a) - ane
(b) - ene
(c) - ol
(d) - one

56. Which of the following groups of enzymes participate in the biogenesis of steroid hormones?
(a) Dehydrogenases
(b) Isomerases
(c) Desmolases
(d) Hydroxylases

57. Which of the following metabolites of cortisol are measured by Porter-Silber methodologies?
(a) Cortolone
(b) Tetrahydrocortisol
(c) 11-keto-etiocholanolone
(d) Cortisone

58. Calculate the osmolality given the following plasma chemistry results:

Na 132 mmol/l   BUN 7 mmol/l
K 6.7 mmol/l   Glucose 16.0 mmol/l
Cl 86 mmol/l HCO_3^- 11 mmol/l

(a) 300.4 mosmol/kg
(b) 308.4 mosmol/kg
(c) 339.4 mosmol/kg
(d) 293.4 mosmol/kg

59. False negative results in a urinary pregnancy test (qualitative human chorionic gonadotrophin (HCG) measurement) can occur when:
(a) the urine is dilute
(b) there is an ectopic pregnancy
(c) there is excess protein in the urine
(d) missed abortion has occurred

60. In the insulin tolerance test (0.1 unit/kg body weight I.V.) increased tolerance may be found in:
(a) Diabetes mellitus
(b) Cushing's syndrome
(c) Pancreatic islet cell tumor
(d) Cases where the blood glucose falls less than 25 per cent and returns rapidly to the fasting level

61. Which of the following drugs may cause urine vanillylmandelic acid (VMA) to be increased in fluorometric and/or colorimetric assay procedures?
(a) Aspirin
(b) Penicillin
(c) Oxytetracycline
(d) Monoamine oxidase (MAO) inhibitors

62. In the laboratory investigation of ovarian function, which of the following are found?
(a) Pituitary gonadotrophins are increased in menopause
(b) 17-ketosteroids (17 KS) are increased in virilizing ovarian tumors
(c) Pregnanediol is decreased in amenorrhoea
(d) Estrogens are increased in primary ovarian hypo-

function

63. Which of the following are true for nephrogenic diabetes insipidus?
    (a) Low urine specific gravity
    (b) Urine output 2 - 4 liters/24 hours
    (c) Urine becomes concentrated when fluids are withheld
    (d) No change in urine volume due to hypertonic NaCl I.V.

64. Which of the following calcium and phosphorus results are found in primary hyperparathyroidism?
    (a) Serum calcium increased and urine calcium decreased
    (b) Serum phosphorus decreased
    (c) Urine phosphorus increased
    (d) Serum and urine calcium levels increased

65. In T_3 thyrotoxicosis, which of the following are found?
    (a) Increased thyroid - stimulating hormone (thyrotrophin) (TSH)
    (b) Decreased thyroxine binding globulin (TBG)
    (c) Normal T_4
    (d) Decreased serum cholesterol

66. Sodium is completely reabsorbed in the kidneys when the level in the plasma falls below:
    (a) 125 mmol/l
    (b) 115 mmol/l
    (c) 100 mmol/l
    (d) 110 mmol/l

67. Calcium is present in the serum in which of the following forms?
    (a) Nondiffusible protein-bound calcium
    (b) Diffusible free ionized calcium
    (c) Diffusible free complexed calcium
    (d) All of the above

68. In the determination of serum magnesium by the Titan yellow method, polyvinyl alcohol is added to:
    (a) increase the sensitivity of the method
    (b) bind phosphates
    (c) provide colloidal particles for dye adsorption
    (d) keep the magnesium hydroxide in solution

69. Iron is mainly absorbed from the:
    (a) stomach
    (b) duodenum
    (c) jejunum
    (d) colon

70. What is the anion gap in a patient with the following blood results?

    Na^+ 139 mmol/l
    K^+ 6.0 mmol/l
    Cl^- 104 mmol/l
    HCO_3^- 16 mmol/l
    pH 7.29
    Ca^{++} 2.7 mmol/l
    Total protein 60 g/l

    (a) 21.7 mmol/l
    (b) 27.7 mmol/l
    (c) 19.0 mmol/l
    (d) 35.0 mmol/l

71. A protein concentration in

plasma of 6.5 g/dl is equivalent to what level of anion concentrations in mmol ion charge/l?
(a) 16
(b) 14.63
(c) 13
(d) 20

72. Given the following plasma results, calculate the per cent saturation:

Plasma iron 125 μg/dl
Unsaturated iron-binding capacity (UIBC) 185 μg/dl
Transferrin 320 mg/dl

(a) 40 per cent
(b) 68 per cent
(c) 39 per cent
(d) 58 per cent

73. Which of the following anticoagulants inhibits thrombin?
(a) Trisodium citrate
(b) Ammonium/potassium oxalate
(c) EDTA
(d) Heparin

74. In intrahepatic jaundice the following test results are found:
(a) feces: urobilin decreased
urine: bilirubin positive
serum: unconjugated bilirubin increased
(b) feces: urobilin decreased or negative
urine: urobilinogen decreased or negative
serum: increased conjugated bilirubin
(c) feces: urobilin increased
urine: bilirubin normal
serum: conjugated bilirubin normal or slightly increased
(d) none of the above

75. Which of the following cannot be used as an anticoagulant in a blood sample collected for uric acid determination by the phosphotungstic acid method?
(a) EDTA
(b) Heparin
(c) Potassium oxalate
(d) None of the above

76. In the Technicon Autoanalyzer[R] procedure using diacetyl monoxime for blood urea nitrogen (BUN) measurement, the addition of thiosemicarbazide serves to:
(a) remove ammonia from the system
(b) intensify the color of the reaction product
(c) deproteinize
(d) help urease hydrolysis

77. In the D-xylose tolerance test, 25 g of D-xylose is given orally in water. A 5-hour urine and bloods at 1/2, 1 and 2 hour intervals are collected. The results are usually found to be normal in:
(a) Postgastrectomy state
(b) Steatorrhoea due to pancreatic disease
(c) Malabsorption in the jejunum
(d) Cirrhosis of the liver

78. An inulin clearance test is limited in its clinical application because it is:
(a) time consuming
(b) uncomfortable to the patient
(c) expensive
(d) all of the above

79. In prerenal azotemia the:
    (a) urine:serum creatinine ratio is greater than 14:1
    (b) urine sodium is less than 10 mEq/l
    (c) urine urea:BUN ratio is greater than 14:1
    (d) the urine sediment is normal

80. At sea level, room air has the following pCO_2 and pO_2 values:
    (a) pCO_2 0 mmHg, pO_2 100 mmHg
    (b) pCO_2 40 mmHg, pO_2 100 mmHg
    (c) pCO_2 40 mmHg, pO_2 150 mmHg
    (d) pCO_2 0 mmHg, pO_2 150 mmHg

81. Which of the following is the electrical symbol for a half wave rectifier?

    (a)

    (b)

    (c)

    (d)

82. Calculate the low density lipoprotein cholesterol given the following test results:

    Triglyceride (TG) 263 mg/dl
    Total cholesterol (C) 218 mg/dl
    High density lipoprotein cholesterol (HDLC) 37 mg/dl

    (a) 90 mg/dl
    (b) 181 mg/dl
    (c) 128 mg/dl
    (d) 158 mg/dl

83. In the method for 5-hydroxy-indole acetic acid (5-HIAA)

determination in urine, using 1-nitroso-2-naphthol and nitrous acid as the color reagents, keto acids are removed by:
    (a) extracting into chloroform
    (b) forming phenylhydrazones
    (c) extracting into ethyl acetate
    (d) adsorbing them onto alumina

84. Which of the following amino acids contain sulphur?
    (a) Cystine
    (b) Cysteine
    (c) Methionine
    (d) Ornithine

85. The total pressure of a mixture of gases is equal to the sum of the partial pressures exerted by each of the component gases. This is the law of:
    (a) Boyle
    (b) Charles
    (c) Dalton
    (d) Beer

86. The Porter-Silber reaction requires the presence of which chemical structure?
    (a) Aromatic ring
    (b) 17 keto-
    (c) 17, 21-dihydroxy-20-keto
    (d) 11 oxy-

87. Sudan III is used to stain:
    (a) glycoprotein
    (b) lipid
    (c) protein
    (d) LDH isoenzymes

88. An isobestic point is a point where:
    (a) proteins have a net negative charge
    (b) proteins are neutral

(c) two spectra absorption curves for two pigments intersect

(d) an enzyme reaction becomes linear

89. The name Kjeldahl is associated with what assay or technique?
    (a) Electrophoresis
    (b) Bilirubin assay
    (c) Protein nitrogen assay
    (d) Ultracentrifugation

90. The measurement of $Hb-A_{1C}$ may be useful in the investigation of:
    (a) sickle cell anemia
    (b) hemolytic anemia
    (c) diabetes mellitus
    (d) hemochromatosis

91. δ-Aminolevulinic acid is the direct precursor of:
    (a) porphyrins
    (b) cholesterol
    (c) methyl dopa
    (d) phenylalanine

92. Prostatic acid phosphatase can be inhibited by:
    (a) fluoride
    (b) manganese
    (c) tartrate
    (d) citrate

93. In examining *normal* oral glucose tolerance test results, the 2-hour blood sample level is usually:
    (a) equal to the 1-hour level
    (b) higher than the fasting level
    (c) lower or equal to the fasting level
    (d) higher than the 1-hour level

94. In severe hemolytic jaundice, which of the following test results are usually found?

(a) urine: urobilinogen increased, bilirubin positive
    feces: urobilin decreased
    blood: increased unconjugated bilirubin

(b) Urine: urobilinogen normal, bilirubin negative
    feces: urobilin normal
    blood: increased conjugated bilirubin

(c) Urine: urobilinogen large increase
    feces: urobilin large increase
    blood: increased unconjugated bilirubin

(d) Urine: increased bilirubin
    feces: urobilin negative
    blood: increased conjugated bilirubin

95. In the red blood cell, the enzyme carbonic anhydrase catalyzes:
    (a) the exchange of bicarbonate ion for chloride ion
    (b) the formation of carbonic acid from CO_2 and H_2O
    (c) the reaction of oxygen with reduced Hb
    (d) the reaction with the proteinate ion

96. If in a population study, the mean potassium was found to be 4.30 mEq/l, if 1 standard deviation (SD) was found to be 0.15, what percentage of the population will have a value greater than 4.6 mEq/l?
    (a) 97.5 per cent
    (b) 4.6 per cent
    (c) 2.3 per cent
    (d) 68.2 per cent

97. The point at which proteins carry a net zero electric charge is called the:
    (a) isobestic point
    (b) point of electrophoretic neutrality
    (c) isoelectric point
    (d) none of the above

98. In uncompensated metabolic acidosis, the following would be observed:
    (a) pH decreased, HCO_3^- increased
    (b) pH decreased, HCO_3^- decreased
    (c) pH increased, HCO_3^- decreased
    (d) pH increased, HCO_3^- increased

99. In an acute myocardial infarction, the enzyme that first shows elevated activity is:
    (a) lactate dehydrogenase (LD)
    (b) alkaline phosphatase (ALP)
    (c) creatine kinase (CK)
    (d) alanine aminotransferase (ALT)

100. The reagent used in Pandy's test for measuring excess globulin in cerebrospinal fluid (CSF) is:
    (a) Trichloroacetic acid
    (b) Sulphosalicylic acid
    (c) Phenol
    (d) none of the above

101. Triglyceride is the main constituent of:
    (a) Chylomicron
    (b) beta-lipoprotein
    (c) prebeta-lipoprotein
    (d) (a) and (c) are correct

102. Which of the following migrate in the alpha-1-globulin region when serum proteins undergo electrophoresis?
    (a) Lipoprotein
    (b) Thyroxine binding globulin (TBG)
    (c) Haptoglobin
    (d) Glycoprotein

103. A plasma glucose concentration 180 mg/dl expressed in S.I. units is:
    (a) 1.0 mmol/l
    (b) 9.0 mmol/l
    (c) 10.0 mmol/l
    (d) 100.0 mmol/l

104. The normal bicarbonate ion to carbonic acid ratio in the body is:
    (a) 20:1
    (b) 1:10
    (c) 1:20
    (d) 5:12

105. The rate of oxidation of methanol compared to the rate for ethanol is:
    (a) the same
    (b) less
    (c) more

106. The two enzymes used in the Clinistix(R) test strip for urine glucose are:
    (a) glucose dehydrogenase, glucose oxidase
    (b) glucose oxidase, peroxidase
    (c) glucose dehydrogenase, peroxidase
    (d) none of the above

107. If a patient has normal intestinal mucosa and a normal length of intestine, what are the prerequisites for absorption of fat?
    (a) Pancreatic lipase
    (b) Conjugated bile salts
    (c) Alkaline intestinal pH

(d) All of the above

108. An exudate has an exudate
      protein to serum protein
      ratio of:
      (a) 1:1
      (b) > 0.6
      (c) < 0.2
      (d) 2:1

109. Which of the following tests
      may sometimes be used in
      medico-legal investigations
      of seminal fluid origins?
      (a) Acid phosphatase deter-
           minations on vaginal
           aspirations
      (b) The presence of A, B
           or H blood group sub-
           stances in fluids or
           stains on clothing
      (c) The Hektoen Precipitin
           Test
      (d) All of the above

110. Which of the following urinary
      casts would usually form in
      the urine of a patient suf-
      fering from kidney disease
      resulting from diabetes
      mellitus?
      (a) Hyaline
      (b) Granular
      (c) Fatty
      (d) Red blood cell

111. How much 5.0 M H_2SO_4 would
      be required to neutralize
      180 ml of 0.6 N NaOH?
      (a) 21.6 ml
      (b) 0.09 ml
      (c) 10.8 ml
      (d) 20.0 ml

112. Convert 470 mg/dl of Na^+ to
      mEq/l:
      (a) 15.6 mEq/l
      (b) 204 mEq/l
      (c) 0.5 mEq/l
      (d) 20.4 mEq/l

113. Thiamine is the chemical
      name for which of the fol-
      lowing vitamins?
      (a) Vitamin A
      (b) Vitamin B_2
      (c) Vitamin B_1
      (d) Vitamin D_3

114. Cyanocobalamin is the
      chemical name for which
      of the following vitamins?
      (a) Vitamin K
      (b) Vitamin E
      (c) Vitamin C
      (d) Vitamin B_{12}

115. Serum alkaline phosphatase
      is usually increased in:
      (a) Paget's disease
      (b) Rickets
      (c) Hyperparathyroidism
      (d) Hypophosphatasia

116. Following heating at 56°C
      for 10 minutes of a serum
      sample, the alkaline phos-
      phatase isoenzyme likely
      to be present is:
      (a) liver isoenzyme
      (b) bone isoenzyme
      (c) placental isoenzyme
      (d) intestinal isoenzyme

117. The optimum pH range for
      the prostatic isoenzyme
      of acid phosphatase is:
      (a) 4.2 - 4.6
      (b) 4.8 - 5.1
      (c) 4.2 - 4.4
      (d) 3.8 - 4.1

118. Serum acid phosphatase
      can be increased in:
      (a) Gaucher's disease
      (b) sickle cell disease
      (c) myelocytic leukemia
      (d) carcinoma of the
           prostate

119. Factors involved in

physiological jaundice of the newborn include:
- (a) the rate of production of bilirubin is greater in neonates than in adults
- (b) the level of Y receptor-carrier protein is low in the neonate
- (c) glucuronic acid and uridine diphosphate glucuronyl transferase (UDPGT) are relatively deficient in the neonate
- (d) bilirubin reabsorption from the gut is greater in the neonate than in adults

120. A didymium filter is used to:
- (a) filter out pyrogens in water supplies
- (b) select wavelengths in continuous flow instruments
- (c) verify wavelength settings in broad bandpass instruments
- (d) remove certain interfering chromogens in urine

121. Which serum enzyme may be useful in the differential diagnosis of hepatobiliary disease in pregnancy?
- (a) Alkaline phosphatase
- (b) Gamma-glutamyl transferase
- (c) 5′-Nucleotidase
- (d) Lactic dehydrogenase isoenzymes

122. An automated assay for serum 5′-nucleotidase requires the addition of the metallic ion:
- (a) cobalt
- (b) chromium
- (c) nickel
- (d) manganese

123. Gamma-glutamyl transferase usually exhibits normal serum activity in:
- (a) Paget's disease
- (b) renal failure
- (c) prostatic malignancy
- (d) muscle diseases

124. The temperature of a flame in a flame photometer using a propane/air gas mixture is approximately:
- (a) 3100°C
- (b) 1900°C
- (c) 2850°C
- (d) 2250°C

125. Alpha particles are:
- (a) nuclei of helium atoms
- (b) negatively charged electrons
- (c) positively charged protons
- (d) electromagnetic radiations of very short wavelengths

126. In a continuous flow analyzer, which of the following influence the quantity of solute that passes through the membrane?
- (a) The duration of contact of the two solutions
- (b) The area of contact
- (c) The temperature at which the dialysis occurs
- (d) All of the above

127. In copper reduction methods for glucose analysis, the reaction depends on:
- (a) the time and temperature of heating
- (b) the concentration of

reagents
- (c) the alkalinity
- (d) all of the above

128. The Rosalki and Tarlow method for the determination of gamma-glutamyl transferase uses which of the following substrates?
- (a) Gamma-glutamyl-amino-proprionitrile
- (b) Gamma-glutamyl-gamma-naphthylamine
- (c) Gamma-glutamyl-p-nitroanilide
- (d) None of the above

129. Amylase in human serum has a pH optimum at:
- (a) 8.3 - 8.5
- (b) 6.9 - 7.0
- (c) 4.8 - 5.1
- (d) 10.0 - 10.2

130. Calcitonin is produced by which endocrine gland?
- (a) Ovary
- (b) Thyroid
- (c) Anterior pituitary
- (d) Posterior pituitary

131. In macroamylasemia, amylase complexes with what protein in the serum?
- (a) IgA
- (b) IgM
- (c) Transcortin
- (d) Haptoglobin

132. The chemical nature of gastrin is such that it is a:
- (a) polypeptide
- (b) glycoprotein
- (c) protein
- (d) nonapeptide

133. Potassium is reabsorbed in the kidney in the:
- (a) narrow descending loop of Henle
- (b) distal convoluted tubule
- (c) proximal convoluted tubule
- (d) wide ascending loop of Henle

134. Which of the following hormones help control serum calcium levels?
- (a) Parathyroid hormone (PTH)
- (b) Thyroxine (T_4)
- (c) Calcitonin
- (d) Vitamin D compounds

135. An amylase method that follows the decrease in substrate (starch) concentration is known as:
- (a) a chrommometric procedure
- (b) a saccharogenic assay
- (c) an amyloclastic method
- (d) a dye-labelled method

136. In adrenogenital syndrome, the most common enzyme deficiency is:
- (a) at the 11-hydroxylation stage
- (b) the lack of side chain degrading enzyme
- (c) the absence of 3-β-ol dehydrogenase
- (d) at the 21-hydroxylation stage

137. Parathyroid hormone is responsible for:
- (a) inhibiting bone re-absorption of calcium
- (b) mobilizing calcium from bone
- (c) increasing the synthesis of 1,25 dihy-droxycholecalciferol ($1,25(OH)_2D_3$)
- (d) increasing renal absorption of calcium

138. Hyperphosphatemia may be found in:
     (a) renal failure
     (b) Fanconi syndrome
     (c) hypoparathyroidism
     (d) hypervitaminosis D

139. In electrophoresis of serum proteins, transferrin migrates with which protein fraction?
     (a) Albumin
     (b) $Alpha_2$-globulin
     (c) $Alpha_1$-globulin
     (d) Beta-globulin

140. In acute pancreatitis, the increase in serum amylase begins in:
     (a) 3 - 6 hours
     (b) 20 - 30 hours
     (c) 48 - 72 hours
     (d) 6 - 10 hours

141. Certain corticosteroids react with phenylhydrazine in the presence of alcohol and sulphuric acid to form a yellow pigment. This reaction is used in what method?
     (a) Guthrie Test
     (b) Berthelot reaction
     (c) Porter-Silber methods
     (d) Lange Test

142. Serum iron will be decreased and total iron binding capacity (TIBC) increased in:
     (a) nephrosis
     (b) hemochromatosis
     (c) iron deficiency anemia
     (d) hepatitis

143. Which of the following have been used as a substrate for lipase activity?
     (a) Corn oil
     (b) β-naphthyl laurate
     (c) N-methylindoxyl myristate
     (d) Olive oil

144. The reaction between 17-ketosteroids and m-dinitrobenzene in alcoholic alkali to produce a reddish-purple color is known as the:
     (a) Liebermann-Burchardt reaction
     (b) Zimmerman reaction
     (c) Neeld-Pearson procedure
     (d) Porter-Silber reaction

145. Most of the copper that is ingested is:
     (a) absorbed by the upper small intestine
     (b) lost through the stool
     (c) transported to the blood to be bound by an $alpha_1$-globulin
     (d) stored in the erythrocytes

146. Which of the following drugs cause a decrease in plasma uric acid?
     (a) Allopurinol
     (b) Probenecid
     (c) Thiazides
     (d) Radiopaque contrast media

147. Which of the following equations are correct versions of the Henderson-Hasselbalch equation?

     (a) $pH = pK - \log \dfrac{(HCO_3^-)}{(CO_2)}$

     (b) $pH = pK + \log \dfrac{Total\ CO_2 - 0.03 pCO_2}{0.03 pCO_2}$

     (c) $pH = pK + \log \dfrac{(HCO_3^-)}{a \times pCO_2}$

     (d) $pH = pK - \log \dfrac{(pCO_2)}{(HCO_3^-)}$

148. Serum lipase is usually increased in:
    (a) acute pancreatitis
    (b) mumps
    (c) perforated peptic ulcer
    (d) opiate induced spasm of pancreatic duct sphincter

149. Luteinizing hormone (LH) has which of the following actions?
    (a) Secretion of progesterone
    (b) Dispersion of pigment granules
    (c) Aids in parturition
    (d) Causes muscle contraction

150. Trypsin activity is stimulated by which of the following ions?
    (a) Calcium
    (b) Magnesium
    (c) Cobalt
    (d) Manganese

151. Parathyroid hormone (PTH) has which of the following actions?
    (a) Glycogenolysis
    (b) Lipogenesis
    (c) Regulates calcium and phosphorus metabolism
    (d) Elevates blood pressure

152. The most important buffer system in plasma is the:
    (a) phosphate buffer system
    (b) protein buffer system
    (c) bicarbonate/carbonic acid buffer system
    (d) hemoglobin buffer system

153. The dibucaine number is a measure of the activity of what enzyme?

    (a) Uropepsin
    (b) Ceruloplasmin
    (c) Cholinesterase
    (d) Sorbitol dehydrogenase

154. Progesterone has which of the following actions?
    (a) Secretion of estrogen
    (b) Inhibition of secretions
    (c) Preparation for ovum implantation
    (d) Initiation of milk secretion

155. Compensatory mechanisms used by the body in acid-base disturbances are:
    (a) blood buffer systems
    (b) respiratory mechanisms
    (c) renal mechanisms
    (d) all of the above

156. Which of the following enzymes is routinely assayed in urine?
    (a) Alkaline phosphatase
    (b) Creatine kinase
    (c) Amylase
    (d) Uricase

157. Low estrogen levels are found at what stage of a 28-day menstrual cycle?
    (a) 12 - 14th day
    (b) Beginning of the cycle
    (c) 20th day
    (d) 24th day

158. The level of glucose in cerebrospinal fluid (CSF) is approximately what fraction of the glucose level in blood?
    (a) 1/2
    (b) Equal to blood
    (c) 2/3
    (d) 1/4

159. In bacterial meningitis

the following cerebrospinal
fluid (CSF) results may be
seen:
  (a) protein increased,
      sugar decreased, white
      blood cell count (WBC)
      increased
  (b) protein increased,
      sugar increased, white
      blood cell count (WBC)
      decreased
  (c) protein decreased,
      sugar decreased, white
      blood cell count (WBC)
      increased
  (d) protein decreased,
      sugar increased, white
      blood cell count (WBC)
      decreased

160. In nephrotic syndrome which
of the following changes are
seen on serum protein electrophoresis?
  (a) Increased $alpha_2$-
      globulin
  (b) Decreased gamma-
      globulin
  (c) Decreased albumin
  (d) All of the above

161. A sudden change in the acid-
base status of a patient
causes which of the following regulatory mechanisms
to respond the quickest to
the change?
  (a) Respiratory mechanism
  (b) Renal mechanism
  (c) Blood buffer system
  (d) None of the above

162. The serum lipoprotein fraction that carries most of the
cholesterol is the:
  (a) alpha-lipoprotein
  (b) beta-lipoprotein
  (c) prebeta-lipoprotein
  (d) chylomicron

163. Possible sources of error in

turbidimetric urine protein
tests are:
  (a) x-ray contrast media
  (b) tolbutamide metabolite
  (c) strongly alkaline
      urine
  (d) all of the above

164. A serum creatinine concentration of 1.7 mg/dl expressed
in S.I. units is:
  (a) 34 mmol/l
  (b) 1.5 mmol/l
  (c) 0.15 mmol/l
  (d) 3.4 mmol/l

165. Ketone bodies may appear in
the urine of:
  (a) diabetics
  (b) hospitalized patients
  (c) people on carbohydrate-
      free diets
  (d) all of the above

166. An increase in serum cholesterol usually occurs in:
  (a) hypothyroidism
  (b) nephrotic syndrome
  (c) obstructive biliary
      tract disease
  (d) all of the above

167. Following myocardial infarction the activity of LD_2
isoenzyme in comparison to
LD_1 isoenzyme is:
  (a) increased
  (b) decreased
  (c) the same

168. The enzyme, Δ^5-3beta-hydroxy
sterol dehydrogenase isomerease,
converts:
  (a) Dehydroepiandrosterone
      sulphate (DHEAS) to
      16-alpha-hydroxy-DHEAS
  (b) 16-alpha-hydroxy-DHEAS to
      16 alpha OH
      dehydroepiandrosterone
      (DHEA)
  (c) 16-alpha-hydroxy-DHEA to

16 alpha OH androstene-
dione
(d) 16 alpha OH androstene
dione to estriol

169. The presence of acetoacetic acid
in a urine sample tested by
the ferric chloride test will
produce which of the following color changes?
(a) Deep gold-yellow or
green
(b) Purple
(c) Red or red-brown
(d) Gray precipitate that
changes to black

170. The presence of homogentisic
acid in a urine sample tested by the ferric chloride
test will produce which of
the following colors?
(a) Blue or green, fades
quickly
(b) Mauve
(c) Purple-pink
(d) Red

171. A serum calcium concentration
of 10 mg/dl expressed in S.I.
units is:
(a) 10.0 mmol/l
(b) 2.5 mmol/l
(c) 5.0 mmol/l
(d) 1.25 mmol/l

172. In the blood, free fatty
acids are carried mostly by:
(a) α_1 globulin
(b) beta-globulin
(c) albumin
(d) gamma-globulin

173. Urinary porphyrins are found
to be increased in most cases
of:
(a) congenital erythropoietic
porphyria
(b) acute intermittent
porphyria
(c) porphyria cutanea tarda

(d) all of the above

174. Detection and quantitation
of ethanol in body fluids
has been successfully
carried out by:
(a) dichromate chemical
reactions
(b) enzymatic analysis
(c) gas chromatography
(d) all of the above

175. The biochemical defect
involved in Gilbert's
disease is:
(a) inhibition of glucuronyl transferase ac-
tivity by a compound
in the mother's serum
(b) defective transport
of direct bilirubin
from the hepatocyte
into the bile canali-
culus
(c) defective transport
of bilirubin from
the plasma to the
hepatocyte
(d) inability to conju-
gate bilirubin

176. Which of the following
enzymes shows an increase
in activity in reconstituted
lyophilized commercial control serum?
(a) Creatine kinase
(b) Amylase
(c) Alkaline phosphatase
(d) Aldolase

177. Increased chorionic gonadotrophins are found in
the urine in:
(a) Seminoma
(b) Chorioepithelioma
of the testicle
(c) Hydatidiform mole
(d) all of the above

178. A serum phosphorus concen-

tration of 4.7 mg/dl ex-
pressed in S.I. units is:
  (a) 2.35 mmol/l
  (b) 9.40 mmol/l
  (c) 4.70 mmol/l
  (d) 1.50 mmol/l

179. Which of the following reagents for the detection
of occult blood in the feces
can give a false-positive
reaction because of meat in
the diet?
  (a) Ortho-toluidine
  (b) Benzidine
  (c) (a) and (b) are correct
  (d) Neither (a) nor (b)

180. The half-life of a drug is
the time required for the
serum concentration of the
drug to:
  (a) decrease to a level
       of half of the dose
       given
  (b) decrease by 50 per
       cent
  (c) produce half the
       required chemical
       response
  (d) reach half the
       required therapeutic
       level

181. The approximate upper limit
in serum for cholesterol in
the 50 yr.[+] age group is:
  (a) 250 mg/dl
  (b) 140 mg/dl
  (c) 320 mg/dl
  (d) none of the above

182. The creatine kinase (CK)
isoenzyme usually found to
be elevated following a myocardial infarction is:
  (a) CK-MM
  (b) CK-MB
  (c) CK-BB
  (d) none of the above

183. Urobilinogen in feces is
decreased in:
  (a) complete biliary
       obstruction
  (b) oral antibiotic
       therapy altering
       intestinal bacterial
       flora
  (c) cachexia
  (d) hemolytic anemias

184. A serum uric acid concentration of 6.7 mg/dl ex-
pressed in S.I. units is:
  (a) 6.7 mmol/l
  (b) 0.40 mmol/l
  (c) 25.08 mmol/l
  (d) 0.04 mmol/l

185. One hour after stimulation
with histamine, a gastric
aspiration with an acid
concentration of 0 mEq
could indicate:
  (a) gastritis
  (b) gastric carcinoma
  (c) achlorhydria
  (d) all of the above

186. The approximate upper limit
in serum for triglyceride
in the 50 yr.[+] age group is:
  (a) 140 mg/dl
  (b) 150 mg/dl
  (c) 190 mg/dl
  (d) none of the above

187. A serum cholesterol concentration of 232 mg/dl ex-
pressed in S.I. units is:
  (a) 6.0 mmol/l
  (b) 1.7 mmol/l
  (c) 12.0 mmol/l
  (d) 0.6 mmol/l

188. The measurement of serum
gastrin may be indicated
in which of the following?
  (a) Patients with re-
       current ulceration
       after surgery for

duodenal ulcer
  (b) Patients with duodenal
       ulcer for whom elective
       gastric surgery is
       planned
  (c) Basal acid secretion
       >10 mEq/hr in patients
       with intact stomachs
  (d) All of the above

189. Plasma renin activity (PRA)
      is increased in:
  (a) erect posture for 4
       hours
  (b) low sodium diet
  (c) estrogen-containing
       oral contraceptives
  (d) primary aldosteronism

190. Decreased levels of serum
      cholinesterase activity can
      be observed in:
  (a) pulmonary embolisms
  (b) muscular dystrophy
  (c) chronic hepatitis
  (d) pregnancy

191. The pancreozymin-secretion
      test measures the effect,
      after intravenous (IV)
      administration of pancreo-
      zymin and secretin, of
      changes in:
  (a) the volume and
       bicarbonate concen-
       tration of duodenal
       fluid
  (b) the amylase concen-
       tration of duodenal
       fluid
  (c) the level of serum
       lipase and amylase
  (d) all of the above

192. The Watson-Schwartz test
      for urinary urobilinogen
      and porphobilinogen uses
      which of the following
      reagents?
  (a) Concentrated HCl
  (b) Copper sulphate

  (c) p-nitrobenzenediazonium
  (d) p-dimethylaminobenzaldehyde
       (PABA)

193. The trough concentration of
      a drug is:
  (a) usually measured just
       before the next dose
  (b) measured to make sure
       that the serum concen-
       tration is more than
       the minimum effective
       concentration
  (c) measured to make sure
       that the drug is being
       eliminated from the
       body at a known rate
  (d) sometimes measured
       for all of the above
       reasons

194. Suxamethonium is a drug
      used in surgery as a muscle
      relaxant. In patients with
      a low serum activity, or an
      abnormal variant of a par-
      ticular enzyme, the drug
      may not be metabolized
      quickly enough and the
      patient may experience a
      prolonged apnea attack.
      What is the enzyme?
  (a) b-Glucuronidase
  (b) Cholinesterase
  (c) Ornithine carbamoyl-
       transferase
  (d) Glucose-6-phosphate
       dehydrogenase

195. Which of the following
      drugs may cause urinary
      17 ketosteroids to be
      increased?
  (a) Penicillin
  (b) Estrogens
  (c) Phenothiazines
  (d) Chloramphenicol

196. A particular enzyme is
      often monitored in agri-
      cultural workers working

with organo-phosphorus insecticides. What is the enzyme?
- (a) Cholinesterase
- (b) Lipase
- (c) Amylase
- (d) Trypsin

197. Barbiturates may be classified as to the duration of hypnotic action after average oral dose. A duration of 3 - 6 hours for amobarbital would indicate it was what type of barbiturate?
- (a) Long acting
- (b) Intermediate acting
- (c) Short acting
- (d) Ultrashort acting

198. Polyuria occurs when the 24-hour urine volume exceeds:
- (a) 1500 ml
- (b) 2500 ml
- (c) 4000 ml
- (d) 1200 ml

199. The normal range for urobilinogen in a 24-hour urine sample is:
- (a) 1.0 - 4.0 mg/24 hours
- (b) negative
- (c) 10 - 150 mg/24 hours
- (d) none of the above

200. The normal range for ketones measured in a 24-hour urine sample, by a qualitative test procedure, would be:
- (a) negative
- (b) less than 0.5 g/24 hours
- (c) 4.5 - 8.0
- (d) 1.0 - 1.6 g/24 hours

201. What percentage of serum cholesterol is present in the form of esters?
- (a) 60 - 75 per cent
- (b) 10 - 20 per cent
- (c) 90 per cent
- (d) 20 - 40 per cent

202. Which of the following drugs may cause urinary 17-hydroxycorticosteroids to be increased?
- (a) Oral contraceptives
- (b) Erythromycin
- (c) Quinidine
- (d) Chlordiazepoxide (Librium)

203. Which disease is characterized by low levels of copper and ceruloplasmin, injury to the cerebral basal ganglia and Kayser-Fleischer rings?
- (a) Tay-Sachs disease
- (b) Wilson's disease
- (c) Addison's disease
- (d) Reye's syndrome

204. The serum activity of alpha-hydroxybutyrate dehydrogenase (HBD) is thought to represent the lactate dehydrogenase (LD) activity of which isoenzymes?
- (a) LD_3
- (b) LD_5
- (c) LD_2
- (d) LD_1 and LD_2

205. A high urine specific gravity (> 1.030) could be found in which of the following conditions?
- (a) Diabetes mellitus with glycosuria
- (b) Vomiting
- (c) Diabetes insipidus
- (d) Nephrosis with proteinuria

206. How many milliliters of a 17.6 per cent solution of Na_2SO_4 would be required to prepare 450 ml of an 0.75 M solution?
- (a) 744 ml

(b)   422 ml
(c)   480 ml
(d)   272 ml

207. The colloidal complex
      heteropoly blue is formed
      in the reaction for the
      measurement in serum of:
      (a)   triglyceride
      (b)   cholesterol
      (c)   phospholipid
      (d)   HDL-cholesterol

208. Calculate the absorbance
      equivalent a transmission
      of 64 per cent:
      (a)   1.799
      (b)   2.143
      (c)   0.201
      (d)   none of the above

209. What is the pH of a solution
      of 0.143 M H_2SO_4?
      (a)   0.544
      (b)   1.456
      (c)   1.544
      (d)   None of the above

210. Isocitrate dehydrogenase
      (ICD) is found in high con-
      centration in:
      (a)   liver
      (b)   heart
      (c)   skeletal muscle
      (d)   all of the above

211. Inhibitors of isocitrate
      dehydrogenase (ICD) are:
      (a) Cu^{2+}
      (b) Hg^{2+}
      (c) Mn^{2+}
      (d) Co^{2+}

212. In adrenogenital syndrome
      due to 11-B-hydroxylation
      deficiency, which of the
      following results are found?
      (a)   Plasma ACTH increased
      (b)   Plasma cortisol de-
            creased

(c)   Hypokalemia mild
(d)   Mild increase in
      plasma deoxycorti-
      costerone

213. The adult therapeutic range
      for digoxin in serum is:
      (a)   0.9 - 2.0 ng/ml
      (b)   2.0 - 3.0 ng/ml
      (c)   > 3.0 ng/ml
      (d)   < 1.0 ng/ml

214. Increased activity of
      isocitrate dehydrogenase
      (ICD) is found in:
      (a)   parenchymal liver
            disease
      (b)   neonatal biliary duct
            atresia
      (c)   myocardial infarction
      (d)   pulmonary infarction

215. Significant quantities of
      the enzyme sorbitol dehy-
      drogenase (SDH) are found
      in which tissues:
      (a)   liver
      (b)   skeletal muscle
      (c)   prostate
      (d)   kidney

216. A pH of 5.7 when expressed
      as hydrogen ion concentra-
      tion ($[H^+]$) has a value of:
      (a) 6.001×10^{-5}
      (b) 8.732×10^{-7}
      (c) 4.732×10^{-4}
      (d) 1.995×10^{-6}

217. In the Neeld-Pearson pro-
      cedure for the determina-
      tion of vitamin A, the
      color formed by reacting
      trichloroacetic acid with
      the π-electrons in the
      conjugated double bonds
      of vitamin A, is:
      (a)   green
      (b)   blue
      (c)   red

(d) yellow

218. In adrenal hyperplasia due
      to pituitary dysfunction
      the:
      (a) level of 17-hydroxycor-
           ticosteroids (17 OHKS)
           in the urine is normal
      (b) plasma cortisol is de-
           creased after dexameth-
           azone suppression of 8
           mg/day
      (c) level of 17 OHKS after
           ACTH stimulation is
           increased
      (d) baseline level of
           plasma cortisol is
           decreased

219. The predominant form of folic
      acid present in human serum
      is:
      (a) tetrahydrofolic acid
      (b) N^5 - formyl-tetrahydro-
           folic acid
      (c) N^5 - methyl-tetrahydro-
           folic acid
      (d) dihydrofolic acid

220. The causes of pathological
      jaundice in the newborn may
      include:
      (a) impaired transport of
           bilirubin
      (b) impaired conjugation
           of bilirubin
      (c) impaired excretion
      (d) excess production of
           bilirubin

221. Lithium is added to standards,
      blanks and tests in some flame
      photometry systems because:
      (a) it has a high emission
           intensity
      (b) it is normally absent
           from biological fluids
      (c) it emits at a wavelength
           removed from Na and K
      (d) it acts as a radiation
           buffer to minimize the

      effects of mutual
      excitation

222. Which of the following
      interferences occur in
      atomic absorption spec-
      trophotometry?
      (a) Chemical interfer-
           ence
      (b) Ionization interfer-
           ence
      (c) Matrix interference
      (d) All of the above

223. Salicylate intoxication
      produces a respiratory
      alkalosis as plasma levels
      of salicylate rise. How
      long after rising plasma
      levels does this alkalosis
      occur?
      (a) 15 - 30 minutes
      (b) 30 - 60 minutes
      (c) 2 - 4 hours
      (d) $>$ 5 hours

224. Aspartate aminotransferase
      (AST) may be elevated in:
      (a) myocardial infarction
      (b) musculoskeletal
           diseases
      (c) liver disease
      (d) diabetic ketoacidosis

225. Calculate the pH of an
      0.023 M NaOH solution:
      (a) 12.362
      (b) 1.638
      (c) 8.638
      (d) none of the above

226. The organism Lactobacillus
      casei is commonly used in
      the assay of:
      (a) phenylalanine
      (b) vitamin B_{12}
      (c) folic acid
      (d) streptomycin

227. Nephelometric measurements
      differ from turbidimetric

measurements in that:
   (a) a diffraction grating
       is used instead of an
       interference filter
   (b) tests are read at high-
       er wavelengths
   (c) light scattered by the
       small particles is
       measured at right angles
       to the beam incident on
       the cuvette
   (d) they are less precise

228. Which of the following pro-
     cesses are responsible for
     the absorption of gamma rays?
   (a) The photoelectric
       effect
   (b) The Compton effect
   (c) Pair production
   (d) All of the above

229. Malate dehydrogenase (MD) is
     used in the aspartate amino-
     transferase (AST) reaction
     mixture to convert:
   (a) L-glutamate to alpha-
       oxoglutarate
   (b) L-glutamate to L-
       aspartate
   (c) L-malate to L-glutamate
   (d) oxalacetate to L-malate

230. In attempting to distinguish
     between primary and secondary
     aldosteronism it is usually
     found that:
   (a) plasma renin activity
       (PRA) is markedly de-
       creased in primary
       and normal or increased
       in secondary
   (b) urinary 17-hydroxy-
       corticosteroids (17 OHKS)
       are usually normal in
       both
   (c) primary is usually due
       to a tumor
   (d) all of the above

231. The Reinsch test is used to

screen in body fluids
for the presence of:
   (a) mercury
   (b) arsenic
   (c) bismuth
   (d) all of the above

232. Creatine +ATP $\overset{CK}{\rightleftharpoons}$ creatine
     phosphate +ADP
     The optimum pH for the CK
     reaction above is:
   (a) 6.8 - 6.9
   (b) 7.3
   (c) 9.0
   (d) 11.2

233. In distinguishing between
     pheochromocytoma and neuro-
     blastoma which of the fol-
     lowing urine test results
     are found?
   (a) vanillylmandelic acid
       (VMA) increased in both
   (b) Catecholamines increased
       in both
   (c) Homovanillic acid (HVA)
       is normal in pheochromo-
       cytoma and increased in
       neuroblastoma
   (d) All of the above

234. In alkaline ferricyanide
     glucose methods the fol-
     lowing substances inter-
     fere with the reaction
     by increasing the apparent
     glucose result:
   (a) calcium ions
   (b) creatinine
   (c) phosphates
   (d) uric acid

235. Calcitonin is responsible
     for:
   (a) increasing renal
       excretion of phos-
       phates
   (b) inhibiting bone
       reabsorption of
       calcium
   (c) increasing intestinal

(d) increasing reabsorp-
tion of calcium from
bone

(at top, continued) absorption of calcium

236. Calculate the pH of a buffer
solution prepared by mixing
7 ml of 0.18 M acetic acid
with 3 ml of 0.18 M sodium
acetate assuming no volume
change on mixing:
(a) 5.11
(b) 4.93
(c) 4.37
(d) none of the above
(Ka for acetic acid = 1.82
x 10^{-5})

237. Which of the following clotting factors are involved
with vitamin K metabolism?
(a) Thrombin
(b) Factor VII
(c) Factor X
(d) All of the above

238. In the method for serum
calcium using o-cresolphthalein complexone, 8-hydroxy-
quinoline is added to:
(a) bind preferentially
with phosphate and
prevent the formation
of calcium phosphate
(b) bind with magnesium
(c) chelate the calcium
(d) alter the pH of the
solution and enhance
final color develop-
ment

239. The Michaelis-Menten (Km)
constant is:
(a) the concentration of
substrate giving one-
half maximum enzyme
velocity
(b) the temperature of
optimum enzyme
velocity

(c) the pH of optimum
enzyme activity
(d) the concentration of
substrate giving
twice maximum enzyme
velocity

240. If a patient has an increase
in norepinephrine blood
levels without an increase
in epinephrine, the type
of tumor present is probably:
(a) a ganglioneuroma
(b) an extra-adrenal pheochromocytoma
(c) an argentaffinoma
(d) neuroblastoma

241. Riboflavin deficiency in
humans may cause which of
the following symptoms?
(a) Angular stomatitis
(b) Disturbances in
vision
(c) Dermatitis
(d) All of the above

242. In the ferrozine method
for iron and iron binding
capacity (IBC) determina-
tion, the presence of
thiourea:
(a) causes dissociation
of the iron-transferrin
complex
(b) enhances color development
(c) prevents precipitation
of proteins
(d) binds copper

243. Calculate the pH of a
buffer solution containing
0.07 M acetic acid and
0.16 M sodium acetate:
(a) 5.099
(b) 4.381
(c) 5.619
(d) 4.901
(Ka for acetic acid = 1.82
x 10^{-5})

244. Which of the following techniques have been used in clinical laboratories for the separation of creatine kinase (CK) isoenzymes?
    (a) DEAE-sephadex column chromatography
    (b) Chemical inhibition
    (c) Electrophoresis
    (d) The use of anti-MM antiserum

245. Measurement of red blood cell glutathione reductase activity is a good indicator of the blood level of which vitamin?
    (a) Folic acid
    (b) Vitamin B_6
    (c) Vitamin B_2
    (d) Lipoic acid

246. Serum aldolase (ALD) may be increased in:
    (a) Duchenne muscular dystrophy
    (b) acute myocardial infarction
    (c) carcinoma of the prostate
    (d) neurogenic muscular atrophy

247. The measurement of red blood cell transketolase activity is a useful method for assessing deficiency of which vitamin?
    (a) Thiamine
    (b) Riboflavin
    (c) Ascorbic acid
    (d) Folic acid

248. In a zero-order reaction, the reaction velocity is:
    (a) proportional to one-third the enzyme concentration
    (b) proportional to the square of the substrate concentration
    (c) independent of substrate concentration
    (d) proportional to the square root of the enzyme concentration

249. Serum copper may be increased in:
    (a) anemias
    (b) hemochromatosis
    (c) collagen diseases
    (d) nephrosis

250. Serum leucine aminopeptidase (LAP) is a useful enzyme to measure:
    (a) as a sensitive indicator of choledocholithiasis
    (b) on no occasion
    (c) as an indicator of liver metastases in anicteric patients
    (d) to diagnose biliary tract obstruction

SECTION B: HEADINGS

For each numbered word or phrase, select one heading that is most closely related to it.

(1) (a) Congenital erythropoietic porphyria (CEP)
     (b) Hepatic porphyria (HP)
     (c) Erythropoietic protoporphyria (EP)

251. Marked increase in porphobilinogen.
     ANSWER: _____

252. Rare condition due to excess production of free uroporphyrin I by marrow red blood cells.
     ANSWER: _____

253. Urine uroporphyrin and coproporphyrin show increase but fecal and red blood cell

protoporphyrin and coproporphyrin are increased.
ANSWER: _____

254. Symptoms may be precipitated by barbiturates or alcohol.
ANSWER: _____

255. Onset usually occurs before the age of two with extreme photosensitivity.
ANSWER: _____

(2) (a) Primary hyperaldosteronism
    (b) Secondary hyperaldosteronism
    (c) Cushing's syndrome
    (d) 17-hydroxylase deficiency
    (e) Renal tubular acidosis

256. Serum sodium normal
Serum potassium decreased
Serum renin increased
Serum aldosterone normal
Normotensive.
ANSWER: _____

257. Serum sodium normal or decreased
Serum potassium decreased
Serum renin decreased
Serum aldosterone normal
Hypertensive.
ANSWER: _____

258. Serum sodium normal or increased
Serum potassium decreased
Serum renin decreased
Serum aldosterone increased
Hypertensive.
ANSWER: _____

259. Serum sodium normal or increased
Serum potassium decreased
Serum renin increased
Serum aldosterone increased
Hypertensive.
ANSWER: _____

260. Serum sodium normal
Serum potassium decreased
Serum renin decreased
Serum aldosterone decreased
Hypertensive.
ANSWER: _____

(3) (a) Urobilinogen
    (b) Urine bilirubin
    (c) BUN
    (d) Urobilin
    (e) Ketone bodies

The following questions (261 - 265) indicate reagents to be used in the determination of (a) to (e) above.

261. Zinc acetate.
ANSWER: _____

262. Diacetylmonoxime.
ANSWER: _____

263. Sodium nitroprusside.
ANSWER: _____

264. Fouchet's reagent.
ANSWER: _____

265. Ehrlich's reagent.
ANSWER: _____

(4) (a) serum calcium 4 mmol/l
    (b) pH 7.50, pCO_2 30.0
    (c) serum phosphorus 9 mg/dl
    (d) gamma globulin 5.4 g/dl
    (e) pH 7.38, pCO_2 60.0

266. Hypoparathyroidism.
ANSWER: _____

267. Multiple myeloma.
ANSWER: _____

268. Hyperparathyroidism.
ANSWER: _____

269. Hypocapnia
ANSWER: _____

270. Chronic hypercapnia.
ANSWER: _____

SECTION C: TRUE OR FALSE

*Mark the following statements
either TRUE (T) or FALSE (F).*

271. Phosphorescence is another
name for fluorescence.

272. - C - N - This structure
     ‖ | is known as the
     O   H   peptide linkage.

273. A glass filter has a wider
band width than a prism.

274. The normal adult fecal color
is due to biliverdin.

275. A blood sample left at room
temperature for 3 hours
shows no loss of acid phosphatase activity.

276. Aldosterone is one of the
factors in the regulation
of plasma sodium.

277. When lithium is excited in
a flame, the color produced
is red.

278. Cloudy urine is usually due
to urates in alkaline urine.

279. Hemoglobin is precipitated
from urine that is 80 per
cent saturated with ammonium
sulphate.

280. Calcium oxalate is the most
commonly formed constituent
of urinary calculi.

281. Plasma creatinine does not
adequately reflect early
renal damage.

282. The level of estrogen in
urine in the first trimester
of pregnancy is higher than
the level of chorionic gona-

dotrophin.

283. Increased secretion of parathyroid hormone does not
cause increased intestinal
absorption of calcium.

284. Fluorescence is not affected
by temperature.

285. Antidiuretic hormone controls
the reabsorption of water by
the distal tubules in the
kidney.

286. Bile acids are produced in
the liver from cholesterol.

287. Alcohol can be esterified
with acids.

288. A refractometer can be used
to measure the protein concentration of cerebrospinal
fluid (CSF).

289. If 95 per cent confidence
limits are established for
a particular method then
1 in 20 test results will
form outside of the acceptable limits.

290. O-toluidine reacts with
pentoses.

291. Enterokinase is present in
pancreatic juice.

292. Cholecystokinin is found in
gastric juice.

293. Red blood cell acid phosphatase is inhibited by
L-tartrate ions.

294. Patients suffering from
pernicious anemia lack
the intrinsic factor.

295. The liver and heart muscle

are the main sites of trans-amination.

296. The color change of ferric ion with phenylpyruvic acid is a result of reduction of ferric ion to ferrous ion.

297. Xanthochromia refers to a yellowish color of the spinal fluid.

298. The phenolsulfonphthalein (PSP) excretion test is a measure of renal blood flow.

299. Hematuria is usually absent in chronic glomerulonephritis.

300. The conversion of an alpha sugar to its beta form is known as mutarotation.

301. Tyrosine can be formed in the liver from phenylalanine.

302. Calcitonin is produced mainly in the thymus gland.

303. Any increase in serum phosphorus is associated with a decrease in serum calcium.

304. Calciferol is the biologically active form of vitamin D.

305. Perchloric acid interferes with the enzymatic method for pyruvate.

306. Pyruvate standard solutions should be prepared fresh because pyruvate polymerizes in solution.

307. A base is a proton donor.

308. Urea is oxidized to ammonium carbonate by urease.

309. Creatinine amidohydrolase can be used to convert creatine to creatinine.

310. When fluid intake is restricted in cases of neurogenic polyuria, the urine will concentrate to above 900 mOsm/kg.

311. If NaOH is added to a pulverized renal stone and heated, then lead acetate is added and heated; a black precipitate indicates the presence of cystine.

312. In the Jendrassik-Grof bilirubin method, the sodium acetate accelerates the coupling of bilirubin with diazotized sulfanilic acid.

313. Sorbitol dehydrogenase is increased in chronic hepatitis.

314. In the Diagnex blue test for gastric analysis, the patient is given an azure A resin.

315. Xylose is not a pentose.

316. Retinol is another name for vitamin A.

317. A combination of an enzyme plus a coenzyme is called an apoenzyme.

318. A glycerophosphatide is a complex lipid containing phosphorus and frequently nitrogen.

319. The most sensitive biochemical response to lead

intoxication is a decrease in red blood cell delta aminolevulinate (ALA) dehydratase activity.

320. The alkali denaturation test is used to identify sickle cell hemoglobin (HbS).

321. In edema, water accumulates in all body compartments.

322. By definition, polyuria is a urine excretion of greater than 3 liters/24 hours.

323. The principal causes of hypoalbuminemia are liver disease, malnutrition and renal disease.

324. Approximately 5 per cent of total body potassium is contained in the plasma.

325. Hydrogen ions entering the cell are balanced by potassium ions leaving the cell in order to maintain electroneutrality.

326. There is a good correlation between hypokalemia and potassium deficiency.

327. Serum potassium concentration is directly related to serum hydrogen ion concentration.

328. A decreased serum lactate/pyruvate ratio is seen in anoxia.

329. Tidal volume, or the inspired volume of a single breath, is approximately 550 ml in adults.

330. Sodium aluminum silicate is also known as Lloyd's reagent.

331. A decrease in pressure in the afferent arterioles in the kidney causes the release of renin from the juxtaglomerular cells.

332. Porphyrins are tripyrrole ring compounds.

333. The liver does not normally synthesize gamma globulin.

334. The Hollander test is one in which insulin-induced hypoglycemia is used as a vagal stimulus for gastric acid measurement.

335. Releasing hormones of the hypothalamus are designated with the suffix -tropin.

336. Random urine samples containing reducing substances can be obtained from approximately 20 per cent of healthy individuals.

337. The mineral component of bone is mainly calcium carbonate.

338. A deficiency in the enzyme p-hydroxyphenylpyruvic acid oxidase is thought to be the cause of tyrosinemia.

339. In humans, the enzyme uricase oxidizes uric acid to allantoin.

340. Lipoprotein X is a complex of phospholipid, unesterified cholesterol, protein and triglyceride.

341. Kwashiorkor is a disease caused by a diet that is very low in protein and carbohydrate.

342. Pulmonary surfactant is a phospholipid-protein complex.

343. Lesch-Nyhan syndrome is caused by a sphingomyelinase deficiency.

344. Increased serum levels of serum carcinoembryonic antigen are found in 60 per cent - 80 per cent of patients with carcinoma of the gastrointestinal tract.

345. High density lipoprotein levels are inversely proportional to serum triglyceride concentration.

346. The process whereby one type of specialized cell is transformed into a type that is abnormal is known as metaplasia.

347. L-Phenylalanine inhibits intestinal, placental and bone isoenzymes of alkaline phosphatase.

348. All immunoglobulins have a similar structure consisting of two identical heavy chains and two identical light chains.

349. Waldenström's macroglobulinemia is a monoclonal gammopathy involving IgM-producing cells.

350. Normally, 55 per cent of the total body potassium is intracellular.

351. Acidosis, high pCO_2 and decreased red blood cell 2,3-diphosphoglycerate (2,3-DPG) will all shift the oxygen dissociation curve to the right.

352. Tamm-Horsfall protein is a glycoprotein which comes from either renal interstitial tissue or from tubular cells.

353. If cardiac output is inadequate, acidosis due to the formation of lactic acid from aerobic glycolysis may be found.

354. Fetal hemoglobin (HbF) consists of two alpha and two beta peptide chains.

355. The reserve bilirubin binding capacity of serum albumin is less in neonates.

356. Bile acid synthesis is a major metabolic pathway for the removal of cholesterol from the body.

357. Dumping syndrome refers to the rapid entry of hypotonic fluid into the duodenum.

358. The control of follicle-stimulating hormone (FSH) and luteinizing hormone (LH) by the hypothalamus appears to be due to gonadoliberin.

359. Neonatal hypothyroidism is due to thyroid dysgenesis.

360. Glucocorticoids inhibit insulin release.

361. Glucose tolerance factor (GTF) is an organic chromium compound that potentiates the action of insulin.

362. A decreased ionized calcium level in serum will

cause a decrease in para-
thormone (PTH) secretion.

363. The reabsorptive ability
of the proximal renal
tubule is affected in
Fanconi syndrome.

364. A primary increase in serum
albumin concentration may
be found in certain meta-
bolic diseases.

365. Proteinase inhibitor (Pi)
typing is a genetic classification system for alpha-
1-antitrypsin deficiencies.

366. A complete absence of plasma
cells is found in Bruton's
disease (X-linked agamma-
globulinemia).

367. Plasma obtained from a blood
sample containing ethylene
diamine tetraacetic acid
(EDTA) is often preferred
to serum for lipoprotein
analysis because EDTA prevents the peroxidation of
lipoproteins by heavy metals.

368. Analphalipoproteinemia, also
known as Bassen-Komzweig
disease, is due to an inability to synthesize normal
amounts of HDL apoproteins.

369. The main acute phase reaction
proteins are alpha-1-anti-
trypsin, C-reactive protein,
haptoglobin and ceruloplasmin.

SECTION D: MISSING WORDS

Fill in the missing word(s).

370. The S.I. unit of mass is the
_____.

371. If the concentration of
a standard cannot be
determined directly from
the volume of the solution
and the weight of the solute,
the standard is a _____
one.

372. In the case of the acidosis,
the renal mechanism causes
an _____(a)_____ excretion of
_____(b)_____ and conservation
of _____(c)_____.

373. The glycoprotein that acts on
the bone marrow to increase
the rate of red cell production is called _____.

374. When the molecules of the
solute in solution are in
equilibrium with the excess
undissolved molecules, the
solution is said to be
_____.

375. The S.I. unit of time is the
_____.

376. Substances are transported
through the cell by two
main processes called
_____(a)_____ and _____(b)_____.

377. Phosphate and citrate buffers
are often known as _____
buffers.

378. The S.I. unit of electric
current is the _____.

379. The major sources of the
heat-stable fraction of
alkaline phosphatase are
_____(a)_____ , _____(b)_____
and _____(c)_____.

380. The common logarithm of a
number is the exponent or
power to which _____
must be raised to give that

number.

381. In the oxyhemoglobin dissociation curve, increasing
pH shifts the curve to the
_____.

382. The 5 stages of cell mitosis
are ____(a)___ , ____(b)___ ,
____(c)___ , ____(d)___ and
____(e)___ .

383. A commonly used preservative
in a 24-hour urine collection
for vanillylmandelic acid (VMA)
is ____(a)___ ml of ___(b)____ .

384. The S.I. unit of temperature
is the _____.

385. The main lipid fractions
elevated in patients with
biliary obstruction are
____(a)___ and __(b)___ .

386. The substrate used in the
Bessey, Lowrg and Brock
procedure for the assay of
alkaline phosphatase is

_____.

387. In a solution, as the concentration increases __(a)__ ,
the per cent transmission
decreases ___(b)__ .

388. The basic compounds used to
form deoxyribonucleic acid
(DNA) are ____(a)___ ,
____(b)___ , ____(c)___ ,
____(d)___ , ____(e)___ ,
and ____(f)___ .

389. To verify wavelength calibration on narrow half band-
width spectrophotometer a
_____ oxide glass
filter may be used.

390. The normal range for blood

pH is ____(a)___ to ___(b)___ :
pCO_2 ____(c)___ to ___(d)___ ,
pO_2 ____(e)___ to ___(f)___ .

391. When light falls on certain
metals, electrons flow in
proportion to the intensity
of the light. Detectors
using this principle are
called _____.

392. The S.I. unit of luminous
intensity is the _____.

393. In an electrophoretic system,
the potential that exists
between the negative fixed
ions on the surface of the
support and the cloud of
positive ions around them
is called the ___(a)___ or
___(b)___ potential.

394. The Golgi complex is involved in the formation
of cytoplasmic organelles
called _____.

395. In uncontrolled diabetes,
excess degradation of
____(a)_____ by beta-
oxidation in liver cells
results from an excess
mobilization of fatty
acids from _____(b)___ .
This causes acetyl CoA to
form increased amounts of
____(c)___ , ___(d)___ and
____(e)___ .

396. In electrophoresis, the
movement of solvent and
its solutes relative to
the fixed support is called

_____.

397. The S.I. unit for an amount
of substance is the _____.

398. A special redox electrode

called a quinhydrone electrode is used to measure _____.

399. The antibiotic used in making potassium-selective electrodes is _____.

400. When blood pH falls, the plasma potassium ion concentration tends to _____.

401. In a cell, ribosomes are composed mainly of _____ which takes part in the synthesis of protein in the cell.

402. The technique of amperometry is based on the measurement of the __(a)__ flowing through an electrochemical cell when a constant __(b)__ __(c)__ is applied to the electrodes.

403. The S.I. unit for enzyme activity is __(a)__ and for enzyme concentration __(b)__.

404. Foam cells are found in the bone marrow and spleen in Types __(a)__ and __(b)__ hyperlipoproteinemia.

405. A Clark electrode is used to measure _____.

406. In the intestinal mucosal cell lipids are transformed into __(a)__ and __(b)__. The __(c)__ are transferred via the thoracic duct to the blood stream.

407. The amount of electricity passing between two electrodes in an electrochemical cell can be measured by the technique known as _____.

408. The S.I. unit of length is the _____.

409. In chromatography, the ratio of the distance the spot has moved to the distance the solvent has moved is known as the _____ value.

410. Beta particles can be negatively charged electrons called __(a)__, or positively charged particles called __(b)__.

411. The presence of protein and lipid on the surface of the cell membrane makes the membrane _____.

412. Carbon dioxide can be transported in the plasma in 3 forms. They are as __(a)__, __(b)__ and __(c)__.

413. The fluor most commonly used as a gamma ray detector is _____.

414. The standard procedure for measuring protein by assaying the nitrogen content is known as the _____ technique.

415. All lipids in plasma circulate in combination with _____.

416. The four chemicals in biuret reagents are __(a)__, __(b)__, __(c)__ and __(d)__.

417. Gamma glutamyltransferase may be elevated in all forms of _____ disease.

418. _____ (HABA) is a dye

used in the determination
of serum albumin.

419. Antibodies belong to a
group of proteins called
_____.

SECTION E: SPECIAL QUESTIONS

*Match the enzyme in COLUMN A with the main organ(s) from which the
enzyme arises, or the disease of interest, in COLUMN B.*

Question 420

COLUMN A	COLUMN B
1. 5' Nucleotidase	(a) Carcinoma of the prostate
2. Cholinesterase	(b) Post anesthetic respiratory disease
3. Lipase	(c) Liver, heart
4. Alkaline phosphatase	(d) Pancreas
5. Lactate dehydrogenase	(e) Heart, muscle, brain
6. Amylase	(f) Copper metabolism defect
7. Alanine aminotransferase	(g) Liver
8. Acid phosphatase	(h) Liver, heart, red blood cells
9. Creatine kinase	(i) Liver, bone, placenta
10. Ceruloplasmin	(j) Pancreas, salivary glands

421. *Fill out the following chart of the familial hyperlipoproteinemia phenotypes, based on the Fredrickson classification:*

Type	Appearance	Cholesterol Concentration	Triglyceride Concentration	Predominant Band(s) on Electrophoresis
I				
IIa				
IIb				
III				
IV				
V				
Normal				

INC = Increased   APPEARANCE = Creamy <u>OR</u>

DEC = Decreased   Clear <u>OR</u>

NORM = Normal   Turbid

422. *Fill in the missing steps (blocks) in the heme synthesis pathway.*

/Continued...

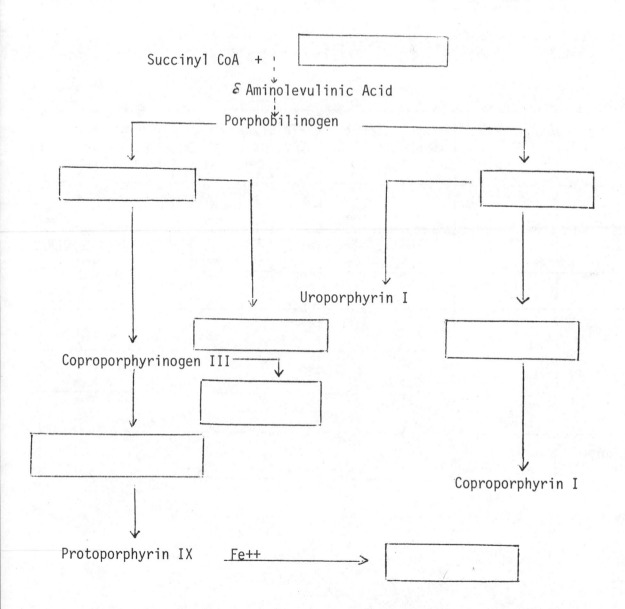

Succinyl CoA + [ ]

δ Aminolevulinic Acid

Porphobilinogen

Uroporphyrin I

Coproporphyrinogen III

Coproporphyrin I

Protoporphyrin IX   Fe++   ⟶   [ ]

423. Case History
      A middle-aged man arrived at the Emergency Department in a
      collapsed condition. He had a known history of diabetes
      mellitus and had been sick with a "stomach upset" for the
      past three days. He had decreased his insulin intake because
      of his illness. When his wife went to him in the evening she
      found him unconscious with deep, rapid respirations. On
      examination at the hospital he was found to have a blood
      pressure of 100/70, a pulse rate of 115 beats/minute and
      very dry mucous membranes. He was unresponsive to stimuli.

      Bloods were sent to the laboratory and the following results
      obtained:-

pH 7.19

pCO_2 16 mm Hg

HCO_3^- 6 mmol/l

Na^+ 133 mmol/l

K^+ 5.9 mmol/l

Plasma Acetone $^{+++}$
Hematocrit 0.59
Glucose 27.8 mmol/l

1. Explain the elevated blood glucose.

2. Why was the pH low, and why were there increased amounts of plasma acetone?

3. Explain the rapid, deep breathing.

424. *Fill in the following chart with the laboratory results observed in the investigation of thyroid function in various conditions:*

Condition	Laboratory Blood Tests				
	T_4	TSH	T_3	T_3Uptake	TBG
Hyperthyroidism					
Hypothyroidism					
Pregnancy					
Estrogen Therapy					

T_4 = Total serum thyroxine

TSH = Thyroid stimulating hormone

T_3 = Tri-iodothyronine

TBG = Thyroxine-binding-globulin

I = Increase
D = Decrease
N = Normal

425. *Fill in the following chart with the laboratory results observed in the investigation of Cushing's syndrome after the use of the various suppression or stimulation tests:*

PC   = Plasma Cortisol
170HCS = 17-hydroxycorticosteroids)
KGS   = Ketogenic steroids   ) in urine
17KS   = 17 ketosteroids   )

N = Normal, I = Increase, D = Decrease, NC = No Change,
SI = Slight Increase

Test	Adrenal Lesion				
	None	Hyperplasia	Adenoma	Carcinoma	Extra-adrenal tumor

Basal level
  PC
  170HCS
  KGS
  17KS					

ACTH stimulation
  PC
  170HCS
  KGS
  17KS					

Metyrapone
  170HCS
  KGS
  17KS					

Dexamethasone suppression
  2 mg/day
  PC
  170HCS
  KGS
  17KS					

Dexamethasone suppression
  8 mg/day
  PC
  170HCS
  KGS
  17KS					

426. *Fill in the following chart with the laboratory results*
      observed in the investigation of the following liver
      diseases.

Disease	Laboratory Blood Tests								
	ALP	ASAT	A1AT	IgA	IgM	IgG	ANF	MA	SMA
Portal Cirrhosis									
Primary Biliary Cirrhosis									
Chronic Active Hepatitis									

ALP = Alkaline phosphatase   ANF = Antinuclear factor
ASAT = Aspartate aminotransferase   MA = Mitochondrial antibodies
A1AT = Alanine aminotransferase   SMA = Smooth muscle antibodies

ANSWERS

SECTION A: MULTIPLE CHOICE

1. (d) Alkalosis can result
         from hyperventilation
         and acute vomiting.

2. (e) Hydrogen ion concentra-
         tion, temperature, sub-
         strate concentration and
         cofactors all govern the
         rate of enzyme reactions.

3. (b) The normal range for
         cerebrospinal fluid (CSF)
         protein from a lumbar
         region spinal tap is 15 -
         45 mg/dl.

4. (c) The total content of fat
         in a stool sample should
         be less than 6 g/day given
         that the patient has been
         on a diet containing 60 -
         150 g of fat/day.

5. (b) Cholesterol acts as an
         alcohol and reacts with
         strong, concentrated acids
         with colored substances
         known as polyenes being
         produced. Acetic acid
         and acetic anhydride are
         used as solvents and de-
         hydrating agents and sul-
         phuric acid as an oxidiz-
         ing agent. The reaction
         is enhanced by the addi-
         tion of ferric ion. This
         is the principle of the
         Leibermann-Burchardt re-
         action.

6. (d) It is thought that amni-
         otic fluid lipids origi-
         nate from developing
         respiratory tract tissue.
         It has been found that
         measurement of lecithin,
         sphingomyelin and other
         lipids may indicate the
         maturity of fetal lung.
         The lecithin to sphingo-
         myelin ratio is used as
         an index of lung maturity
         with a mature ratio being
         greater than 2.0.

42

7. (d) A lack of phytanate alpha-
         oxidase and subsequent
         build-up of phytanic acid
         which has the effect of
         blocking beta-oxidation
         of fatty acids is seen in
         Refsum's disease.

8. (d) Lysophosphatidyl choline,
         phosphatidyl ethanolamine
         and sphinogomyelin are
         all typical phospholipids
         found in serum.

9. (a) Serum IgG has a concentra-
    (b) tion of 600 - 1800 mg/dl,
    (d) shows major antibacterial
         activity and has a half-
         life of 23 days. Proteins
         can be differentiated due
         to different densities by
         use of an ultracentrifuge.
         The Svedberg coefficient,
         or S value, increases in
         value with increasing
         density. Thus IgG has an
         S value of 7S, IgM has an
         S value of 19S, and IgA
         is variable with values
         between 7S and 11S.

10. (a) A serum bilirubin concen-
         tration of 16.0 mg/dl $\equiv$
         274 mmol/l when expressed
         in S.I. units.

11. (d) The creatinine clearance
         is calculated as follows:

         $$C = \frac{U \times V}{S} \text{ ml/min}$$

         Where C = Creatinine
                   clearance
               U = Urine creatinine
               V = 24-hour urine
                   volume in ml
                   excreted/minute
                   of collection
               S = Serum creatinine

$$C = \frac{60 \times 900}{1.8 \times 1440}$$

$$= 21 \text{ ml/min}$$

12. (d) The molar extinction
         coefficient can be
         calculated as follows:

         $$A = Edc$$

         Where A = absorbance
               E = molar extinction
                   coefficient
               d = length of light
                   path in cm
               c = molar concentra-
                   tion of the sub-
                   stance in solu-
                   tion

         $$c = 4.53 \text{ mg/l}$$

         $$= \frac{4.53 \times 10^{-3}}{585} \text{ moles/l}$$

         $$= 7.74 \times 10^{-6} \text{ M}$$

         $$E = \frac{A}{d \times c}$$

         $$= \frac{0.468}{1 \times 7.74 \times 10^{-6}}$$

         $$= \frac{4.68 \times 10^{5}}{7.74}$$

         $$= 60500$$

13. (a) A Torr is equal in pressure
         to 1 atmosphere at sea
         level.

14. (d) The pk value of the hy-
         drogen ion concentration
         in normal blood at 37°C
         is 6.10.

15. (c) Oxygen moves into the
         blood from the lungs by

the action of passive diffusion.

16. (b) A patient with a blood level of 100 - 150 mg/dl of ethanol should exhibit euphoria, loss of inhibitions and prolonged reaction times. If there is no evidence of intoxication, increased tolerance should be considered.

17. (b) Concentration of albumin is calculated as follows:

(100 - 71)% of 6.7 g/dl

= 29% of 6.7 g/dl

= 1.9 g/dl

18. (b) An orange-red color due to the formation of cuprous ions is formed by the reaction between cupric ions and glucose in the presence of heat and alkali. This is the principle of the copper reduction method for urine glucose.

19. (d) Epithelial cells, white blood cells and neutral fat globules may all be found in small numbers in a normal feces sample.

20. (d) The Zollinger-Ellison syndrome is a condition where G cells, usually in the pancreatic islets, produce large amounts of gastrin. In this condition, acid secretion by the stomach is very high.

21. (b) A transudate protein con-
    (c) centration is usually less than 3.0 g/dl.

22. (a) The sweat chloride concentration is usually between 60 and 120 mEq/l.

23. (d) "Shake" or "Foam" test, Nile-blue stain and creatinine concentration can all be used to indicate fetal maturity.

24. (b) A clear and straw-colored synovial fluid, with a good mucin clot, and usually without a fibrin clot is found in non-flammatory conditions. A turbid yellow sample, with a fibrin clot and a fair to poor mucin clot is found in acute inflammatory conditions. A xanthochromic sample, with a variable mucin clot and usually without a fibrin clot is found in hemorrhagic conditions.

25. (c) Seminal fluid analysis
    (d) on a normal sample will produce the following results:
    The volume is greater than 3 ml, the sperm count is greater than 5×10^7/ml, greater than 60 per cent of the sperms are motile, greater than 50 per cent of the sperms have normal morphology.

26. (a) Ammonium biurate, triple
    (b) phosphate and amorphous
    (c) phosphate crystals can all be found in normal alkaline urine. Calcium oxalate crystals can be found in normal acid urine.

27. (b) Osmolality is the measure of the number of solute particles per unit of solvent.
Refractive index is the ratio of the velocity of light in air to the velocity of light in solution.

28. (a) A normal solution contains 1 gram-equivalent weight of the solute in 1 liter of solution.
A molar solution contains 1 mole of the solute in 1000 ml of solvent.

29. (c) 1 g of $BaCl_2 \cdot 2H_2O$ is equivalent to:

$$\frac{BaCl_2}{BaCl_2 \cdot 2H_2O} = \frac{137.3 + 71}{137.3 + 71 + 36}$$

$$= \frac{208.3}{244.3}$$

$$= 0.853 \text{ g } BaCl_2$$

Therefore:
25g $BaCl_2 \cdot 2H_2O$ =
21.32g $BaCl_2$

30. (d) Standard error = $\dfrac{S}{\sqrt{N}}$

31. (c) R.C.F. = $1.118 \times 10^{-5} \times r \times N^2$
= $1.118 \times 10^{-5} \times 12 \times 8000^2$
= $1.118 \times 10^{-5} \times 12 \times (8 \times 10^3)^2$
= $1.118 \times 1.2 \times 6.4 \times 10^3$
= 8586

32. (c) The mode is the most frequently occurring value. The median is equal to the middle value of a series of numbers; the mean is equal to the sum of the values divided by the number of values; the coefficient of variation is equal to the standard deviation of the series divided by the mean.

33. (a)
    (b) An ideal analytical procedure should be accurate, precise, sensitive and specific.
    (c)
    (d)

34. (a) The fat soluble vitamins
    (b) are A, D, E and K.
    (c)

35. (a) Para-nitrophenylphos-
    (b) phate, beta-glycero-
    (d) phosphate, phenylphos-
         phate and phenolphtha-
         lein monophosphate
         have all been used as
         substances in the assay
         of alkaline phosphatase.

36. (d) Ceruloplasmin is the metalloprotein enzyme responsible for transporting copper.

37. (d) Thirty per cent of the LD activity in lung is LD_3.

38. (c) Wilson's disease is a disorder in copper metabolism. Decreased cystathionine synthetase in the liver is seen in homocystinuria Increased cystine and lysine in the urine is seen in cystinuria Increased serum CK may be found in Duchenne muscular dystrophy.

39. (c) L-aspartate + alpha oxoglutarate

$$\text{AST} \quad \text{Oxaloacetate} +$$
$$\underset{\text{p-5-p}}{\rightleftarrows} \quad \text{L-glutamate}$$

40. (c) Free bilirubin in the serum is attached to albumin.

41.   Any two of the following criteria should be present to establish a diagnosis of cystic fibrosis:
      (a) characteristic lung pathology
      (b) pancreatic insufficiency
      (c) increased sweat electrolytes
      (d) family history

42. (d) Photocells, thermocouples and quartz crystals can all generate electrical charges.

43. (a) A micron (μ) is 10^{-6}m

44. (d) An Allen correction adjusts for interfering substances

    Example: $A_{corr} = A_{300} - \dfrac{(A_{280} + A_{320})}{2}$

    Where A = absorbance and 280, 300 and 320 refer to the wavelengths at which substance was read.

45. (c) Narrow bandpass filters isolate emission energy at a given wavelength.

46. (a) The rate of migration in
    (b) an electrophoretic system
    (c) depends on the net charge
    (d) on the molecule and the strength of the electric field, the size and shape of the molecule, the nature of the supporting medium and the temperature of operation.

    The equation for the driving force is:

    $$F = (X)(Q) = \frac{E \cdot Q}{d}$$

    F = the force exerted on an ion
    X = the current field strength (V/cm)
    Q = the net charge on the ion
    E = the voltage applied (V)
    d = the width, or distance across, the electrophoretic membrane (cm)

47. (a) When a solute is dis-
    (b) solved in a solvent,
    (c) the osmotic pressure
    (d) is increased, the vapor pressure of the solution is lowered below that of the pure solvent, the boiling point of the solution is raised above that of the pure solvent and the freezing point of the solution is lowered below that of the pure solvent.

48. (d) Thermal conductivity, flame ionization and electron capture detectors have all been used on gas chromatographs.

49. (c) The mass number is the sum of the number of protons and neutrons in the nucleus and is represented by the letter A.

50. (a) Growth hormone, epine-
    (b) phrine and thyroxine
    (d) all can increase glu-
         cose levels.

51. (d) The formula for glycer-
         aldehyde is COH - CHOH -
         CH$_2$OH.
         The formula for a furan
         is

$$
\begin{array}{c}
O \\
HC \diagup \diagdown CH \\
\| \qquad \| \\
CH\text{--}CH
\end{array}
$$

         for an aldehyde is
         - CHOH - COH and for
         D-glucose is
         COH - (CHOH)$_4$ - CH$_2$OH

52. (d) The formula for cysteine
         is HSCH$_2$CHNH$_2$COOH. The
         formula for cystine is
         S - CH$_2$CHNH$_2$COOH
         |
         S - CH$_2$CHNH$_2$COOH

         for alanine is
         CH$_3$CHNH$_2$COOH and for a
         Zwitterion formula is

$$
R\text{---}\underset{\underset{H}{|}}{\overset{\overset{NH_3^+}{|}}{C}}\text{---}C\diagup^{\displaystyle O}_{\diagdown O^-}
$$

53. (d) The prefix for femto is
         10^{-15}. The prefix used
         for tera is 10^{12}, for
         nano 10^{-9}, and for pico
         10^{-12}.

54. (a) Prolactin acts on mammary
         glands to initiate milk
         secretion. Thyrotrophin
         acts on the thyroid to
         stimulate formation and
         secretion of thyroid
         hormone. Relaxin acts

on the symphysis pubis
as a relaxant to aid
in child birth. Glucagon
acts in the liver as a
glucose source in glyco-
genolysis.

55. (a) The suffix for a saturated
         hydrocarbon is - ane. The
         suffix for an hydroxyl
         group is - ol, for a ketone
         group - one, and for an
         unsaturated hydrocarbon
         - ene.

56. (a) Dehydrogenases, isomerases,
    (b) desmolases and hydroxylases
    (c) all participate in the bio-
    (d) genesis of steroid hormones.

57. (b) Tetrahydrocortisol and
    (d) cortisone are measured
         by Porter-Silber meth-
         odologies.

58. (b) Many different formulas
         have been proposed for
         the calculation of plasma
         osmolality. The following
         one has been used in the
         calculation:

         2Na mmol/l + 2 K mmol/l
         + Urea mmol/l
         + Glucose mmol/l =
         Osmolality mosmol/kg

         BUN x $\frac{60}{28}$ = UREA

         $\therefore$ 7 x $\frac{60}{28}$ = 15 mmol/l

         (2 x 132) + (2 x 6.7) +
         (15) + (16) = 308.4 mosmol/kg

         The usual normal range quoted
         is 280 - 295 mosmol/kg.

59. (a) False negative results may
    (b) occur with dilute urine,
    (d) in ectopic pregnancy and

with missed abortion. Proteinuria (excess protein in the urine) usually causes false positive results.

60. (a) Increased tolerance in
    (b) an insulin tolerance test may be found in diabetes mellitus and Cushing's syndrome. A decreased tolerance is generally found in the presence of a pancreatic islet cell tumor. A blood glucose falling to less than 25 per cent of the fasting level and rapidly returning to the fasting level indicates increased tolerance. A normal response is a fall to 50 per cent of the fasting level within 20 - 30 minutes and a return to the fasting level within 90 - 120 minutes.

61. (a) Aspirin, penicillin and
    (b) oxytetracycline may all
    (c) cause an increase in urine VMA. MAO inhibitors may cause a decrease in urine VMA.

62. (a) In the investigation of
    (b) ovarian function it is
    (c) found that in menopause, pituitary gonadotrophins are increased, 17 KS are increased in virilizing ovarian tumors and preg-nanediol is decreased in amenorrhea. Estrogens are decreased in primary ovarian hypofunction.

63. (a) In nephrogenic diabetes
    (d) insipidus (NDI), the patient has low urine specific gravity (usually less than 1.004) and there is no change (decrease in normal person) in urine volume due to hypertonic (3%) NaCl I.V. Normal urine output in N.D.I. is 5 - 15 liters/day, and the urine does not become concentrated when fluids are withheld.

64. (b) In primary hyperpara-
    (c) thyroidism, serum and
    (d) urine calcium levels are increased, urine phosphorus is increased and serum phosphorus is decreased. Urinary calcium is decreased in hypoparathyroidism.

65. (c) In T_3 thyrotoxicosis
    (d) the patient has a normal T_4 and a decreased serum cholesterol. The thyroid-stimulating hormone (thyrotrophin) (TSH) is decreased and the thyroxine binding globulin (TBG) is increased.

66. (d) Sodium is completely re-absorbed when the plasma level drops below 110 mmol/l.

67. (d) Calcium is present in serum in the following forms:

    Nondiffusible protein-bound calcium 45 per cent
    Diffusible ionized calcium 50 per cent
    Diffusible complexed cal-cium 5 per cent

68. (a) Polyvinyl alcohol is
    (d) added to the Titan Yellow method of magnesium de-termination to keep the magnesium hydroxide form-

ed in solution and to
increase the sensitivity
of the method (by a fac-
tor of 2).

69. (b) Iron is mainly absorbed
    (c) from the duodenum and
         the jejunum.

70. (c) The usual formula for
         calculating the anion
         gap is:

A.G. = $Na^+ - (Cl^- + HCO_3^-)$
     = $139 - (104 + 16)$
     = $139 - 120$
A.G. = 19 mmol/l

This result is elevated.
The normal ranges for
Na^+, Cl^- and HCO_3^- may
vary depending on each
laboratory's reference
range, but the usual
reference range quoted
for anion gap is 5 - 15
mmol/l.

71. (b) A protein concentration
         of 6.5 g/dl is equivalent
         to 14.63 mmol ion charge/l
         of anion.
         Protein concentration
         (in g/dl) x 2.25 = mmol
         ion charge/l.

72. (a) The percentage saturation
         can be calculated as fol-
         lows:

Per cent saturation =
serum iron x 100
 TIBC

Total iron-binding capacity
(TIBC)
= serum iron + unsaturated
iron-binding capacity(UIBC)

Therefore: Per cent satura-

tion = $\dfrac{125 \times 100}{310}$
     = 40 per cent

73. (d) Heparin inhibits thrombin.
         Trisodium citrate is used
         in coagulation studies;
         ammonium/potassium oxalate
         cannot be used as an anti-
         coagulant if potassium
         determinations are to be
         made. EDTA removes cal-
         cium from the plasma.

74. (a) In intrahepatic jaundice,
         urobilin is decreased in
         the feces, urine bili-
         rubin is positive and
         the unconjugated bili-
         rubin in the serum is
         increased.

75. (c) Potassium oxalate can-
         not be used to anti-
         coagulate blood for
         uric acid measurement
         because potassium phos-
         photungstates form
         which are insoluble,
         resulting in turbidity.
         Heparin and EDTA can
         be used as the anti-
         coagulant.

76. (b) Thiosemicarbazide serves
         to intensify the color
         of the reaction product
         in the diacetyl monoxime
         BUN procedure on the
         Technicon Autoanalyzer[R].
         Pentavalent arsenic,
         other polyvalent ions
         and ferric ion can also
         be added to intensify
         the color.

77. (a) The D-xylose absorption
    (b) test is usually normal
    (d) in postgastrectomy state,
         steatorrhoea due to pan-
         creatic disease and

cirrhosis of the liver. The results are usually decreased in jejunal malabsorption (less than 4 g in a 5-hour urine - normal : greater than 5 g).

78. (d) An inulin clearance test is generally not used because it is time consuming, expensive and uncomfortable to the patient.

79. (a)
    (b) In prerenal azotemia the urine:serum creatinine ratio is greater
    (d) than 14:1, the urine sodium is less than 10 mEq/l and the urine sediment is normal.

80. (d) At sea level room air has a pCO_2 of 0 mmHg and a pO_2 of 150 mmHg.

81. (b) The symbol for a phototube is

for a variable resistor

and for electrical ground

82. (c) Low density lipoprotein cholesterol (LDL cholesterol) is calculated as follows:

LDL Cholesterol = Total cholesterol - (High density lipoprotein cholesterol + $\frac{Triglyceride}{5}$)

= 218 - $(37 + \frac{263}{5})$ mg/dl

= 218 - 90 mg/dl

= 128 mg/dl

83. (b) The urine sample is treated with dinitrophenylhydrazine which will react with any keto acids to form phenylhydrazones. The urine is then extracted with chloroform to remove indole acetic acid. Sodium chloride is then used to saturate the aqueous phase. The 5-hydroxyindole acetic acid is then extracted into ether and then into a buffer of pH 7.0 for the color reaction with 1-nitroso-2-naphthol and nitrous acid.

84. (a)
    (b) Cystine, cysteine and methionine all contain
    (c) sulphur. Ornithine does not.

85. (c) Dalton's law states: "The total pressure of a mixture of gases is equal to the sum of the partial pressures exerted by each of the component gases."

86. (c) The Porter-Silber method for the determination of corticosteroids is based upon a reaction between certain corticosteroids and phenylhydrazine in the presence of alcohol and sulphuric acid. A yellow pigment is formed. A 17, 21-dihydroxy-20-keto structure on the steroid is required for the reaction.

87. (b) Sudan III is used to stain lipid.

88. (c) An isobestic point

is a point where two spectral absorption curves for two pigments intersect.

89. (c) In the Kjeldahl nitrogen technique the proteins are precipitated with trichloroacetic acid or tungstic acid. The non-protein nitrogen (NPN) is removed with the supernatant. The organic matter in the washed precipitate is then oxidized by hot refluxing sulphuric acid. Certain catalysts, e.g., copper sulphate, selenium, may be added. The nitrogen is converted to an ammonium salt which is then reacted with Nessler's reagent (a double iodide of mercury and potassium). A yellow to orange-brown is formed.
Svedberg coefficients are a measure of ultra-centrifugation, the Van den Berg technique is a method for bilirubin measurement and Tiselins was involved in early electrophoresis methodologies.

90. (c) In 1958, three minor components of normal human hemoglobin were identified. These were entitled; HbA_{1a}, HbA_{1b} and HbA_{1c}. These glycosylated hemoglobins have faster electrophoretical mobility than HbA. They have a carbohydrate complex attached to the N-terminal valine of the beta globin chain. Their physiological function is

unsure but it has been shown that the carbohydrate complex is added non-enzymatically after the formation of HbA and throughout the life span of the mature red blood cell. The attachment of the carbohydrate occurs slowly and depends on the circulating level of blood glucose, so that the glycosylated hemoglobin level is thought to be representative of the time-averaged blood glucose level. A commonly used method for quantitation of glycosylated hemoglobins is cation exchange chromatography.

91. (a) δ-Aminolevulinic acid is the direct precursor of porphyrins.

92. (c) Prostatic acid phosphatase can be specifically inhibited by tartrate.

93. (c) In an oral glucose tolerance test performed on a normal person, the two-hour blood sample has a glucose level that is usually lower than or equal to the fasting level.

94. (c) In severe hemolytic jaundice urobilinogen in the urine shows a large increase, urobilin in the feces shows a large increase and there is increased unconjugated bilirubin in the blood.

95. (b) In the red blood cell

carbonic anhydrase cata-
lyzes the formation of
carbonic acid from CO_2
and H_2O.

96. (c) In a Gaussian distribution 1 standard devia-
tion (SD) includes 34.1
per cent of the popula-
tion and 2 SD includes
34.1 per cent plus an
additional 13.6 per cent
of the population. There-
fore 2 SD includes 47.7
per cent of the popula-
tion. As a Gaussian
distribution is distri-
buted equally on each
side of the mean value
(i.e., 50 per cent of
the population on each
side of the mean), in
the example given, 2.3
per cent of the popula-
tion will have a potas-
sium value greater than
4.60 mEq/l (50 - 47.7
per cent).

97. (c) The point at which proteins carry a net zero
charge is called the
isoelectric point.

98. (b) In uncompensated metabolic acidosis, both
the pH and HCO_3^- are
decreased.

99. (c) In myocardial infarction,
creatine kinase (CK) is
the enzyme that first
shows elevation.

100. (c) A saturated aqueous solution of phenol is used
to make up Pandy's rea-
gent.

101. (d) Triglyceride is the main

constituant of chylo-
micron and prebeta-
lipoprotein (very low
density lipoprotein -
VLDL).

102. (a) Lipoprotein, thyroxine
(b) binding globulin and
(d) glycoprotein all migrate
in the alpha-1-globulin
region. Two other im-
portant proteins migrat-
ing in this region are
transcortin and alpha-
1-antitrypsin. Hapto-
globin migrates in the
alpha-2-globulin region
along with macroglobulin,
ceruloplasmin and other
glycoproteins.

103. (c) A plasma glucose concentration of 180 mg/dl =
10.0 mmol/l in S.I. units.

104. (a) The normal bicarbonate
ion to carbonic acid
ratio in the body is
20:1.

105 (b) Methanol is oxidized
at one seventh the
rate of ethanol. There-
fore, because of its
slow elimination, re-
peated small doses may
accumulate to produce
toxic effects.

106. (b) The chemical reactions
taking place in the
Clinistix $^{(R)}$ test
strip for urine glucose
are:

Glucose + O_2 (air)
$\xrightarrow[\text{Oxidase}]{\text{Glucose}}$ Gluconic acid
+ H_2O_2

H_2O_2 + Chromogen
$\xrightarrow{\text{Peroxidase}}$ Oxidized Chromogen
blue + H_2O

107. (d) Pancreatic lipase, conjugated bile salts and
an alkaline intestinal
pH are all required for
fat absorption.

108. (b) The exudate protein to
serum protein ratio is
generally greater than
0.6.

109. (d) Acid phosphatase measurements are made on vagi-
nal aspirations because
seminal fluid has an
acid phosphatase concen-
tration several thousand
times the level of other
body fluids. If an in-
dividual has the dominant
secretor gene he will
secrete the A, B or H
blood group substances
in other body fluids.
Thus the presence of
these substances can be
tested for in body
fluids or stains on
clothing. The Hektoen
precipitin test utilizes
specific antiserum ob-
tained by immunizing
suitable animals with
human semen. It is
specific for human semen
and can be used to iden-
tify semen stains on
clothing.

110. (c) Fatty casts indicate
tubular fatty changes.
They are frequently seen in
the nephrotic syndrome,
whatever its cause, and
particularly in diabetic
nephropathy. Hyaline
casts are formed in the
tubules from Tamm-Horsfall
micoprotein. Red blood
cell casts always indi-
cate renal parenchymal

disease. Granular
casts are formed from
epithelial casts in
which the distinct cell
margin has disappeared.
As the epithelical cast
stagnates in the tubule
or moves towards the
renal pelvis, the cells
trapped inside the cast
disintegrate.

111. (c) The volume of 5.0 M
H_2SO_4 required to
neutralize 180 ml of
0.6 N NaOH may be
calculated by the fol-
lowing formula:

Concentration$_{(solution\ 1)}$
x Volume $_{(solution\ 1)}$ =
Concentration $_{(solution\ 2)}$
x Volume$_{(solution\ 2)}$
which can be abbreviated
to:

$$C_1V_1 = C_2V_2$$

5.0 M H_2SO_4, being di-
valent for the hydrogen
ion, is equivalent to
10.0 N H_2SO_4.

$$C_1V_1 = C_2V_2$$
$$10.0 \times x = 0.6 \times 180$$
$$x = \frac{0.6 \times 180}{10.0}$$
$$= 10.8$$

Therefore, the volume of
5.0 M H_2SO_4 required to
neutralize 180 ml of
0.6 N NaOH is 10.8 ml.

112. (b) The formula for con-
verting from a concen-
tration expressed in
mg/l to one in mEq/l
is:

$$mEq/l = \frac{mg/l}{Eq.\ wt.}$$

470 mg/dl = 4700 mg/l
Therefore, the Na^+ concentration in mEq/l is:

$$\frac{4700}{23}$$

= 204

Therefore, 470 mg/dl of Na^+ is equal to 204 mEq/l of Na^+.

113. (c) Vitamin B_1 is known as thiamine. Retinol is vitamin A, riboflavin is vitamin B_2 and cholecalciferol is vitamin D_3.

114. (d) Cyanocobalamin is vitamin B_{12}. Naphthoquinone is vitamin K, tocopherol is vitamin E and ascorbic acid is vitamin C.

115. (a) Alkaline phosphatase
     (b) occurs in high levels
     (c) in intestinal epithelium, kidney tubules, osteoblasts, liver and placenta. In bone it is concerned with the calcification process in bone synthesis. In Paget's disease, the osteoblastic cells try to rebuild bone that is being reabsorbed by the uncontrolled activity of osteoclasts. Levels of serum alkaline phosphatase may be 10 - 25 times normal. In rickets, osteomalacia has occurred before the epiphyses are closed.
     Serum alkaline phosphatase activity of 2 - 4 times normal is seen, dropping to normal with vitamin D therapy. In primary hyperparathyroidism, and less frequently in sec-

ondary hyperparathyroidism, a slight to moderate increase in activity may be seen that is relative to the extent of bone involvement. Hypophosphatasia is a recessive metabolic condition with low levels of alkaline phosphatase. Diagnosis may be assisted by identifying the increased levels of phosphoethanolamine in the urine.

116. (a) Liver, placental and
     (c) intestinal isoenzymes
     (d) of alkaline phosphatase are all more stable to heat than the bone isoenzyme. Following heating a sample for 10 minutes at 56°C most of the bone isoenzyme activity is destroyed. The intestinal isoenzyme is more stable than the liver isoenzyme and the placental isoenzyme, the most stable. Increasing the temperature of incubation to 65°C does not diminish placental alkaline phosphatase activity whereas the activity of all other alkaline phosphatase isoenzymes is completely destroyed. A number of patients with various types of cancers have in their serum an alkaline phosphatase isoenzyme with very similar properties to the placental isoenzyme. This placenta-like fetal form of alkaline phosphatase

is known as the Regan
isoenzyme. It is as
heat stable as the
placental form.

117. (b) The optimum pH range
for the acid phosphatase
prostatic isoenzyme is
4.8 - 5.1.

118. (a) Serum acid phosphatase
(b) may be increased in
(c) Gaucher's disease,
(d) sickle cell anemia,
myelocytic leukemia and
carcinoma of the prostate.

119. (a) The rate of production
(b) of bilirubin, the level
(c) of Y receptor carrier
(d) protein, glucuronic
acid and UDPGT relative
deficiences and bili-
rubin reabsorption from
the gut all may contri-
bute to physiological
jaundice of the newborn.

120. (c) A didymium filter is
used to verify wavelength
settings in broad band-
pass instruments.

121. (b) Serum alkaline phosphatase
(c) is increased in the third
trimester of pregnancy.
This 2 - 3 times increase
is due to enzyme of pla-
cental origin. 5'-
nucleotidase and gamma-
glutamyl transferase are
not increased in pregnan-
cy. Lactic dehydrogenase
isoenzymes IV and V are
sometimes increased if a
mother is carrying an
erythroblastotic child.
Therefore, if an increase
in either gamma-glutamyl
transferase or 5'-

nucleotidase is ob-
served it will be
because of reasons
other than pregnancy.

122. (c) In the automated assay
for 5'-nucleotidase,
serum is reacted with
and without nickel.
The amount of phos-
phorus liberated is
then determined. The
reaction without nickel
represents alkaline
phosphatase plus 5'-
nucleotidase activity
and with nickel, just
the 5'- nucleotidase
activity.

123. (a) The serum activity of
(b) the enzyme gamma-
(d) glutamyl transferase
is usually normal in
Paget's disease, renal
failure and muscle
disease. However, as
high levels of the
enzyme are found in
the prostate, prostatic
malignancy may cause
high serum levels of
gamma-glutamyl trans-
ferase.

124. (b) The temperature of a
propane-air flame is
approximately 1900°C.
The flame temperatures
of the other gas mix-
tures are:

acetylene/oxygen   3100°C
propane/oxygen   2850°C
acetylene/air   2250°C

125. (a) Alpha particles are
nuclei of helium atoms.

126. (d) In a continuous flow
analyzer, factors which

influence the quantity
of solute that passes
through the membrane,
or dialysis, are:

- the duration of
  contact of the two
  solutions
- the area of contact
- the temperature at
  which the dialysis
  occurs
- the thickness and
  porosity of the
  membrane
- the concentration
  gradient across the
  membrane
- the size, shape and
  electrical charge of
  molecules

127. (d) In copper reduction
          blood glucose methods,
          e.g., the Folin-Wu
          method, cupric ions are
          reduced to cuprous ions
          by heating a tungstic
          acid filtrate of whole
          blood with an alkaline
          copper solution. A
          molybdenum blue color
          pigment is produced by
          adding excess phospho-
          molybdic acid to the
          cuprous ions. This
          pigment is read spec-
          trophotometrically.
          These methods depend
          on the time and temper-
          ature of heating, the
          concentration of rea-
          gents and the alkalinity
          of the solution.

128. (c) The substrate used in
          the Rosalki and Tarlow
          method for the measure-
          ment of gamma-glutamyl
          transferase is gamma-

glutamyl-p-nitroanilide.
Buffering in the system
is by use of tris(hydroxy-
methyl)aminomethane and
glycylglycine. Glycylgly-
cine also acts as an ac-
ceptor. Serum is added
to the acceptor/buffer
solution, and the addi-
tion of substrate in
HCl solution initiates the
reaction. The formation
of p-nitroaniline in the
reaction causes an in-
creased absorbance which
is measured at 405 nm.

129. (b) The optimum pH for amy-
          lase in human serum is
          6.9 - 7.0.

130. (b) Calcitonin is produced
          by the thyroid. Follicle-
          stimulating hormone (FSH)
          is produced by the anter-
          ior pituitary, antidiu-
          retic hormone (ADH,
          vasopressin) is pro-
          duced by the posterior
          pituitary and relaxin
          is produced by the
          ovaries.

131. (a) Amylase forms a com-
          plex with IgA in mac-
          roamylasemia.

132. (c) Gastrin is a protein.
          Oxytocin is a nona-
          peptide, thyroid-
          stimulating hormone
          (TSH) a glycoprotein
          and glucagon a poly-
          peptide.

133. (c) Potassium is reabsorbed
          in the kidney in the
          proximal convoluted
          tubule.

134. (a) Serum calcium levels
     (c) are controlled by para-
     (d) thyroid hormone (PTH),
          calcitonin and vitamin
          D compounds.

135. (c) Amyloclastic methods
          follow the decrease in
          substrate (starch) con-
          centration.

136. (d) In the adrenogenital
          syndrome there is an
          inherited lack or de-
          ficiency of enzymes
          that lead to the forma-
          tion of cortisol. The
          most common of these
          enzyme deficiencies is
          in the hydroxylation
          at the C-21 position.
          The activity of the
          adrenal cortex is con-
          trolled through a nega-
          tive feedback process
          which exists between
          the blood levels of
          free cortisol and cor-
          ticotrophin (ACTH).
          With a decrease or lack
          of cortisol, excess
          ACTH is released which
          will stimulate the
          adrenal cortex and cause
          hyperplasia. The con-
          version of cholesterol
          to pregnenolone is
          stimulated by ACTH, so
          that with excess ACTH
          in the circulation there
          will be excess produc-
          tion of the cortisol
          precursors that are
          synthesized ahead of
          the enzyme block. These
          precursors cause excess
          production of androgenic
          steroids which in turn
          cause virilization.

137. (b) Parathyroid hormone (PTH)

     (c) mobilizes calcium
     (d) from the bone, in-
          creases the synthesis
          of 1,25 $(OH)_2D_3$, in-
          creases renal absorp-
          tion of calcium and
          decreases the reab-
          sorption of phos-
          phorus.

138. (a) Hyperphosphatemia
     (c) may be found in renal
     (d) failure, hypoparathy-
          roidism and hypervi-
          taminosis D. Hypo-
          phosphatemia is usually
          found in Fanconi syn-
          drome.

139. (d) Transferrin migrates
          with the beta-globulin.

140. (a) In acute pancreatitis
          the increase in serum
          amylase occurs in 3 - 6
          hours, peaks in 20 - 30
          hours and may persist
          for 48 - 72 hours.
          Urine levels reflect
          serum changes by a
          lag time of 6 - 10
          hours.

141. (c) The Porter-Silber
          method for cortico-
          steroids relies on
          the formation of a
          yellow pigment when
          certain corticoster-
          oids are reacted with
          phenylhydrazine in
          the presence of al-
          cohol and sulphuric
          acid.
          The Guthrie test is
          a bacterial test for
          detecting the disease
          phenylketonuria. The
          Berthelot reaction is
          a procedure for measur-
          ing urea nitrogen by

liberating ammonia from a specimen with urease and reacting the ammonia with phenolhypochlorite in the presence of sodium nitroprusside. The Lange test involves precipitating cerebrospinal fluid (CSF) gamma globulins with a colloidal gold suspension. Several tubes with increasing dilutions of CSF are used and the precipitation pattern produced may be used to implicate certain neurological diagnoses. The procedure has been largely replaced by CSF electrophoresis and immunoelectrophoresis techniques.

142. (c) Serum iron will be decreased and total iron binding capacity (TIBC) will be increased in iron deficiency anemia.

143. (a) Corn oil, beta-naphthyl
     (b) laurate, N-methylindoxyl
     (c) myristate and olive oil
     (d) have all been used as substrates in lipase assays.

144. (b) The reaction between 17-ketosteroids and n-dinitrobenzene in alcoholic alkali is known as the Zimmerman reaction.

145. (b) Most of the copper that is ingested is lost through the stool.

146. (a) Allopurinol, probenecid
     (b) and radiopaque dye can
     (d) all cause a decrease in plasma uric acid. Thiazides can cause an increase in plasma uric acid.

147. (b) The two generally
     (c) accepted forms of Henderson-Hasselbalch equation are:

$$pH = pK + \log \frac{Total\ CO_2 - 0.03\ pCO_2}{0.03\ pCO_2}$$

and

$$pH = pK + \log \frac{(HCO_3^-)}{a \times pCO_2}$$

148. (a) Serum lipase is usually
     (c) increased in acute pan-
     (d) creatitis, perforated peptic ulcer and opiate induced spasm of pancreatic duct sphincter.

149. Luteinizing hormone (LH, interstitial cell-stimulating hormone, ICSH) is involved in the secretion of progesterone. Relaxin aids in paturition, oxytocin causes uterine muscle contraction and melanophore-stimulating hormone (MSH) causes dispersion of pigment granules.

150. (a) Calcium, magnesium,
     (b) cobalt and manganese
     (c) all stimulate trypsin
     (d) activity.

151. Parathyroid hormone (PTH) regulates calcium and phosphorus metabolism. Vasopressin elevates blood pressure, glucagon takes part in glycogenolysis and insulin

in lipogenesis.

152. (c) The most important plasma buffer system for the control of acid/base disturbances is the bicarbonate/carbonic acid system. This system is also present in the red blood cell. The buffer system is effective because of its high concentration and because carbon dioxide can be disposed of or retained in the lungs. The renal tubules are able to increase or decrease the reabsorption of bicarbonate from the glomerular filtrate.

153. (c) The dibucaine number is a measure of the activity of cholinesterase. The fluoride number is another way of expressing the cholinesterase activity.

154. (c) Progesterone prepares the uterus for ovum implantation. Prolactin initiates milk secretion, enterogastrone inhibits secretions in the stomach and follicle-stimulating hormone causes secretion of estrogens.

155. The human body compensates for acid-base disturbances in the following ways:
(1) Blood buffer systems
- the bicarbonate/carbonic acid, plasma protein, phosphate and hemoglobin buffer systems all work by removing or releasing hydrogen ions in response to changes in pH.
(2) Respiratory mechanism
- carbon dioxide can be retained or excreted through the lungs by decreasing or increasing the respiration rate and depth.
(3) Renal mechanism
- the kidney has the ability to excrete variable amounts of acid or base.

156. (c) Amylase is routinely assayed in urine.

157. (b) Low estrogen levels are found at the beginning of the menstrual cycle.

158. (c) CSF glucose is approximately 2/3 the level of the blood glucose.

159. (a) In bacterial meningitis the cerebrospinal fluid (CSF) protein is usually increased, the cerebrospinal fluid (CSF) glucose is decreased and the white blood cell count (WBC) is increased.

160. (d) In nephrotic syndrome, the serum protein electrophoresis changes seen are that the alpha-2

globulin fraction is increased, the gamma-globulin fraction is decreased and the albumin is decreased.

161. (c) The blood buffer system responds the quickest to a change in acid-base status, followed by the respiratory mechanism and the renal mechanism. The most effective blood buffers are the bicarbonate/carbonic acid, plasma protein, phosphate and the hemoglobin buffer systems.

162. (b) Beta-lipoprotein carries most of the cholesterol in serum.

163. (d) If a turbidimetric test is used for urine protein, the presence of x-ray contrast media in the urine can cause a false positive reaction, as can tolbutamide metabolites. A strongly alkaline urine can cause a false negative result.

164. (c) A serum creatinine concentration of 1.7 mg/dl ≡ 0.15 mmol/l when expressed in S.I. units.

165. (d) Diabetics, hospitalized patients and people on carbohydrate-free diets all may have ketone bodies in their urine.

166. (d) An increase in serum cholesterol may be found in hypothyroidism, nephrotic syndrome, and obstructive biliary tract disease.

167. (a) LD_2 isoenzyme shows an increase over LD_1 following a myocardial infarction. This is the so called "flipped ratio."

168. (c) The enzyme, Δ^5-3beta-hydroxysterol dehydrogenase isomerase, converts 16-alpha-hydroxy-DHEA to 16 alpha OH androstenedione.

169. (c) Acetoacetic acid in a urine sample tested by the ferric chloride test will produce a red or red-brown color. Melanin will produce a grey precipitate that changes to black, pyruvic acid produces a deep gold-yellow or green color and salicylates produce a purple color.

170. (a) Homogentisic acid in a urine sample tested by the ferric chloride test will produce a blue or green color that fades quickly. Cyanates produce a red color, phenothiazines produce a purple-pink color and o-hydroxy-phenylacetic acid produces a mauve color.

171. (b) A serum calcium concentration of 10.0 mg/dl ≡ 2.5 mmol/l when expressed in S.I. units.

172. (c) Most of the free fatty

acids in blood are
carried by albumin.

173. (d) Urinary porphyrins are
found to be increased
in most cases of con-
genital erythropoietic
porphyria, acute inter-
mittent porphyria and
porphyria cutanea tarda.

174. (d) In acid solution, ethanol reduces potassium
dichromate and forms a
green salt of chromium.
Alcohol dehydrogenase
can be used in an enzy-
matic procedure. Gas
chromatography can be
used to identify and
quantitate ethanol and
other volatile sub-
stances.

175. (c) In Gilbert's disease
there is defective trans-
port of bilirubin from
the plasma to the hepa-
tocyte. Indirect serum
bilirubin is increased.
In Crigler-Najjar disease
there is inability to
conjugate bilirubin to
bilirubin glucuronide in
hepatic cells. It is a
rare familial autosomal
recessive disease that
is due to a congenital
deficiency or absence
of glucuronyl-transferase.
In Dubin-Johnson syndrome
there is defective trans-
port of direct bilirubin
from the hepatocyte into
the bile canaliculus.
The Lucy-Driscoll syn-
drome is characterized
by inhibition of glucur-
onyl-transferase by a
compound in the mother's
serum. This unidentified

substance is only
present in the last
trimester of pregnancy.

176. (c) Alkaline phosphatase
shows an increase in
activity following
reconstitution of
commercial lyophilized
control sera.

177. (d) Increased chorionic
gonadotrophins are
found in the urine
in seminoma, chorio-
epithelioma of the
testicle and in hyda-
tidiform mole.

178. (d) A serum phosphorus
concentration of 4.7
mg/dl $\equiv$ 1.50 mmol/l when
expressed in S.I. units.

179. (c) When ortho-toluidine and
benzidine reagents are
used for occult blood
testing, false positives
may occur if the patient
has eaten meat within the
previous three days be-
fore the collection of
the feces sample.

180. (b) The half-life of a drug
is the time required
for the serum concen-
tration of the drug to
decrease by 50 per cent.

181. (c) The normal range for
serum cholesterol in
the 50 yr.[+] age group
is approximately 160 -
320 mg/dl.

182. (b) CK-MB is the significant creatine kinase
isoenzyme found to be
elevated following a
myocardial infarction.

183. (a) The urobilinogen content
     (b) of feces is usually in-
     (c) creased in hemolytic
         anemia.

184. (b) A serum uric acid con-
         centration of 6.7 mg/dl
         $\equiv$ 0.40 mmol/l in S.I.
         units.

185. (d) Gastritis, gastric car-
         cinoma and achlorhydria
         all could cause a gas-
         tric aspiration acid
         concentration of 0 mEq
         one hour post stimula-
         tion.

186. (c) The upper limit for
         serum triglyceride in
         the 50 yr.[+] age group
         is approximately 190
         mg/dl.

187. (a) A serum cholesterol con-
         centration of 232 mg/dl
         $\equiv$ 6.0 mmol/l in S.I.
         units.

188. (d) The measurement of serum
         gastrin may be indicated
         in patients with recur-
         rent ulceration after
         surgery for duodenal
         ulcer, patients with
         duodenal ulcer for whom
         elective surgery is plan-
         ned and in patients with
         intact stomachs who have
         a basal acid secretion
         of greater than 10 mEq/
         hour. There will be an
         increase in serum gastrin
         when there is a loss of
         the normal feedback con-
         trol by which gastrin
         normally stimulates acid
         secretion. Gastrin re-
         lease is then inhibited
         by the acid entering the
         antrum of the stomach.

189. (a) Erect posture, low
     (b) sodium diet (especially
     (c) if with reduced plasma
         volume) and estrogen-
         containing oral con-
         traceptives can all
         cause an increase in
         plasma renin activity
         (PRA). Primary aldo-
         steronism results in
         decreased PRA.

190. (a) A decreased activity
     (b) of serum cholinesterase
     (c) is observed in pulmon-
     (d) ary embolism, muscular
         dystrophy, chronic
         hepatitis and pregnancy.

191. (d) The pancreozymin-secretin
         test measures the effect,
         after intravenous admin-
         istration of pancreozymin
         and secretin, of changes
         in the volume and bicar-
         bonate concentration in
         duodenal fluid, the amy-
         lase concentration of
         duodenal fluid and the
         level of serum lipase
         and amylase.

192. (a) The Watson-Schwartz
     (d) test for urinary uro-
         bilinogen and porpho-
         bilinogen uses Ehrlich's
         reagent which is made up
         from p-dimethylaminobenzal-
         dehyde and hydrochloric
         acid.

193. (d) To obtain the trough
         concentration of a drug,
         a sample is usually
         drawn just before the
         next dose. The measure-
         ment is made to make
         sure that the serum con-
         centration is more than
         the minimum effective
         concentration and also

to make sure that the
drug is being eliminated
from the body at a known
rate.

194.   (b)   In succinyldicholine
             (suxamethonium) apnea
             the patient has either
             a low serum activity or
             an abnormal variant of
             cholinesterase. Succinyl-
             dicholine, being similar
             to acetylcholine, is also
             hydrolyzed by cholines-
             terase. If this hydro-
             lysis and destruction
             of the drug is impaired,
             the effect of the drug
             is prolonged.

195.   (a)   Penicillin, phenothiazine
       (c)   and chloramphenicol may
       (d)   all cause an increase in
             urinary 17-ketosteroids.
             Estrogens may cause a
             decrease.

196.   (a)   Many organic phosphorus
             compounds used by agri-
             cultural workers inhibit
             cholinesterase activity.
             Therefore, measuring
             serum activity of cholin-
             esterase in the workers
             assists in monitoring
             possible toxicity due
             to excess exposure of
             the organic phosphorus
             material.

197.   (b)   A barbiturate with a 3 -
             6 hour effect would be
             classified as an inter-
             mediate acting barbi-
             turate. Amobarbital,
             butabarbital and pro-
             barbital are all exam-
             ples of intermediate
             acting barbiturates.

198.   (b)   Polyuria occurs when
             the 24-hour urine
             volume exceeds 2500 ml.
             The commonly accepted
             normal range is 600 -
             2500 ml/24 hours.

199.   (a)   The normal range for
             urobilinogen in a 24-
             hour urine is 1.0 -
             4.0 mg. The normal
             range for protein in
             a 24-hour urine sample
             is 10 - 150 mg. The
             sample is normally
             negative for nitrite
             and bilirubin.

200.   (a)   A qualitative test
             for ketones in a 24-
             hour urine sample
             would normally be
             negative. Glucose
             usually has a concen-
             tration of less than
             0.5 g/24 hours, crea-
             tinine of 1.0 - 1.6
             g/24 hours. The nor-
             mal range for urine
             pH is 4.5 - 8.0 with
             an average of 6.

201.   (a)   Normally, 60 - 75
             per cent of the
             total serum choles-
             terol is in the form
             of esters.

202.   (b)   Erythromycin, quini-
       (c)   dine and chlordiaze-
       (d)   poxide may all cause
             an increase in urinary
             17-hydroxycorticosteroids.
             Oral contraceptives may
             cause a decrease.

203.   (b)   Wilson's disease, or
             hepatolenticular degen-
             eration, is a disease

of copper metabolism and is characterized by low levels of serum copper and ceruloplasmin, injury to the cerebral basal ganglia and Kayser-Fleischer rings (pathology of the cornea typical of the disease and due to the deposition of copper).

204. (d) The serum activity of alpha-hydroxybutyrate dehydrogenase is thought to represent the activity of the lactate dehydrogenase isoenzymes, LD_1 plus LD_2.

205. (a)
     (b) Diabetes mellitus with glycosuria, vomiting
     (d) (causing dehydration), and nephrosis with proteinuria can all cause a high urine specific gravity.

206. (d) A 17.6 per cent Na_2SO_4 solution contains 17.6 g/dl

$$= 176 \text{ g/l}$$

A 1 M Na_2SO_4 solution contains 142 g/l

Therefore: 17.6 per cent Na_2SO_4 is $\frac{176}{142}$ M

$$= 1.24 \text{ M}$$

$$\text{Vol.}_1 \times \text{Conc.}_1 = \text{Vol.}_2 \times \text{Conc.}_2$$

$$X \times 1.24 = 450 \times 0.75$$
$$X = 272 \text{ ml}$$

207. (c) Almost all analytical methods for the measurement of phospholipids measure inorganic phosphorus by the formation of the phosphomolybdate ion, which is then reduced to form the colloidal complex, heteropoly blue.

208. (c) The formula for conversion of transmission to absorbance is:

$$\log_{10}T = 2 - A$$

where T = Transmission
      A = Absorbance

Therefore:
$$A = 2 - \log_{10}T$$
$$= 2 - \log_{10}63$$
$$= 2 - 1.799$$
$$= 0.201$$

209. (a) 1 molecule of H_2SO_4 gives 2 hydrogen ions; therefore the hydrogen ion concentration (H^+) is 0.286.

$$pH = \log_{10} \frac{1}{[H^+]}$$
$$= \log_{10} \frac{1}{0.286}$$
$$= \log_{10} 100 - \log_{10} 28.6$$
$$= 2 - 1.456$$
$$= 0.544$$

210. (d) Isocitrate dehydrogenase (ICD) is found in high concentration in the liver, heart and skeletal muscle. It is also found in high concentration in the kidney, adrenal tissue, platelets

and red blood cells.

211. (a) Isocitrate dehydrogenase
     (b) (ICD) activity is inhi-
         bited by Cu^{2+} and Hg^{2+}.
         Mn^{2+} and Co^{2+} are acti-
         vators of ICD.

212. (a) In adrenogenital syndrome
     (c) due to 11-beta-hydroxy-
     (d) lation deficiency, plasma
         ACTH is increased. The
         hypokalemia and increase
         in plasma deoxycortico-
         sterone increase are
         both mild compared to a
         17-α hydroxylation de-
         ficiency. Plasma cor-
         tisol is usually normal.

213. (a) The adult therapeutic
         range for digoxin in
         serum is 0.9 - 2.0 ng/ml.
         The minimum effective
         concentration has been
         found to be 0.9 ng/ml.

214. (a) Increased isocitrate
     (b) dehydrogenase (ICD)
     (d) activity is found in
         parenchymal liver
         disease, neonatal
         biliary duct atresia
         and pulmonary infarc-
         tion. Increased levels
         are found in myocardial
         infarction only if the
         infarction is accompa-
         nied by congestive
         failure. This results
         in hepatic ischemia.

215. (a) Sorbitol dehydrogenase
     (c) (SDH) is found in signi-
     (d) ficant quantities in the
         liver and to a lesser
         extent in the kidney
         and prostate. Cardiac
         and skeletal muscles
         contain little sorbitol

dehydrogenase (SDH)
activity.

216. (d) The formula relating
         pH and hydrogen ion
         concentration ($[H^+]$)
         is:

$$pH = -\log_{10} [H^+]$$

$$5.7 = -\log_{10} [H^+]$$

Therefore: $\log_{10} [H^+] = -5.7$

$$= 0.3 - 6.0$$

Therefore: $[H^+]$ = antilog 0.3 + antilog (-6.0)

$$= 1.995 \times 10^{-6}$$

217. (b) The Neeld-Pearson pro-
         cedure for the deter-
         mination of vitamin A
         relies upon the reaction
         between trichloroacetic
         acid and the π-electrons
         in the conjugated double
         bonds of vitamin A to
         form a blue color.

218. (b) In adrenal hyperplasia
     (c) due to pituitary dys-
         function, the plasma
         cortisol is decreased
         after dexamethasone
         suppression of 8 mg/day
         and the level of 17-
         hydroxyketosteroid
         (17 OHKS) after adreno-
         corticotrophin (ACTH)
         stimulation is increased.
         The level of 17-hydroxy-
         ketosteroid (17 OHKS)
         in the urine is increased
         and the baseline level
         of plasma cortisol is
         variable (normal or in-
         creased).

219. (c) N^5-methyl-tetrahydrofolic acid is the predominant form of folic acid in human serum.

220. (a) Pathological jaundice
     (b) in the neonate may be
     (c) caused by any of the
     (d) following mechanisms:
          (a) impaired transport of bilirubin due to abnormalities in albumin binding caused by hypoxia, acidosis or drugs (e.g., sulfonamides).
          (b) impaired conjugation of bilirubin which may be associated with the presence of pregnane-3 alpha, 20 beta-diol in maternal breast milk or with certain drugs (e.g., chloramphenicol).
          (c) impaired excretion of conjugated bilirubin due to biliary atresia.
          (d) excess production of bilirubin which may be secondary to hemolysis caused an ABO or Rh incompatibility or a bacterial or viral infection.

221. (a) Lithium is chosen as an
     (b) "internal standard" be-
     (c) cause it has a high
     (d) emission intensity, is normally absent from biological fluids, emits at a wavelength removed from Na and K and acts as a radiation buffer.

222. (d) Chemical interference (e.g., phosphate interference in calcium determinations forming calcium phosphate), ionization interference (e.g., when atoms in the flame become excited instead of only being dissociated) and matrix interferences (e.g., enhancement of light absorption by organic solvents), all may cause interferences in atomic absorption spectrophotometry.

223. (c) The respiratory alkalosis produced by salicylate intoxication lags behind rising plasma salicylate levels by 2 - 4 hours.

224. (a) Aspartate aminotrans-
     (b) ferase (AST) may be
     (c) elevated in myocardial infarction, musculoskeletal disease and liver diseases. It may be falsely decreased in diabetic ketoacidosis because of increased serum lactate consuming the enzyme during the test.

225. (a) An 0.023 M NaOH solution will have an hydroxide concentration of 0.023 M

Therefore: $[OH^-] = 0.023$ M

as $\log_{10} \dfrac{1}{[OH^-]} = pOH$

$pOH = \log_{10} \dfrac{1}{0.023}$

$= \log_{10} \dfrac{100}{2.3}$

$= 2 - 0.362$

$= 1.638$

as $pH = 14 - pOH$

$pH = 14 - 1.638$

$= 12.362$

226. (c) A microbiological assay
for folic acid utilizes
the bacteria Lactobacil-
lus casei. Bacillus
subtilis is used in the
Guthrie test for phenyla-
lanine, Euglena gracilis
is used to assay for
serum levels of vitamin
B_{12} and Bacillus circulans
for the assay of strepto-
mycin (Price, Neilson,
Welch method).

227. (c) An essential difference
between nephelometric
and turbidimetric measurements is that in nephelo-
metry, the light scattered
is measured at right
angles to the incident
beam. The optical arrangement is similar to that
used in fluorimetry.
Nephelometric measurement
systems are usually capable
of more precision than
turbidimetric measurement
systems.

228. (d) The photoelectric effect,
the Compton effect and
pair production are all
responsible for the ab-
sorption of gamma rays.

229. (d) Malate dehydrogenase
(MD) is used in the
aspartate aminotrans-
ferase (AST) reaction

mixture to convert
oxalacetate to L-
malate. This part
of the AST assay
method is shown below:

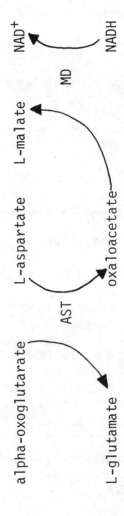

230. (d) Three of the main
distinguishing factors
in differentiating
between primary and
secondary aldosteronism
are the plasma renin
activity (PRA), the
urinary 17-hydroxy-
corticosteroids (17 OHKS)

and the etiology. Tabulated results of the investigation
of the three factors are shown below:

FACTOR	PRIMARY	SECONDARY
PRA	markedly decreased	normal or increased
Urine 17 OHKS	usually normal may be increased in adrenal carcinoma	usually normal
Etiology	usually a tumor	edematous conditions

231. (d) The Reinsch test is used to screen for the presence of
mercury, arsenic, bismuth and antimony. Metallic copper
in the presence of concentrated HCl will reduce the heavy
metal to the elemental form which then deposits on the
copper.

232. (c) The optimum pH for the CK reaction is 9.0. However, in
most CK procedures, the following reactions take place,
for which the optimum system pH is 6.8 - 6.9

Creatine phosphate + ADP $\xrightarrow{CK}$ creatine + ATP

ATP + glucose $\xrightarrow{HK}$ glucose-6-phosphate + ADP

Glucose-6-phosphate + $NADP^+$ $\xrightarrow{GPD}$ 6-phosphogluconate + NAPDH + H^+

233. (d) In distinguishing between a diagnosis of pheochromocytoma
and neuroblastoma, measurements of urinary VMA, catecholamines
and HVA are very useful. Typical results of these assays
are found below:

Urine results	Pheochromocytoma	Neuroblastoma
VMA	Increased	Increased
Catecholamines	Increased	Increased
HVA	Normal	Increased

234. (b)
      (c) Reducing substances such as creatinine and uric acid have
an additive effect on glucose measurements by alkaline
ferricyanide procedures.

235. (a)
      (b) Calcitonin is responsible for increasing renal excretion
of phosphates and inhibiting bone reabsorption of calcium.

236. (c) A buffer solution is prepared by mixing 7 ml of 0.18 M
acetic acid with 3 ml of 0.18 M sodium acetate. The pH
of the buffer is calculated as follows:

Total volume = 10 ml

Concentration of acetic acid = $0.18 \times \dfrac{7}{10}$

= 0.126 M

Concentration of sodium acetate = $0.18 \times \dfrac{3}{10}$

= 0.054 M

$pH = pK_a + \log_{10} \dfrac{Salt}{Acid}$

$pK_a = -\log_{10}K_a$

$= -\log_{10}(1.82 \times 10^{-5})$

$= 5 - 0.26$

$= 4.74$

Therefore:

$pH = 4.74 + \log_{10} \dfrac{0.054}{0.126}$

$= 4.74 - \log_{10} \dfrac{126}{54}$

$= 4.74 - 0.368$

$= 4.37$

237. (d) Thrombin, Factor VII and Factor X are all involved in vitamin K metabolism.

238. (b) In the o-cresolphthalein complexone method for measuring calcium, 8-hydroxyquinoline is added to bind magnesium.

239. (a) The Michaelis-Menten constant is the concen-tration of substrate giving one-half maxi-mum enzyme velocity.

240. (b) If the blood level of norepinephrine is increased and that of epinephrine is normal then the most probable tumor is an extra-adrenal phenochromocytoma.

241. (d) Angular stomatitis, disturbances in vision and dermatitis may all occur in vitamin B_2 (riboflavin) deficiency.

242. (d) In the ferrozine method for the determination of iron and iron binding capacity, thiourea is added to bind copper and prevents the forma-tion of a ferrozine-Cu^+ complex.

243. (a) A buffer solution con-tains 0.07 M acetic acid and 0.16 M sodium acetate. The pH of this buffer is calculated as follows:

$pKa = -\log_{10}Ka$

$= -\log_{10}(1.82 \times 10^{-5})$

$= 5 - 0.26$

$= 4.74$

$pH = pK_a + \log_{10} \dfrac{Salt}{Acid}$

$= 4.74 + \log_{10} \dfrac{0.16}{0.07}$

$= 4.74 + \log_{10} 2.286$

$= 5.099$

244. (a) DEAE-sephadex column
     (b) chromatography, chem-
     (c) ical inhibition, elec-
     (d) trophoresis and anti-
         body/antigen reactions
         have all been used to
         assay serum for creatine
         kinase (CK) isoenzymes.

245. (c) Red blood cell gluta-
         thione reductase activ-
         ity is a good indicator
         of serum riboflavin
         levels.

246. (a) Serum aldolase (ALD) is
     (b) increased in Duchenne
     (c) muscular dystrophy,
         acute myocardial infarc-
         tion and carcinoma of
         the prostate. A normal
         serum aldolase activity
         is found in neurogenic
         muscular dysfunction.

247. (a) In thiamine deficiency
         there is a decrease in
         red blood cell transket-
         olase activity.

248. (c) In a zero-order enzyme
         reaction, the rate of
         the reaction is depen-
         dant only on the enzyme
         concentration and is
         independent of the sub-
         strate concentration.
         This can also be ex-
         pressed by saying that
         the rate of the reac-
         tion is a function of
         the zeroth power
         ($S° = 1$) of the sub-
         strate concentration.

249. (a) Serum copper may be
     (b) increased in anemias,
     (c) hemochromatosis and in
         collagen diseases. It
         is decreased in nephro-
         sis due to the loss of

ceruloplasmin in
the urine.

250. (a) Serum leucine amino-
     (c) peptidase (LAP) is
         a more sensitive
         indicator than alka-
         line phosphatase in
         choledocholiathiasis
         and with liver metastases
         in anicteric patients.

SECTION B: HEADINGS

(1)
251. (a) HP

252. (a) CEP

253. (c) EP

254. (b) HP

255. (a) CEP

(2)
256. (e) Renal tubular acidosis

257. (c) Cushing's syndrome

258. (a) Primary hyperaldosteronism

259. (b) Secondary hyperaldosteronism

260. (d) 17-Hydroxylase deficiency

(3)
261. (d) Urobilin

262. (c) BUN

263. (e) Ketone bodies

264. (b) Urine bilirubin

265. (a) Urobilinogen

266. (c) Serum phosphorus 9.0 mg/dl

267. (d) Gamma globulin 5.4 g/dl   280. True

268. (a) Serum calcium 4.0 mmol/l   281. True

269. (b) pH 7.5, PCO_2 30.0   282. False In the first
                                                    trimester of preg-
270. (e) pH 7.38, PCO_2 60.0   nancy, urinary
                                                    chorionic gonado-
                                                    trophin is at a
                                                    higher level than
SECTION C: TRUE OR FALSE   urinary estrogen.

271. False Phosphorescence occurs   283. False Increased secretion
             when the length of   of parathyroid hormone
             time exceeds 10^{-4} (PTH) causes increased
             seconds from the time   intestinal absorption
             the chemical species   of calcium.
             absorbs the energy
             until the light is   284. False As the temperature
             emitted. Fluorescence   decreases, fluores-
             has a delay time of   cence increases.
             between 10^{-8} to 10^{-4}
             seconds.   285. True

272. True   286. True

273. True   287. True

274. False The color is due to   288. False A refractometer
             urobilin.   cannot be used to
                                                    measure cerebro-
275. False Some of the isoenzymes   spinal fluid (CSF)
             of acid phosphatase   protein concentra-
             (ACP) in serum (espe-   tion.
             cially the prostatic
             isoenzyme) are quite   289. True
             labile so that greater
             than 50 per cent of   290. True
             ACP activity may be
             lost from blood left   291. False Enterokinase is
             standing at room tem-   secreted by the
             perature for 1 hour.   intestinal mucosa.

276. True   292. False Cholecystokinin is
                                                    secreted in the
277. True   intestine.

278. False Urate formation usually   293. False Red blood cell acid
             occurs in acid urine.   phosphatase is in-
                                                    hibited by formal-
279. True   dehyde.

294. True

295. True

296. False The color change is
           due to chelation of
           ferric ion with the
           enol form of phenyl-
           pyruvic acid.

297. True

298. False The PSP excretion test
           is a test of renal
           tubular secretion.

299. True

300. True

301. True

302. False Calcitonin is produced
           mainly in the para-
           follicular cells of
           the thyroid gland and
           to a much lesser degree
           by the parathyroids
           and thymus gland.

303. True

304. False Calciferol is biologi-
           cally inactive.

305. True

306. True

307. False A base is a proton
           acceptor.

308. False Urea is hydrolyzed by
           urease.

309. False Creatinine amidohydro-
           lase is used to con-
           vert creatinine to
           creatine. The creatine
           formed can be measured
           by an enzyme system

using creatine
kinase (CK) to give
a measure of creati-
nine concentration.

310. True

311. True

312. False In the Jendrassik-
           Grof bilirubin
           method sodium ace-
           tate buffers the
           pH of the diazoti-
           zation reaction.

313. False Sorbitol dehydrogenase
           is near zero in chronic
           hepatitis but shows a
           marked increase in
           acute hepatitis.

314. True

315. False Xylose is a pentose.

316. True

317. False An enzyme/coenzyme
           combination is called
           a holoenzyme. An
           apoenzyme is the en-
           zyme protein without
           the cofactor.

318. True

319. True

320. False The alkali denatura-
           tion test is used to
           identify fetal hemo-
           globin (HbF).

321. False In edema, water accum-
           ulates in the extra-
           cellular spaces.

322. True

323. True

324. False   Approximately 0.3 per cent of total body potassium is contained in the plasma.

325. True

326. False   As many factors may cause an extracellular shift of potassium, there is often not a good correlation between hypokalemia and potassium deficiency.

327. True   However, serum potassium is inversely related to pH.

328. False   An increased serum ratio of lactate to pyruvate is seen in anoxia.

329. True

330. True

331. True

332. False   Porphyrins are tetra-pyrrole ring compounds.

333. True

334. True

335. False   Releasing hormones of the hypothalamus are designated with the suffix -liberin.

336. True

337. False   The mineral component of bone is mainly hydroxyapatite ($3Ca_3 (PO_4)_2\ Ca(OH)_2$).

338. True

339. False   Humans do not have the enzyme uricase which would metabolize uric acid to allantoin so that the end of the purine pathway is uric acid.

340. True

341. False   Kwashiorkor is a disease caused by a diet that is low in protein but contains some carbohydrate. A diet low in protein and carbohydrates can cause marasmus.

342. True

343. False   Lesch-Nyhan syndrome is caused by a deficiency of hypoxanthine-guanine phosphoribosyl transferase deficiency.

344. True

345. True

346. True

347. False   L-Phenylalanine has no inhibitory effect on bone (or liver) isoenzymes of alkaline phosphatase.

348. True

349. True

350. False   Normally 95 per cent of body potassium is intracellular.

351. False   An increased level of 2, 3-DPG is needed to shift the oxygen

dissociation curve to
the right.

352. True

353. False The acidosis that
results if cardiac
output is inadequate
is a result of anaer-
obic glycolysis.

354. False HbF consists of two
alpha and 2 gamma
peptide chains.

355. True

356. True

357. False Dumping syndrome is
caused by the rapid
entry of hypertonic
fluid into the duo-
denum. This causes
transfer of water and
electrolytes into the
bowel. It may occur
following gastrectomy.

358. True

359. False Neonatal hypothyroidism may be equally due
to thyroid dysgenesis
or to an enzyme defect.

360. False Glucocorticoids decrease the tissue
response to insulin.

361. True

362. False A decreased ionized
calcium level in serum
will cause an increase
in PTH secretion.

363. True

364. False A primary increase in

serum albumin
concentration is
rarely found in any
condition.

365. True

366. True

367. True Also, chylomicrons
may be trapped in
a serum clot.

368. False Analphalipoproteinemia is known as
Tangier disease.
There is the inability
to synthesize normal
amounts of HDL apopro-
teins.

369. True

SECTION D: MISSING WORDS

370. Kilogram

371. Secondary

372. (a) Increased
     (b) Acids
     (c) Bases

373. Erythropoietin

374. Saturated

375. Second

376. (a) Diffusion
     (b) Active transport

377. Sørensen

378. Ampere

379. (a) Liver
     (b) Placenta

(c)   Intestine

380.   10

381.   Left

382.   (a)   Prophase
       (b)   Prometaphase
       (c)   Metaphase
       (d)   Anaphase
       (e)   Telophase

383.   (a)   10 - 15
       (b)   Concentrated HCl

384.   KELVIN

385.   (a)   Phospholipid
       (b)   Cholesterol

386.   p-Nitrophenylphosphate

387.   (a)   Linearly
       (b)   Logarithmically

388.   (a)   Phosphoric acid
       (b)   Deoxyribose
       (c)   Adenine
       (d)   Guanine
       (e)   Thymine
       (f)   Cytosine

389.   Holmium

390.   Approximate ranges:
       (a) (b)   pH 7.35 - 7.45
       (c) (d) pCO_2 35 - 45 mmHg
       (e) (f) pO_2 80 - 100 mmHg

391.   Barrier layer cells

392.   Candela

393.   (a)   Electrokinetic
       (b)   Zeta

394.   Lysosomes

395.   (a)   Fatty acids
       (b)   Adipose cells
       (c)   Acetoacetic acid

(d)   B-Hydroxybutyric acid
(e)   Acetone

396.   Endosomosis

397.   Mole

398.   pH

399.   Valinomycin

400.   Rise

401.   Ribonucleic acid

402.   (a)   Current
       (b)   Electric
       (c)   Potential

403.   (a)   Mole/Second (mol/s)
       (b)   Katal/Liter (kat/l)

404.   (a)   I
       (b)   V

405. pO_2

406.   (a)   Chylomicrons
       (b)   Triglycerides
       (c)   Chylomicrons

407.   Coulometry

408.   Meter

409. R_f

410.   (a)   Negatrons
       (b)   Positrons

411.   Hydrophilic

412.   (a)   Dissolved CO_2
       (b)   Carbonic acid
       (c)   Carbamino compounds

413.   Sodium iodide

414.   Kjeldahl

415.   Proteins

416. (a) Potassium iodide
      (b) Sodium hydroxide
      (c) Copper sulphate
      (d) Potassium sodium
           tartrate

417. Liver

418. 2-(4'-Hydroxyazobenzene)-
      benzoic acid

419. Immunoglobulins

SECTION E: SPECIAL QUESTIONS

420. 8A, 2B, 5H, 7C, 3D, 6J, 4I, 9E, 1G, 10F

421.

Type	Appearance	Cholesterol Concentration	Triglyceride Concentration	Predominant Band(s) on Electrophoresis
I	Creamy	INC	INC	Chylomicron
IIa	Usually clear	INC	NORM or INC	Beta
IIb	Clear or faintly turbid	INC	INC	Beta Prebeta
III	Turbid	INC	INC	Wide beta
IV	Turbid	INC or NORM	INC	Prebeta
V	Turbid	INC	INC	Chylomicron Prebeta
Normal	Clear	NORM	NORM	Beta

INC = Increased
DEC = Decreased
NOR = Normal

422.

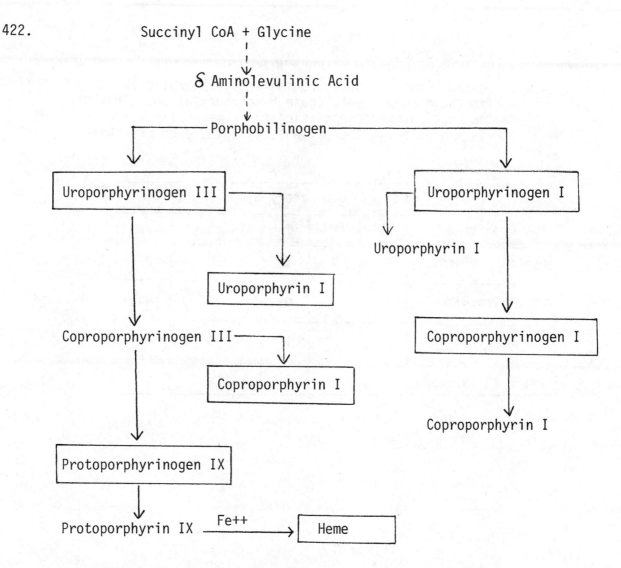

Succinyl CoA + Glycine
↓
δ Aminolevulinic Acid
↓
Porphobilinogen

Uroporphyrinogen III   Uroporphyrinogen I

Uroporphyrin I

Uroporphyrin I

Coproporphyrinogen III   Coproporphyrinogen I

Coproporphyrin I

Coproporphyrin I

Protoporphyrinogen IX

Protoporphyrin IX —Fe++→ Heme

423. 1. A lack of insulin and an excess of cortisol causes the
          following:

          - increased hepatic gluconeogenesis
          - increased mobilization of fatty acids from adipose
            tissue
          - breakdown of proteins
          - decreased uptake of glucose from blood

          All of these may contribute to an elevated blood glucose.

      2. Free fatty acids are transported from adipose tissue to
          the liver where they are broken down to acetyl-CoA.
          Only some of the acetyl-CoA can be oxidized because the
          TCA cycle is not completely functional. The excess
          acetyl-CoA is converted to acetoacetic acid, acetone and

beta-hydroxybutyric acid. This extra source of H^+
lowers the blood pH.

3. Increased blood H^+ concentration acts on carotid and
    aortic chemoreceptors to cause hyperventilation. This
    is the respiratory compensation for a metabolic acidosis
    and is exhibited in the patient by rapid, deep breathing.

424.

Condition	Laboratory Blood Tests				
	T_4	TSH	T_3	T_3Uptake	TBG
Hyperthyroidism	I	D	I	N	D
Hypothyroidism	D	I	D	D	N-I
Pregnancy	I	N	I	D	I
Estrogen Therapy	I	N	I	D	I

425.

Test	Adrenal Lesion				
	None	Hyperplasia	Adenoma	Carcinoma	Extra-adrenal tumor
Basal level					
PC	N	N-I	I	I	I
17OHCS	N	I	I	I	I
KGS	N	I	I	I	I
17KS	N	N-SI	D-N	I	I
ACTH stimulation					
PC	I	I	NC-I	NC	NC-I
17OHCS	I	I	I	NC	I-NC
KGS	I	I	I	NC	I-NC
17KS	I	I	I	NC	I-NC
Metyrapone					
17OHCS	D	D-NC	NC	NC	I
KGS	I	I	I-NC	NC	NC
17KS	N	I	I-NC	NC	NC
Dexamethasone suppression 2 mg/day					
PC	D	NC	NC	NC	NC
17OHCS	D	NC	NC	NC	NC
KGS	D	NC	NC	NC	NC
17KS	D	NC	NC	NC	NC
Dexamethasone suppression 8 mg/day					
PC	D	D	NC	NC	NC
17OHCS	D	D	NC	NC	NC
KGS	D	D	NC	NC	NC
17KS	D	D	NC	NC	NC

426.

Disease	Laboratory Blood Tests								
	ALP	ASAT	A1AT	IgA	IgM	IgG	ANF	MA	SMA
Portal Cirrhosis	MI	SI	N-SI	LI	SI	MI	A	A	V
Primary Biliary Cirrhosis	LI	MI	MI	N	LI	SI	A	P	V
Chronic Active Hepatitis	MI	LI	MI	N	SI	LI	V	V	V

N = Normal   A = Absent
SI = Slight Increase   P = Present
MI = Moderate Increase   V = Variable (may or may not be
LI = Large Increase   present)

MICROBIOLOGY

SHARON LAYNE
M.Sc.
Chief Technologist
Microbiology
TORONTO WESTERN HOSPITAL
TORONTO, ONTARIO, CANADA

QUESTIONS

SECTION A: MULTIPLE CHOICE

*Select the phrase, sentence or
symbol which completes the statement or answers the question.
More than one answer may be
correct in each case.*

1. The number of viable bacteria
   in a specimen can be determined by:
   (a) a microscopic count
       using a bacterial
       counting chamber
   (b) determination of total
       nitrogen content of the
       packed organisms
   (c) calibrated loop streaked
       on a culture plate
   (d) reduction of tetrazolium
       salts by the metabolizing
       organisms.

2. The difference between gram
   positive and gram negative
   bacteria is known to reside
   in the:
   (a) cell wall
   (b) nucleus

   (c) lamellae
   (d) cell membrane

3. Differentiation of enteric
   bacilli is based on:
   (a) cultural appearance
   (b) antigenic structure
   (c) biochemical reactions
   (d) all of the above

4. Food poisoning caused by
   Staphylococcus aureus is
   due to production of:
   (a) hemolysin
   (b) penicillinase
   (c) enterotoxin
   (d) leukocidin

5. The majority of gonococcal
   infections occur in the
   genital tract, but the
   organisms can give rise to:
   (a) septicemia
   (b) arthritis
   (c) osteomyelitis
   (d) all of the above

6. Organisms of the *Klebsiella*,
   Enterobacter and *Serratia*

group:
(a) are nonmotile
(b) give a positive Voges-
     Proskauer reaction
(c) ferment lactose
(d) produce pigment on
     MacConkey agar

7. In the slide coagulase test,
    clumping of staphylococci in
    saline and without plasma is
    indicative of:
    (a) a pathogenic *Staphylococcus*
    (b) presence of free coagulase
         only
    (c) presence of bound coagu-
         lase only
    (d) autoagglutination

8. A test which may give a false
    positive reaction if the organ-
    ism is growing on blood agar:
    (a) oxidase
    (b) optochin
    (c) catalase
    (d) coagulase

9. Characteristically, *Strepto-
    coccus faecalis* shows all
    the following properties except:
    (a) resistance to 60°C for
         30 minutes
    (b) growth in presence of 40
         per cent bile
    (c) negative catalase reac-
         tion
    (d) sensitive to penicillin

10. Toxigenic strains of *Coryne-
    bacterium diphtheriae* may be
    identified by:
    (a) agglutination with speci-
         fic antisera
    (b) Nagler reaction
    (c) Elek reaction
    (d) brown halo on Tinsdale
         agar

11. The satellite phenomenon demon-
    strated by *Haemophilus influenzae*
    indicates that staphylococci

produce:
(a) X factor
(b) V factor
(c) hemolysins
(d) hyaluronidase

12. Skin scraping for fungus
    examination should be sent:
    (a) in formalin
    (b) in alcohol
    (c) in transport medium
    (d) in folded paper

13. Standard autoclaving con-
    ditions are:
    (a) 10 lbs/sq. inch at
         80°C - 15 minutes
    (b) 15 lbs/sq. inch at
         110°C - 15 minutes
    (c) 20 lbs/sq. inch at
         125°C - 20 minutes
    (d) 15 lbs/sq. inch at
         121°C - 15 minutes

14. Salmonella infection is
    transmitted by:
    (a) ingestion
    (b) inhalation
    (c) person to person con-
         tact
    (d) inoculation

15. The term "thermolabile"
    means:
    (a) activated by heat
    (b) insensitive to heat
    (c) produces heat
    (d) sensitive to heat

16. Most bacteria are:
    (a) psychrophiles
    (b) mesophiles
    (c) thermophiles
    (d) cryophiles

17. Effective sterilization
    using a hot air oven
    requires:
    (a) 100°F for 30 minutes
    (b) 260°F for 2 hours
    (c) 160°C for 1 hour

(d) 121°C for 20 minutes

18. Bacterial spores:
    (a) stain gram positive
    (b) are metabolically
         active
    (c) resist heat better
         than vegetative cells
    (d) occur in gram negative
         cells

19. Zero growth rate is observed
    in:
    (a) lag phase
    (b) logarithmic phase
    (c) exponential phase
    (d) stationary phase

20. "Fractional" sterilization is
    known as:
    (a) inspissation
    (b) Pasteurization
    (c) Tyndallization
    (d) fractionation

21. The diameter of a staphylococ-
    cus is approximately:
    (a) 0.8 micron
    (b) 2 microns
    (c) 8 microns
    (d) 0.05 micron

22. The antistreptolysin O test
    is an example of:
    (a) agglutination
    (b) complement fixation
    (c) neutralization
    (d) flocculation

23. The intermediate host for
    Taenia solium is:
    (a) dog
    (b) pig
    (c) man
    (d) cow

24. The site of infection in sub-
    acute bacterial endocarditis
    is:
    (a) blood stream

(b) meninges
(c) mouth
(d) valves of the heart

25. The purpose of resazurin
    in thioglycollate broth
    is to:
    (a) indicate production
         of acid
    (b) inhibit aerobic
         organisms
    (c) remove oxygen
    (d) indicate presence
         of oxygen

26. If 0.35 ml of N/10 NaOH
    is required to adjust the
    pH of 10 ml of medium,
    for 1 liter of medium using
    1N NaOH you would need:
    (a) 35 ml
    (b) 3.5 ml
    (c) 7 ml
    (d) 0.35 ml

27. In the microscope, light
    rays are focused on the
    object to be observed by
    means of the:
    (a) diaphragm
    (b) condenser
    (c) objective
    (d) eyepiece

28. The ovum of *Diphyllobothrium
    latum* is:
    (a) circular with a thick
         shell
    (b) thin walled and oper-
         culate
    (c) thick walled with a
         plug at each end
    (d) tuberculate

29. The melting and gelling
    points of agar are respec-
    tively:
    (a) 80°C, 37°C
    (b) 100°C, 45°C
    (c) 60°C, 40°C

(d) 120°C, 60°C

30. In subactue bacterial endo-
     carditis, the most likely
     causative agent is:
     (a) *Streptococcus pyogenes*
     (b) *Streptococcus pneumoniae*
     (c) viridans streptococci
     (d) *Staphylococcus aureus*

31. The etiologic agent of botu-
     lism is:
     (a) gram negative
     (b) anaerobic
     (c) *Clostridium bifermentans*
     (d) *Clostridium tetani*

32. A substrate incorporated into
     media to demonstrate hydrogen
     sulphide production by certain
     bacteria is:
     (a) ferrous ammonium sulphate
     (b) sodium thioglycollate
     (c) para-aminobenzoic acid
     (d) potassium phosphate

33. Steam, as a sterilizing agent,
     acts by:
     (a) splitting the cell wall
     (b) coagulation of protein
     (c) inactivation of enzymes
     (d) oxidation of protein

34. Many difficulties in micro-
     bial identification are due
     to:
     (a) use of an impure culture
     (b) use of abbreviated
          schemata
     (c) lack of sensitive tests
     (d) lack of appropriate
          media

35. Tetrazolium compounds are
     used in some media to indicate:
     (a) sterility
     (b) resistance
     (c) bacterial growth
     (d) reduced oxygen levels

36. To determine whether the
     attack on carbohydrates by
     an organism is by oxidation
     or fermentation, the method
     used is that described by:
     (a) Cowan and Steel
     (b) Edwards and Ewing
     (c) Hugh and Leifson
     (d) Scott and Bailey

37. Demonstration of high or
     steadily increasing concen-
     trations of antistreptolysin O
     in a patient's serum:
     (a) indicates recent
          group A streptococcal
          infection
     (b) indicates recent
          viridans streptococcal
          infection
     (c) is diagnostic of acute
          rheumatic fever
     (d) is diagnostic of rheu-
          matoid arthritis

38. The following features are
     characteristic of *Nocardia
     asteroides* except:
     (a) aerobic
     (b) partially acid-fast
     (c) gram positive
     (d) anaerobic

39. The production of acetoin
     in which of the following
     tests is a basis for dif-
     ferentiation of *Enterobacter
     aerogenes* from *Escherichia
     coli*:
     (a) methyl red test
     (b) Voges-Proskauer test
     (c) citrate test
     (d) malonate test

40. The concentration of ethyl
     alcohol (in aqueous mixture)
     which produces maximum
     bactericidal effect is:
     (a) 95 per cent

(b)   85 per cent
(c)   70 per cent
(d)   60 per cent

41. A small amount of agar is
     incorporated into thiogly-
     collate broth to:
     (a) allow separation of
          organisms
     (b) demonstrate motility
     (c) decrease rate of dif-
          fusion of oxygen into
          the medium
     (d) act as carbon source

42. In this test a positive reac-
     tion is produced when the pH
     falls below 4.5:
     (a) urease test
     (b) methyl red test
     (c) Voges-Proskauer test
     (d) lysine decarboxylase
          test

43. Beta lactamase is:
     (a) an enzyme produced by
          penicillin-sensitive
          Staphylococcus aureus
     (b) the active part of the
          penicillin molecule
     (c) an enzyme which in-
          activates penicillin
     (d) a by-product of lactose
          fermentation

44. Enteric streptococci:
     (a) fail to hydrolyze escu-
          lin
     (b) grow in the presence of
          bile salts
     (c) are soluble in bile
          salts
     (d) belong to Lancefield
          group B

45. Tryptophane broth is used to:
     (a) stop overgrowth of
          Staphylococcus aureus
     (b) indicate fermentation
          of a carbohydrate

(c) prevent swarming of
     Proteus.
(d) test for indole forma-
     tion

46. The ONPG test:
     (a) is always negative
          if an organism has
          a TSI with acid butt
          and alkaline slant
     (b) would differentiate
          between *Shigella* and
          Escherichia
     (c) is always positive
          if an organism ferments
          lactose
     (d) is always negative if
          an organism does not
          ferment lactose

47. Virulence tests should be
     done on *Corynebacterium
     diphtheriae* isolated from
     throat cultures:
     (a) to differentiate
          *Corynebacterium
          diphtheriae* from *C.
          xerosis*
     (b) to confirm biochemical
          reactions
     (c) not all strains of
          C. diphtheriae are
          toxigenic
     (d) to confirm a positive
          FA screen

48. *Listeria monocytogenes*:
     (a) is a gram variable
          bacillus
     (b) is motile at 42°C
     (c) is motile at room
          temperature
     (d) is motile at room
          temperature and 35°C

49. Which of the following is
     an example of a broad-
     spectrum antibiotic?
     (a) erythromycin
     (b) colistin

(c)   nystatin
(d)   tetracycline

50.   Many prepared bacterio-
      logical plating media
      can be stored for some
      time if:
      (a)   condensation is pre-
            vented
      (b)   restrict reheating
      (c)   moisture is retained
      (d)   the media are kept
            in the dark

51.   The bacterial cell wall:
      (a)   is an impermeable
            barrier
      (b)   is thinner in gram
            positive bacteria
            than in gram negative
      (c)   makes up to 40 per
            cent of the dry weight
            of the cell
      (d)   is permeable to mole-
            cules as large as
            nucleotides

52.   Bacterial spores will be
      killed by a temperature of:
      (a)   100 °C for 15 minutes
      (b)   121°C for 15 minutes
      (c)   160°F for 10 minutes
      (d)   160°F for 30 minutes

53.   Transplants from one area to
      another of the same indivi-
      dual are referred to as:
      (a)   isografts
      (b)   autografts
      (c)   homografts
      (d)   heterografts

54.   Salmonella food poisoning
      may be due to:
      (a)   *Salmonella typhimurium*
      (b)   *Salmonella enteritidis*
      (c)   neither of the above
      (d)   both of the above

55.   *Bacillus anthracis*:

(a)   causes anthracosis
(b)   causes "wool-sorters"
      disease
(c)   forms spores which
      are heat sensitive
(d)   is an anaerobic bacil-
      lus

56.   *Mycobacterium tuberculosis*
      when grown on solid media
      appears:
      (a)   smooth, moist colony
      (b)   metallic sheen
      (c)   dry, heaped colony
      (d)   brightly pigmented

57.   Typing of *Streptococcus
      pneumoniae* is accomplished
      by:
      (a)   bile solubility of
            the organism
      (b)   transformation of
            specific types
      (c)   use of type specific
            antisera
      (d)   capsular staining

58.   Characteristically *Neisseria
      meningitidis*:
      (a)   is a gram positive
            intracellular diplo-
            coccus
      (b)   is a facultative
            anaerobe
      (c)   ferments glucose,
            maltose and sucrose
      (d)   none of the above

59.   All the following statements
      describe *Clostridium tetani*
      except:
      (a)   blood agar is hemolysed
      (b)   vegetative forms in
            young cultures are
            motile
      (c)   spores are centrally
            located
      (d)   spores are located at
            one end

60. *Haemophilus influenzae*:
    (a) is motile
    (b) is never encapsulated
    (c) grows better on choco-
         late agar than blood
         agar
    (d) is the causative agent
         of influenza

61. Freshly isolated strains re-
    quire an atmosphere of 10
    per cent carbon dioxide:
    (a) *Brucella abortus*
    (b) *Brucella melitensis*
    (c) *Brucella suis*
    (d) none of the above

62. The sensitivity of anaerobes
    to oxygen is related to which
    of the following?
    (a) absence of flagella
    (b) presence of enzymes
         with sulfhydryl groups
    (c) absence of superoxide
         dismutase
    (d) absence of lipopoly-
         saccharide

63. Endotoxins composed of lipo-
    polysaccharides are found in:
    (a) *Salmonella typhi*,
         Enterobacter aerogenes
         and *Escherichia coli*
    (b) *Salmonella*, *Shigella*
         and *Clostridia*
    (c) *Streptococcus pyogenes*,
         Shigella and *Salmonella*
    (d) all of the above

64. All of the following may be
    dependent on the environment
    of a bacterial cell except:
    (a) presence or absence of
         capsules
    (b) presence or absence of
         beta galactosidase
         activity
    (c) presence or absence of
         flagella
    (d) presence or absence
         of ribosomes

65. Penicillin would be most
    active in bacterial cells
    during:
    (a) lag phase
    (b) stationary phase
    (c) exponential phase
    (d) decline phase

66. Which of the following
    elements of the disc dif-
    fusion antibiotic suscepti-
    bility test most affects
    the zone of inhibition:
    (a) pH of the medium
    (b) inoculum size
    (c) thickness of the agar
    (d) percentage of agar in
         the medium

67. *Enterobius vermicularis* is
    also known as:
    (a) tapeworm
    (b) liver fluke
    (c) pinworm
    (d) whip worm

68. All members of the family
    Enterobacteriaceae ferment:
    (a) mannitol
    (b) glucose
    (c) sucrose
    (d) dulcitol

69. Oval or club-shaped macro-
    conidia usually produced
    in groups of three are
    characteristic of:
    (a) *Microsporum*
    (b) *Trichophyton*
    (c) *Epidermophyton*
    (d) *Candida*

70. The end product in a posi-
    tive test for this enzyme
    is phenylpyruvic acid.
    The enzyme is:
    (a) diphenylpyruvate
         decarboxylase
    (b) phenylalanine deaminase
    (c) diphenylpyruvate
         deaminase

(d) diphenyalanine deaminase

71. Bacitracin discs used in the identification of strepto-cocci:
(a) contain 10 units of bacitracin per disc
(b) inhibit the growth of Lancefield group A streptococci
(c) size of inhibition zone is not significant
(d) may also be used for antibiotic sensitivity test

72. N-acetyl-l-cysteine is:
(a) a mucolytic agent
(b) a mounting medium for mycology
(c) a preservative for feces
(d) a reducing agent when culturing anaerobes

73. Dermatophytes are fungi which:
(a) infect the keratinized areas of the body
(b) require complex media for growth
(c) invade subcutaneous tissues
(d) characteristically have two growth forms in culture

74. Which of the following com-pressed gases is a potential explosion hazard in the lab-oratory?
(a) nitrogen
(b) carbon dioxide
(c) hydrogen
(d) helium

75. Trophozoites of *Entamoebae histolytica*:
(a) contain club-shaped chromatoidal bars
(b) may contain ingested erythrocytes

(c) contain up to four nuclei
(d) have radial striations

76. A phenylalanine positive enteric organism:
(a) belongs to the genus *Proteus*
(b) belongs to the genus *Providencia*
(c) belongs to the genus *Morganella*
(d) all of the above

77. A hospital acquired *Staphy-lococcus aureus* wound in-fection should be treated with:
(a) penicillin
(b) ampicillin
(c) oxacillin
(d) gentamicin

78. Gram stain of foul smelling pus from a brain abscess shows tiny gram positive cocci in chains. This is suggestive of:
(a) beta-hemolytic streptococci - not Lancefield group A
(b) viridans streptococci
(c) anaerobic streptococci
(d) *Streptococcus faecalis*

79. Phosphates in bacteriological media act as:
(a) reducing agents
(b) oxidizing agents
(c) buffers
(d) sources of nitrogen

80. In size *Trichomonas vaginalis* is most closely comparable to:
(a) *Rickettsia*
(b) yeast cell
(c) polymorphonuclear leukocyte
(d) red blood cell

81. Whether cultured at 36°C or

at room temperature, which of
the following always produces
yeast-like colonies:
(a) *Blastomyces dermatitidis*
(b) *Cryptococcus neoformans*
(c) *Coccidioides immitis*
(d) *Paracoccidioides brasi-
     liensis*

82. Synergy of antibiotic drug
     combinations occurs if the
     activity of:
     (a) two drugs in combination
          is greater than the sum
          of both effects
     (b) the combination is greater
          than either drug alone but
          less than that obtained by
          doubling the concentration
          of either
     (c) the effect of combined drugs
          is equal to that of either
          drug alone
     (d) the combination is less
          than that obtained with
          either drug alone

83. Meningitis due to *Haemophilus
     influenzae* occurs most fre-
     quently in:
     (a) adolescents
     (b) middle-age men
     (c) young women
     (d) infants under two months

84. *Streptococcus pneumoniae* may
     be differentiated from the
     viridans streptococci by:
     (a) lysis by surface active
          agents
     (b) inulin fermentation
     (c) failure to grow in the
          absence of blood
     (d) none of the above

85. At least two substances make
     up staphylocoagulase and they
     are:
     (a) bound coagulase and
          citrate
     (b) prothrombin and free

          coagulase
     (c) free coagulase and
          bound coagulase
     (d) free coagulase and
          fibrin

86. The highest incidence of
     chronic carriers of *Salmonella
     typhi* is found among:
     (a) young men
     (b) middle-age women
     (c) middle-age men
     (d) young women

87. The usual source of comple-
     ment for complement fixation
     tests is:
     (a) human serum
     (b) rabbit serum
     (c) horse serum
     (d) guinea pig serum

88. Aerogenic implies:
     (a) growth in carbon
          dioxide
     (b) gas production
     (c) growth in the absence
          of oxygen
     (d) carbon dioxide required
          for growth

89. An organism which charac-
     teristically contains
     metachromatic granules is:
     (a) *Bacillus subtilis*
     (b) *Mycobacterium
          tuberculosis*
     (c) *Corynebacterium diph-
          theriae*
     (d) *Actinomyces israelii*

90. The enzyme responsible for
     opacity in serum or egg
     yolk media is:
     (a) coagulase
     (b) lecithinase
     (c) decarboxylase
     (d) oxidase

91. The division of hemolytic
     streptococci into serologic

groups depends on group specific cellular antigens which
are:
  (a) M proteins
  (b) T proteins
  (c) C polysaccharides
  (d) mucopeptides

92. Typical strains of *Salmonella typhi*:
  (a) produce acid and gas
       from glucose
  (b) are ONPG positive
  (c) are nonmotile
  (d) produce a weakly posi-
       tive hydrogen sulphide
       reaction in triple sugar
       iron agar

93. In the nitrate reduction test,
    a red color which develops
    only after the addition of
    zinc dust indicates:
  (a) nitrite reduced to
       nitrate
  (b) nitrate not reduced
  (c) nitrate reduced beyond
       nitrite
  (d) nitrogen gas present

94. A disinfectant will be more
    effective when applied to
    objects if:
  (a) temperature is lowered
  (b) pH is neutral
  (c) no organic material is
       present
  (d) surface tension is in-
       creased

95. The test which is most use-
    ful in differentiating *Salmon-
    ella enteritidis* from *Citro-
    bacter freundii* is:
  (a) citrate utilization
  (b) methyl red test
  (c) ONPG test
  (d) indole test

96. Iodine belongs to which one
    of the following groups of

disinfectants:
  (a) phenolics
  (b) halogens
  (c) quaternary ammonium
       compounds
  (d) aldehydes

97. The exclusion of *Ascaris lumbricoides* infection
    requires:
  (a) macroscopic examina-
       tion of feces for
       mature parasites
  (b) microscopic examina-
       tion of fresh worm
  (c) examination of Scotch ®
       tape preparations
  (d) microscopic examina-
       tion of a number of
       fecal samples collected
       at 2 - 3 day intervals

98. The mechanism by which hypo-
    chlorite acts is through:
  (a) protein denaturation
  (b) oxidation
  (c) hydrolysis
  (d) inactivation of enzymes

99. A culture of *Clostridium perfringens* on an anaerobic
    blood plate is characterized
    by:
  (a) a zone of alpha hemo-
       lysis
  (b) a single zone of beta
       hemolysis
  (c) a double zone of alpha
       hemolysis
  (d) a double zone of beta
       hemolysis

100. The CAMP test utilizes:
  (a) a blood plate
  (b) an egg yolk plate
  (c) antitoxin soaked filter
       paper
  (d) optochin discs

101. Two members of the family
     Enterobacteriaceae are

characteristically nonmotile.
They are:
(a) *Shigella* and *Escherichia coli*
(b) *Klebsiella* and *Serratia*
(c) *Klebsiella* and *Escherichia coli*
(d) *Klebsiella* and *Shigella*

102. It is necessary to use a cap allowing air exchange when using triple sugar iron agar. This is:
(a) to allow fermentation of the carbohydrates
(b) to allow oxidation of the carbohydrates
(c) to allow oxidation of peptones
(d) to allow gas to escape

103. *Klebsiella pneumoniae*:
(a) is anaerogenic
(b) produces large amounts of gas fermentation of carbohydrates
(c) has peritrichous flagella
(d) is oxidase positive

104. *Mycobacterium tuberculosis*:
(a) is very heat resistant
(b) is relatively resistant to effects of alkali
(c) is inhibited by low concentrations of malachite green
(d) is fluorescent under ultraviolet light

105. Diseases of animals transmissible to man are called:
(a) vectors
(b) communicable diseases
(c) zoonoses
(d) endogenous diseases

106. *Candida albicans* may be identified by the production of:
(a) blastospores and pseudomycelium
(b) chlamydospores and germ tubes
(c) microconidia and macroconidia
(d) arthrospores and germ tubes

107. Essential ingredients of the carbol fuchsin solution used in the Ziehl-Neelsen stain are:
(a) basic fuchsin and phenol
(b) acid fuchsin and phenol
(c) basic fuchsin and potassium hydroxide
(d) none of the above

108. Aerosols containing infectious material may be produced when using:
(a) centrifuges
(b) rubber stoppered tubes
(c) wire loops
(d) all of the above

109. Specimens useful for the isolation of *Brucella* should include:
(a) blood
(b) bone marrow
(c) lymph node biopsies
(d) all of the above

110. The growth of *Clostridium perfringens* in tissues is enhanced by the production of:
(a) lecithinase C
(b) enterotoxin
(c) leukocidin
(d) beta hemolysis

111. Capsules of *Streptococcus pneumoniae* are:
(a) necessary for virulence
(b) useful only for typing purposes
(c) only produced in vivo

(d)   only produced on
      chocolate agar

112. Tetanus and diphtheria are
      prevented by:
      (a)   passive immunization
            with antitoxin
      (b)   active immunization
            by vaccine
      (c)   acquiring the disease
      (d)   passive immunization
            with toxoid

113. *Proteus, Pseudomonas* and
      Serratia organisms:
      (a)   are gram negative
            bacteria
      (b)   are often refractory
            to many antibiotics
      (c)   produce nosocomial
            disease
      (d)   all of the above

114. The *Neisseria* genus is char-
      acterized by:
      (a)   bile solubility
      (b)   oxidase positivity
      (c)   alpha hemolysis
      (d)   anaerobic growth

115. *Shigella:*
      (a)   cause disease in humans
            only
      (b)   are nonmotile; have no
            H antigens
      (c)   are nonlactose fermen-
            ters
      (d)   all of the above

116. The most satisfactory medium
      for isolation of pathogenic
      fungi is:
      (a)   brain heart infusion
            agar
      (b)   Sabouraud's dextrose
            agar
      (c)   chocolate agar
      (d)   Tinsdale's medium

117. In typhoid fever, the organ-
      ism is found very early in

the disease in the:
      (a)   feces
      (b)   blood
      (c)   spinal fluid
      (d)   urine

118. The single best test for
      biochemical identification
      of *Mycobacterium tuberculosis*
      is:
      (a)   nitrate reduction
      (b)   niacin
      (c)   catalase
      (d)   pigment production

119. *Bacteroides fragilis* is:
      (a)   the most numerous
            micro-organism in
            the intestine
      (b)   a gram negative rod
      (c)   anaerobic
      (d)   all of the above

120. The causative organism of
      actinomycosis is:
      (a)   acid fast
      (b)   anaerobic
      (c)   grows on Sabouraud's
            agar
      (d)   none of the above

121. Gram stain of an infected
      wound caused by a cat bite
      showed gram negative cocco-
      bacilli. The most likely
      isolate will be:
      (a)   *Haemophilus influenzae*
      (b)   *Brucella abortus*
      (c)   *Pasteurella multocida*
      (d)   *Pseudomonas aeruginosa*

122. The best combination of
      media for isolation of a
      pathogen from cloudy cere-
      brospinal fluid with a
      high polymorphonuclear
      count would be:
      (a)   aerobic and anaerobic
            blood plates
      (b)   aerobic blood plate,
            thioglycollate broth

(c) chocolate agar incubated
     in 10 per cent CO_2,
     brain heart infusion
     broth
(d) blood agar plate,
     MacConkey

123. A fluid medium which inhibits
     commensal organisms but al-
     lows the multiplication of
     pathogens during the first
     24 hours is:
     (a) a selective medium
     (b) an enrichment medium
     (c) an enriched medium
     (d) a synthetic medium

124. In the tube coagulase test:
     (a) a positive test is
          shown by turbidity
     (b) bound coagulase is
          tested for
     (c) a negative test can
          be detected in two
          hours
     (d) free coagulase is
          tested for

125. Specimens for serological
     investigation are best
     collected:
     (a) at the first sign
          of illness
     (b) when the patient is
          in the acute stage of
          illness
     (c) when the patient is
          in the convalescent
          stage of illness
     (d) both (b) and (c)

126. Discs containing ethylhydro-
     cupreine hydrochloride may
     be used to:
     (a) characterize the enter-
          ococci
     (b) group beta-hemolytic
          streptococci
     (c) differentiate *Strepto-
          coccus pneumoniae* from
          viridans streptococci

(d) differentiate vari-
     ous strains of pneu-
     mococci

127. In the performance of the
     tube coagulase test, oxa-
     lated plasma is preferable
     to citrated plasma because:
     (a) staphylococci can
          utilize oxalate
     (b) some bacteria uti-
          lize citrate
     (c) oxalate is more solu-
          ble than citrate
     (d) some bacteria utilize
          oxalate

128. The *Hafnia* group of organ-
     isms shows temperature vari-
     ation in the MR/VP tests
     so that:
     (a) MR negative and VP
          positive at 22°C
     (b) MR positive at 22°C
          and MR negative at
          37°C
     (c) MR positive and VP
          negative at 22°C
     (d) MR negative and VP
          negative at 22°C

129. When using an anaerobic
     jar, it is important to
     include an indicator of
     anaerobiosis such as:
     (a) thioglycollate
     (b) methylene blue
     (c) pyrogallol
     (d) vacuum gauge

130. False negative coagulase
     tests with staphylococci
     may be the result of
     lysis of the coagulase-
     induced clot by:
     (a) hyaluronidase
     (b) leukocidin
     (c) staphylokinase
     (d) free coagulase

131. The organisms formerly

known as *H. pertussis*, *H. parapertussis*, and *H. bronchiseptica* are now included in the genus *Bordetella* because they:
- (a) do not require the growth factors found in blood
- (b) require hemin
- (c) require DPN factors
- (d) are all isolated on Bordet-Gengou medium

132. Usually glucose, maltose and sucrose will be sufficient to differentiate *Corynebacterium diphtheriae* from related corynebacteria. The fermentation pattern of the former in the above sugars in the order given is:
- (a) - - -
- (b) + - +
- (c) + + +
- (d) + + -

133. The gel strength of an agar medium is not affected by:
- (a) size of the dish into which it is poured
- (b) the number of times it is remelted
- (c) the pH at which it is sterilized
- (d) the concentration in which it is used

134. Liquefaction of sputa for tuberculosis culture may be accomplished by any of the following except:
- (a) sodium hydroxide
- (b) N-acetyl cysteine in NaOH
- (c) trisodium phosphate
- (d) sodium hypochlorite

135. A selective medium for the isolation of *Neisseria gonorrhoeae* from contaminated specimens is:

- (a) soy-peptone medium
- (b) Thayer-Martin medium
- (c) Hugh-Leifson medium
- (d) Blair-Carr medium

136. A technique most extensively used for epidemiologic studies of *Staphylococcus aureus* is:
- (a) serologic grouping
- (b) phage typing
- (c) differences in susceptibility to penicillin
- (d) hemolysis on blood agar

137. The palladium catalysts used in many anaerobic jars are readily inactivated by:
- (a) H_2/CO_2 mixtures
- (b) dessication
- (c) moisture
- (d) warm air

138. The streptococci generally associated with urinary tract infections in man belong to Lancefield group:
- (a) D
- (b) C
- (c) A
- (d) F

139. *Listeria monocytogenes* should be considered when small gram positive bacilli from hemolytic colonies and:
- (a) colonies are transparent
- (b) organisms show tumbling motility at 37°C
- (c) organisms show tumbling motility at 25°C
- (d) a positive bile esculin reaction is obtained

140. The genus *Bacteroides*

consists of gram negative
anaerobic bacilli. Which
species produces a black
colony on laked blood agar?
- (a) *B. disiens*
- (b) *B. ovatus*
- (c) *B. asaccharolyticus*
- (d) *B. melaninogenicus*

141. A feature of *Alcaligenes
faecalis* which distinguishes
it from other gram negative
bacilli is:
- (a) failure to utilize
carbohydrates
- (b) ability to grow on
the usual enteric
isolation media
- (c) failure to produce
spores
- (d) sensitivity to heat

142. The most important cause of
epidemic ringworm of the
scalp in school children is:
- (a) *Microsporum audouini*
- (b) Tinea capitis
- (c) *Microsporum canis*
- (d) Tinea pedis

143. India ink is useful for
demonstrating:
- (a) chlamydospores
- (b) spores
- (c) capsules
- (d) granules

144. Scotch ℞ tape preparation
is a useful diagnostic tool
for demonstrating eggs of:
- (a) *Enterobius vermicularis*
- (b) *Trichuris trichiura*
- (c) *Ancylostoma duodenale*
- (d) *Taenia* species

145. In the interpretation of the
Davidsohn differential test,
the heterophile antibodies
will:
- (a) not be absorbed by

guinea pig kidney
but will by beef
erythrocytes
- (b) be absorbed by guinea
pig kidney and by
beef erythrocytes
- (c) be absorbed by guinea
pig kidney but not by
beef erythrocytes
- (d) not be absorbed by
either guinea pig
kidney or beef ery-
throcytes

146. The most distinctive property of complement is:
- (a) mode of reactivity
- (b) inactivation by mild
heat
- (c) absence from human
serum
- (d) none of the above

147. Egg based media are commonly used for the isola-
tion of:
- (a) *Brucella abortus*
- (b) *Corynebacterium
diphtheriae*
- (c) *Bordetella pertussis*
- (d) *Mycobacterium tuberculosis*

148. The site at which protein
synthesis takes place in
bacteria is:
- (a) cell wall
- (b) cytoplasmic membrane
- (c) ribosome
- (d) nucleus

149. The filtering material in
a Millipore ℞ filter is
made of:
- (a) cellulose acetate
- (b) asbestos
- (c) porcelain
- (d) sintered glass

150. Gram negative cells differ

from gram positive cells in
that gram negative cells:
- (a) have a higher lipid
  content
- (b) are less permeable to
  the crystal violet-
  iodine complex
- (c) are less permeable to
  alcohol
- (d) have a greater affinity
  for the counterstain

151. The reagent used in the oxidase test is:
- (a) cysteine hydrochloride
- (b) tetramethyl-p-phenylene
  diamine hydrochloride
- (c) paradimethylaminobenzal-
  dehyde
- (d) alpha naphthylamine

152. If all the air has not been
expelled from an autoclave
set at 121°C:
- (a) a temperature of less
  than 121°C will result
- (b) condensation will occur
  on the glassware
- (c) a temperature greater
  than 121°C will result
- (d) boiling of liquid media
  will occur

153. Yeast extract is added to
culture media:
- (a) to enhance the hemolytic reactions of
  bacteria
- (b) to act as a detoxifying
  agent
- (c) to provide a readily
  available source of
  vitamin B
- (d) to make medium selective
  for *Candida albicans*

154. A precipitate formed due to
the combination of toxin and
antitoxin in optimal proportions is the basis of:
- (a) Lancefield grouping

- (b) antistreptolysin
  O titration
- (c) Flek test
- (d) Nagler reaction

155. Which of the following
antimicrobial agents is
classified as an amino-
glycoside?
- (a) gentamicin
- (b) clindamycin
- (c) chloramphenicol
- (d) sulfonamide

156. Durham tubes are used:
- (a) to demonstrate
  motility
- (b) to detect gas production
- (c) to detect toxigeni-
  city
- (d) to identify *Candida
  albicans*

157. The purpose of a transport
medium such as Stuart's
or Amies' is to:
- (a) support the growth
  of fastidious organ-
  isms such as *Neisseria
  gonorrhoeae*
- (b) inhibit undesirable
  organisms in a speci-
  men
- (c) maintain viability
  of various bacteria
  present in a speci-
  men
- (d) all of the above

158. Sodium polyanethol sulfo-
nate (Liquid ®) is used
as:
- (a) a liquefying agent
- (b) a surface active agent
- (c) an antimicrobial agent
- (d) an anticoagulant

159. In clinical microbiology,
lactobacilli are most
commonly isolated from:

(a) vaginal swabs
(b) urine specimens from infants
(c) feces
(d) ear swabs

160. Immersion oil is used in microscopy because it:
(a) protects the surface of high power objectives
(b) protects the adhesive that holds the lens in the objective
(c) has a refractive index close to that of glass
(d) makes the use of a coverglass unnecessary

161. In a positive Nagler reaction:
(a) the organism would produce lecithin which causes opacity in the medium
(b) the antitoxin would inhibit the opacity on one side of the medium, but opacity would be present on the other side
(c) the antitoxin would cause opacity in the medium
(d) growth occurs on both sides of the plate

162. Which of the following characteristics does not apply to *Neisseria gonorrhoeae*?
(a) bean-shaped morphology
(b) humans are the only natural hosts
(c) produces acid from maltose
(d) catalase positive

163. The following are characteristics of *Shigella sonnei* except:
(a) nonmotile
(b) anaerogenic
(c) ONPG positive

(d) produces trace amount of H_2S

164. Small translucent colonies with a zone of beta hemolysis were isolated from a throat culture. Which of the following tests would be useful for identification?
(a) Gram stain
(b) bile solubility
(c) bacitracin susceptibility
(d) Elek Test

165. *Klebsiella pneumoniae*:
(a) is frequently nonlactose fermenting
(b) produces blue color on Simmons citrate agar
(c) is peritrichous
(d) produces ornithine decarboxylase

166. Protozoan parasites include:
(a) *Entamoeba coli* and *Giardia lamblia*
(b) *Enterobius vermicularis* and *Entamoeba coli*
(c) *Trichomonas vaginalis* and *Trichuris trichiura*
(d) *Enterobius vermicularis* and *Trichuris trichiura*

167. The best solution for decontamination of a blood spill on the laboratory bench is:
(a) alcoholic solution of iodine
(b) 5 per cent phenol
(c) 70 per cent alcohol
(d) strong hypochlorite solution

168. A bacterial colony turns dark blue-black when a 1 per cent solution of tetramethyl-para-phenylene-

diamine dihydrochloride is
applied. The organism is
thus:
  (a) phenylanine positive
  (b) *Escherichia coli*
  (c) oxidase positive
  (d) catalase positive

169. Of the following indicators,
      which will be yellow at pH
      6.0?
        (a) phenol red
        (b) phenol phthalein
        (c) neutral red
        (d) cresol green

170. *Streptococcus agalactiae* is
      recognized as a cause of neo-
      natal infections. To which
      Lancefield group does it be-
      long?
        (a) A
        (b) B
        (c) C
        (d) G

171. The characteristic cell type
      found in the cerebrospinal
      fluid in bacterial menin-
      gitis is:
        (a) polymorphonuclear
             leukocyte
        (b) monocyte
        (c) lymphocyte
        (d) eosinophil

172. The concentration of blood
      recommended for use in blood
      agar is:
        (a) 2 - 3 per cent
        (b) 3 - 5 per cent
        (c) 5 - 8 per cent
        (d) 1 - 3 per cent

173. The term "stationary phase"
      is the stage in the growth
      cycle where:
        (a) dying population is
             greater than vegetative
             population

  (b) vegetative cell
       population equals
       the dying population
  (c) the cells have not
       yet started to multi-
       ply
  (d) none of the above

174. A thermostable substance
      may be said to be:
        (a) inactivated by heat
        (b) activated by heat
        (c) unaffected by heat
        (d) produces heat

175. Identification of anaerobic
      bacteria may be accomplished
      by:
        (a) electrophoresis
        (b) radial diffusion
        (c) chromatography
        (d) hypertrophy

176. An organism may be said to
      be eugonic when it:
        (a) grows poorly
        (b) grows rapidly
        (c) grows slowly
        (d) grows luxuriantly

177. The term "capneic" refers
      to:
        (a) incubation under
             decreased oxygen
             tension
        (b) incubation under
             increased oxygen
             tension
        (c) incubation under
             hydrogen-nitrogen
             atmosphere
        (d) incubation under
             increased CO_2 tension

178. *Corynebacterium diphtheriae*:
        (a) is resistant to peni-
             cillin
        (b) is motile
        (c) produces spores
        (d) may be club shaped

179. As a quality control measure, which of the following pairs of organisms would be suitable for positive and negative reactions for the stated test?
    (a) phenylalanine deaminase: *Proteus vulgaris* and *Providencia stuartii*
    (b) glucose fermentation: *Staphylococcus aureus* and *Streptococcus pyogenes*
    (c) oxidase test: *Pseudomonas aeruginosa* and *Aeromonas hydrophila*
    (d) Voges-Proskauer: *Citrobacter freundii* and *Enterobacter cloacae*

180. In which of the following clinical conditions is a direct gram stain of the clinical specimen least useful?
    (a) gas gangrene
    (b) pulmonary tuberculosis
    (c) salmonellosis
    (d) gonorrhoeae

181. The ability to break down hydrogen peroxide is characteristic of:
    (a) *Streptococcus pyogenes*
    (b) *Clostridium perfringens*
    (c) *Staphylococcus epidermidis*
    (d) *Streptococcus pneumoniae*

182. Which of the following pairs are used in preparation of the MacFarland standard used in Kirby-Bauer susceptibility testing?
    (a) barium chloride and hydrochloric acid
    (b) barium chloride and distilled water
    (c) barium sulphate and distilled water
    (d) barium chloride and sulphuric acid

183. Which one of the following methods of sterilization would be most efficient for use with plastic Petri plates?
    (a) ultraviolet irradiation
    (b) ethylene oxide
    (c) autoclave
    (d) boil for 20 minutes

184. *Pasteurella multocida*:
    (a) is a strict anaerobe
    (b) shows satellitism
    (c) is a small gram negative coccobacillus
    (d) requires increased CO_2 for growth

185. Bacteria which show an oxidative reaction in carbohydrate media include:
    (a) *Staphylococcus aureus*
    (b) *Streptococcus faecalis*
    (c) *Staphylococcus epidermidis*
    (d) *Pseudomonas aeruginosa*

186. Recognition of *Campylobacter* species in the laboratory includes:
    (a) a positive oxidase reaction
    (b) characteristic curved and S shaped bacilli
    (c) species differentiation by temperature of growth
    (d) all of the above

187. Lowenstein-Jensen medium:
    (a) is prepared by inspissation
    (b) contains glycerol
    (c) contains potato flour
    (d) all of the above

188. Members of the genus *Acinetobacter*:

(a)   ferment carbohydrates with trace amounts of gas
(b)   are oxidase positive
(c)   are aerobic gram negative coccobacilli
(d)   are anaerobic gram negative bacilli

189. Vancomycin, colistin and nystatin are frequently added to media used to isolate *Neisseria gonorrhoeae* in order to:
(a)   inhibit normal commensals
(b)   increase the sensitivity of the oxidase test
(c)   enhance the growth of *Neisseria gonorrhoeae*
(d)   bring about "chocolating" of the blood added to the media

190. When sterilizing by means of an autoclave:
(a)   materials should be packed in as tightly as possible
(b)   superheated steam is used because it is a very effective sterilizing agent
(c)   time should begin when the chamber pressure gauge registers the desired pressure
(d)   none of the above

191. The most primitive form of gene transfer in bacteria occurs by:
(a)   transduction
(b)   conjugation
(c)   transformation
(d)   cell fusion

192. Facultative anaerobes:
(a)   are unable to grow in the presence of molecular oxygen
(b)   require no oxygen
(c)   grow with equal facility in the presence or absence of oxygen
(d)   require an excess of oxygen

193. Which one of the statements regarding bacterial spores is incorrect?
(a)   they are unusually dehydrated
(b)   they are metabolically active
(c)   they are formed within certain gram positive cells
(d)   they do not take ordinary stains

194. Organisms that can use only molecular oxygen as the final acceptor because they lack the enzymes of the other reductive pathway are referred to as:
(a)   obligate aerobes
(b)   obligate anaerobes
(c)   facultative anaerobes
(d)   strict anaerobes

195. Antibacterial agents may affect cells by:
(a)   protein denaturation
(b)   disruption of the cell membrane or wall
(c)   chemical antagonism
(d)   all of the above

196. Flagella distributed over the entire cell is known as:
(a)   amphitrichous
(b)   peritrichous
(c)   monotrichous
(d)   lophotrichous

197. Disinfectants and antiseptics:
    (a) are both used for living tissue
    (b) are the same
    (c) are not the same
    (d) destroy all bacteria

198. Symbiosis is most accurately described as a:
    (a) relationship in which one is benefited and the other is unaffected
    (b) relationship in which only the host benefits
    (c) relationship in which both organisms benefit
    (d) relationship in which one species depends on the other for survival

199. What is the colony count if a 0.1 ml sample of a 1/100 dilution of urine produces 65 colonies when plated on nutrient agar?
    (a) 6500 organisms/ml
    (b) 6.5 organisms/ml
    (c) 650,000 organisms/ml
    (d) 65000 organisms/ml

200. In microscopy, chromatic aberration means:
    (a) inability of the optical system to resolve two neighboring points as separate entities
    (b) breakup of light into its component parts resulting in a hazy image fringed with color
    (c) the bending of light rays as they pass from one medium to another
    (d) none of the above

201. *Bacillus stearothermophilus*

is commonly used as a control organism for which sterilization method?
    (a) moist heat at 121°C for 15 minutes
    (b) dry heat at 160°C for 60 minutes
    (c) steam at 100°C for 30 minutes on 3 successive days
    (d) filtration using Seitz filter

202. What volume of serum is present in 1 ml of 10^{-3} dilution of serum?
    (a) 0.0001
    (b) 0.03
    (c) 0.01
    (d) 0.001

203. The magnification obtained with the oil immersion objective and a 10 X eyepiece is approximately:
    (a) 4000 times
    (b) 1000 times
    (c) 400 times
    (d) 100 times

204. *Salmonella* may be differentiated from *Shigella* on the basis of:
    (a) one is a strict aerobe
    (b) gram stain
    (c) motility
    (d) spore shape

205. Fluorescent microscopy for *Mycobacterium tuberculosis* depends on:
    (a) "sandwich" fluorescent antibody technique
    (b) direct fluorescent antibody technique
    (c) indirect fluorescent antibody technique
    (d) none of the above

206. The use of the stained smear in parasitology has one advantage in that it best demonstrates a particular stage which may not be seen by other methods. Which stage is this?
     (a) trophozoite
     (b) cyst
     (c) larval
     (d) proglottid

207. *Clostridium perfringens* may cause:
     (a) tetanus
     (b) gas gangrene
     (c) food poisoning
     (d) more than one of the above

208. Approximately 20 per cent of the population are carriers of *Neisseria meningitidis*. What type of specimen should be collected to detect carriage of this organism?
     (a) external nares
     (b) throat
     (c) CSF
     (d) feces

209. *Moraxella* species, when isolated on a Thayer-Martin plate, may be confused with *Neisseria*. This is because they are:
     (a) resistant to penicillin
     (b) oxidase positive
     (c) fermentative
     (d) gram negative cocci

210. *Leptospira* species:
     (a) are transmitted to man by rodents or other small animals
     (b) are eukaryotic organisms
     (c) can only be seen by electron microscopy
     (d) are obligate aerobes

211. Prepackaged cake mix was found to be contaminated by *Salmonella*. The most likely source of the organism was:
     (a) food processing personnel
     (b) dried milk
     (c) the dried eggs
     (d) flour

212. A gram negative bacillus was isolated from the blood cultures of a patient on intravenous therapy. The organism had yellow pigment and no decarboxylase activity. The identification is most likely to be:
     (a) *Acinetobacter calcoaceticus*
     (b) *Enterobacter agglomerans*
     (c) *Flavobacterium*
     (d) *Enterobacter cloacae*

213. Flagella stain of *Pseudomonas aeruginosa* shows:
     (a) cilia
     (b) no flagella
     (c) peritrichous flagella
     (d) a single polar flagellum

214. Indole production by *Escherichia coli* is dependent upon:
     (a) a source of tryptophan in the medium
     (b) a source of tryptose in the medium
     (c) anaerobic incubation
     (d) pH

215. *Vibrio parahemolyticus* requires which of the following substances for growth?
     (a) blood
     (b) menadione
     (c) salt
     (d) hemin

216. When gram staining a film of *Staphylococcus aureus*,

you omitted the iodine solution. What color would you
see in the cocci?
   (a) pink
   (b) purple
   (c) colorless
   (d) pink and purple

217. Mycoplasma can be differentiated from true bacteria
because they:
   (a) do not cause disease
      in man
   (b) lack lipopolysaccharide
      in their cell envelope
   (c) both of the above
   (d) neither of the above

218. Three of the following organisms share an important common characteristic. Which
organism is the exception?
   (a) beta-hemolytic strep-
      tococcus
   (b) *Staphylococcus aureus*
   (c) *Bacillus subtilis*
   (d) *Corynebacterium diphtheriae*

219. The role of *Corynebacterium*
phage in toxin production is
that it:
   (a) provides genetic mater-
      ial for synthesis of
      toxin
   (b) protects the organism
      from lysis by other
      phage
   (c) controls the amount of
      iron in the medium
   (d) none of the above

220. Which of the following tests
best separates *Salmonella*
from *Arizona*?
   (a) citrate utilization
   (b) malonate utilization
   (c) indole
   (d) motility

221. Which of the following
organisms is not part of
normal flora of the res-
piratory tract?
   (a) viridans streptococci
   (b) *Staphylococcus epidermidis*
   (c) *Streptococcus pneumoniae*
   (d) *Bordetella pertussis*

222. Hepatitis due to hepatitis
B surface antigen is:
   (a) frequently seen in
      drug addicts
   (b) a complication of
      Weil's disease
   (c) caused by the same
      virus as infectious
      mononucleosis
   (d) a sequela of amebic
      hepatitis

223. A major advantage of phase
microscopy is:
   (a) it is cheaper than
      light microscopy
   (b) a structural feature
      can be better observed
      in living cells
   (c) it equalizes the re-
      fractive index of the
      specimens
   (d) a structural feature
      can be better observed
      in stained preparations

224. The organism referred to as
B.C.G. is:
   (a) the cause of atypical
      pulmonary disease in
      man
   (b) an bovine strain of
      *Mycobacterium tuber-
culosis*
   (c) a spore bearing organ-
      ism
   (d) a normal inhabitant
      of the intestine

225. Dimorphism is a property of:
    (a) *Actinomycetes*
    (b) *Nocardia*
    (c) fungi
    (d) *Corynebacteria*

226. Infection of a sensitive
    bacterial culture with a
    temperate bacteriophage
    can result in:
    (a) lysogeny
    (b) vegetative phage pro-
        duction
    (c) either of the above
    (d) neither of the above

227. *Herpesvirus hominis* is:
    (a) the cause of smallpox
    (b) an RNA virus
    (c) noninfectious for man
    (d) none of the above

228. The traditional serologic
    test for syphilis depends
    on antibody reacting with
    antigen derived from bovine:
    (a) liver
    (b) heart
    (c) spleen
    (d) brain

229. The quellung reaction is seen
    with which organism?
    (a) *Streptococcus*
    (b) *Staphylococcus*
    (c) penumococcus
    (d) *Escherichia coli*

230. The word *Escherichieae* refers
    to which of the following
    classification terms?
    (a) genus
    (b) tribe
    (c) family
    (d) order

231. Chemolithotrops are bacteria
    that:
    (a) utilize inorganic com-
        pounds as energy sources
    (b) utilize organic com-

pounds as energy
sources
    (c) both of the above
    (d) neither of the above

232. V factor has been identi-
    fied as:
    (a) pyridium nuclease
    (b) alpha ketoglutaric
        acid
    (c) ribonuclease
    (d) nicotinamide adenine
        dinucleotide

233. One of the characteristics
    of *Streptococcus pneumoniae*
    is the presence of a capsule.
    Loss of this capsule would
    result in:
    (a) death of the organism
    (b) loss of virulence
    (c) inability to differ-
        entiate the organism
        from viridans strep-
        tococci
    (d) inability to excrete
        waste products from
        cell

234. Phosphates required for
    synthesis of ATP, nucleic
    acids and enzymes by bac-
    terial cells are supplied
    as:
    (a) phospholipids
    (b) polyphosphates
    (c) phosphorous
    (d) free inorganic phos-
        phates

235. Muramic acid is present
    in:
    (a) cell walls of gram
        positive and gram
        negative bacteria
    (b) pili
    (c) protein
    (d) flagella

236. The *Proteus* group is com-
    posed of motile organisms.

which:
- (a) do not grow in KCN broth
- (b) are anaerogenic
- (c) deaminate phenylalanine to phenylpyruvic acid
- (d) produce cytochrome oxidase

237. Fluid media may be used for the growth of anaerobic organisms provided it does not contain which of the following?
- (a) cysteine
- (b) resazurin
- (c) thioglycollic acid
- (d) ascorbic acid

238. The most important feature which distinguishes *Staphylococcus epidermidis* from *Staphylococcus aureus* is its:
- (a) inability to ferment mannitol
- (b) inability to produce coagulase
- (c) absence of beta hemolysis on blood agar
- (d) sensitivity to high salt concentrations

239. An "educated guess" may be made as to which genus a particular anaerobe belongs if one knows its:
- (a) gram stain, spore stain, capsule stain, flagella stain
- (b) gram stain, presence of spores, shape, size
- (c) motility, spore location, size
- (d) shape, microscopic arrangement, flagella stain, gram stain

240. When grown in the dark, yellow to orange pigmentation of the colonies is usually demonstrated by:
- (a) scotochromogens
- (b) photochromogens
- (c) rapid growers
- (d) slow growers

241. The potential fermentative powers of "late lactose fermenters" may be detected by a test named:
- (a) A.T.C.C.
- (b) O.F.
- (c) I.E.P.
- (d) O.N.P.G.

242. Conjugation may result in:
- (a) recombination
- (b) catabolism
- (c) degradation
- (d) synthesis

243. The maintenance of cell shape is determined by:
- (a) the media on which the organism grows
- (b) the cell wall
- (c) the presence of organic nitrogen
- (d) none of the above

244. Media with high oxidation-reduction potentials:
- (a) do not support the growth of obligate aerobes
- (b) do not support the growth of obligate anaerobes
- (c) containing reducing substances
- (d) none of the above

245. A Shick test is a skin test used to show:
- (a) immunity to diphtheria
- (b) susceptibility to diphtheria
- (c) immunity to scarlet fever
- (d) susceptibility to scarlet fever

246. Direct immunofluorescence
      is:
      (a) detection of antigens
           by fluorescent labelled
           antibody
      (b) detection of antibody
           by fluorescent labelled
           antigen
      (c) both of the above
      (d) neither of the above

247. Tinea versicolor is caused
      by:
      (a) *Candida albicans*
      (b) *Microsporum gypseum*
      (c) *Epidermophyton flocco-
           sum*
      (d) *Pityrosporon furfur*

248. The resolution limit of the
      light microscope is:
      (a) 0.001 micron
      (b) 0.2 micron
      (c) 400 nanometers
      (d) 0.001 mm

249. *Salmonella* may be serotyped
      based on:
      (a) O and B antigens
      (b) O and H antigens
      (c) A, B and C antigens
      (d) none of the above

250. The atypical mycobacteria
      resemble *Mycobacterium tuber-
      culosis* in being acid fast
      but differ in:
      (a) biochemical reactions
      (b) growth rate
      (c) pathogenicity for
           guinea pigs
      (d) all of the above

SECTION B: HEADINGS

*For each numbered word or phrase,
select the heading that is most
closely related to it.*

(1) (a) *Mycobacterium tuberculosis*
     (b) *Bordetella portussis*
     (c) *Haemophilus influenzae*
     (d) *Treponema pallidum*
     (e) *Corynebacterium diphtheriae*

251. Isolation requires enriched
      medium made of glycerin,
      potato and blood.
      ANSWER: _____

252. Originally thought to be the
      cause of influenzae and cal-
      led Pfeiffer's bacillus.
      ANSWER: _____

253. Slow growing organism re-
      quiring medium made with
      glycerol, potato and eggs.
      ANSWER: _____

254. Loffler serum slopes used to
      encourage characteristic
      morphology.
      ANSWER: _____

255. Strict human pathogen; usually
      demonstrated by dark field
      microscopy.
      ANSWER: _____

(2) (a) *Neisseria meningitidis*
     (b) *Neisseria gonorrhoeae*
     (c) *Branhamella catarrhalis*
     (d) *Staphylococcus aureus*
     (e) *Staphylococcus epidermidis*

256. Ferments mannitol, salt tol-
      erant and is DNA positive.
      ANSWER: _____

257. Ferments glucose and maltose
      and is oxidase positive.
      ANSWER: _____

258. Salt tolerant, does not fer-
      ment mannitol and is DNA
      negative.
      ANSWER: _____

259. Ferments glucose and is oxi-
     dase positive.
     ANSWER: _____

260. Inert biochemically and is
     oxidase positive.
     ANSWER: _____

(3) (a) *Streptococcus pyogenes*
     (b) *Streptococcus faecalis*
     (c) *Clostridium perfringens*
     (d) *Bacteroides fragilis*
     (e) *Clostridium tetani*

261. Terminal round spores and
     spreading film of growth on
     blood agar.
     ANSWER: _____

262. Frequently vacuolated in
     gram stains and growth is
     stimulated by bile.
     ANSWER: _____

263. Catalase negative, sensitive
     to penicillin and belong to
     group A.
     ANSWER: _____

264. Catalase negative, resistant
     to penicillin and belong to
     group D.
     ANSWER: _____

265. Catalase negative, sensitive
     to penicillin and can be
     typed on basis of toxins
     produced.
     ANSWER: _____

(4) (a) *Epidermophyton floccosum*
     (b) *Trichophyton mentagrophytes*
     (c) *Yersinia enterocolitica*
     (d) *Borrelia vincentii*
     (e) *Yersinia pestis*

266. A cause of gastroenteritis
     in the young.
     ANSWER: _____

267. Associated with "trench

mouth" and diagnosed by
gram stain.
ANSWER: _____

268. Produces many microconidia,
     hyphal spirals and few
     macroconidia.
     ANSWER: _____

269. Causative organism of "Black
     Death" in Europe during 14th
     century.
     ANSWER: _____

270. Produces smooth walled club-
     shaped macroconidia.
     ANSWER: _____

SECTION C: TRUE OR FALSE

*Mark the following statements
either TRUE (T) or FALSE (F).*

271. A common cause of meningi-
     tis in neonates is *Haemo-
     philus influenzae*, group B.

272. A common complication of
     gonorrhea is arthritis.

273. Using a hot air oven at
     180°C for 60 minutes is
     the most effective method
     of sterilization.

274. Penicillin is the anti-
     biotic of choice for treat-
     ment of *Mycoplasma* infec-
     tions.

275. Gram negative bacteria have
     teichoic acid in their cell
     walls.

276. Bacterial spores are gene-
     tically identical to their
     vegetative cells.

277. Saprophytic fungi usually

grow more rapidly in culture media than the pathogenic fungi.

278. Anaerobic organisms are usually isolated in pure culture from most clinical specimens.

279. The macroscopic slide agglutination technique is used particularly in identifying the gram negative intestinal pathogens.

280. The complement fixation test for the detection of antigen or antibody is based in general on the ability of complement to combine with many antigen-antibody aggregates.

281. Subacute bacterial endocarditis is commonly caused by *Staphylococcus aureus*.

282. Bile solubility test is the most reliable test for differentiation of pneumococci from other coccal forms.

283. The cold catalyst in an anaerobic jar need only be changed when the indicator shows the presence of oxygen.

284. A bactericidal agent is an excellent disinfectant as it kills bacteria.

285. *Clostridium perfringens* has spores characteristically located at one end giving the bacterium a drum stick appearance.

286. The irregular clusters of *Staphylococcus aureus* are found characteristically in smears from cultures grown

in broth and on solid media.

287. Cultures for pathogenic fungi may be discarded after two weeks if no growth appears.

288. Scotch ® tape swabs are useful in the diagnosis of infection due to *Ascaris lumbricoides*.

289. The antibody titre of a serum is the highest dilution of a serum which will give a reaction with the antigen.

290. Antistreptolysin O is an antibody found in the serum of patients recently infected with streptococci of Lancefield group B.

291. Identification of *Serratia* species is facilitated by their consistent production of pink to red pigmented colonies.

292. *Listeria* are aerobic motile, gram positive, catalase negative bacilli.

293. Members of the *Citrobacter* and *Arizona* groups closely resemble *Salmonella* in their biochemical reactions.

294. Phenolphthalein, because of its pH range, is a very useful indicator in bacteriology.

295. The presence of phenol in the Ziehl-Neelsen stain appears to facilitate penetration of carbol fuchsin through the mycobacterial lipid.

296. Resistance of bacteria to antimicrobial agents may be transferred from one bacterium to another during conjugation and transformation.

297. The change to gram negative of many old gram positive cultures is due to changes in the plasma membrane.

298. Disruption of the bacterial cell is not necessary for the release of endotoxins and exotoxins.

299. *Clostridium perfringens* does not sporulate in tissues.

300. Penicillin is the antibiotic of choice for infections due to *Staphylococcus aureus*.

301. The catalase test is a quick, simple method for differentiating staphylococci from streptococci.

302. An atmosphere of 5 - 10 per cent carbon dioxide enhances the growth of *Neisseria meningitidis*.

303. Food poisoning due to *Staphylococcus aureus* results from the production of enterotoxin in the food by the organism.

304. The dimple or checker type colony characteristic of *Streptococcus pneumoniae* is due to the heaping up of dead cells at the periphery.

305. Blood cultures are almost always positive when a patient has dysentery due to *Shigella*.

306. The sensitivity of anaerobes to oxygen is due to their lack of two enzymes-catalase and superoxide dismutase.

307. The pathogenicity of *Corynebacterium diphtheriae* is indicated by its growth on Tinsdale agar.

308. Gram stain of cerebrospinal fluid shows the presence of regular shaped gram negative bacilli characteristic of *Haemophilus influenzae*.

309. Atypical mycobacteria do not spread from man to man.

310. Active immunity is that possessed by infants for 2 - 3 months after birth.

311. Boiling for 20 minutes is an adequate process for destroying spores of bacteria and fungi.

312. Ascitic fluid may be added to culture media as an enrichment.

313. B.C.G. vaccine used in immunization against tuberculosis contains dead organisms.

314. Phenylethanol agar is useful in the laboratory because it enhances the growth of certain coliforms.

315. An infection acquired during stay in hospital is referred to as a nosocomial infection.

316. Working with specimens suspected of containing *Mycobacterium tuberculosis*,

one should be careful to
avoid production of aerosols.

317. "Lock jaw" is associated with
infection by *Clostridium
tetani*.

318. *Shigella* are non-lactose fermenters like *Salmonella* and
also like *Salmonella* have O
and H antigens.

319. The principal use of staphylococcal phage typing is
detecting the source of out-
breaks.

320. Steam at 121°C for 20 minutes
is not as effective as hot
air at 180°C for 60 minutes.

321. Prolonged use of antibiotics
may predispose a patient to
supra infection with *Candida
albicans*.

322. Hemolytic reactions of the
enterococci on blood agar
may be alpha, beta or gamma.

323. The reaction on egg yolk
agar by *Clostridium perfringens* is due to the production
of hyaluronidase.

324. Selective isolation of *Staphylococcus aureus* may be accomplished by using a medium
containing mannitol and 10
per cent sodium chloride.

325. Serologic identification of
Haemophilus influenzae is
detected by capsular swelling.

326. "Sulphur granules" may be
seen in specimens of pus
from cases of actinomycosis.

327. In the methyl red test, one

is detecting the alkalin-
ity of the culture.

328. Like the diplococci of
Neisseria, the diplococci
of *Streptococcus pneumoniae*
are lancet shaped.

329. A rapid preliminary identification of *Cryptococcus*
can be made on its ability
to produce an alkaline
reaction on urea.

330. A 10 per cent solution of
sodium hydroxide is used
as a mounting fluid for
skin scrapings.

331. The intracutaneous skin
test for tuberculosis was
introduced by Mantoux
after whom it is named.

332. *Trichophyton* species usually
produce numerous microconidia and small numbers of
macroconidia.

333. Multiple infection of erythrocytes is common with
Plasmodium vivax.

334. Carbohydrate fermentation
by colon bacilli results
in the formation of pyruvic
acid.

335. Incubation at 37°C or room
temperature of *Candida
albicans* always results in
yeast-like colonies.

336. A common fungal laboratory
contaminant that is green
in color with a brush-like
spore bearing structure
is *Penicillium*.

337. Staphylococcal infections
can be prevented by vac-

cination.

338. The macroconidia of *Microsporum* species are characteristically thick-walled, rough and multicelled.

339. Diagnosis of brucellosis involves culturing blood, bile, lymph and sputum.

340. *Neisseria meningitidis* is easy to culture in the laboratory because it is aerobic and quite resistant to low temperatures.

341. Bacteria that grow at temperatures between 10°C - 20°C are called mesophiles.

342. *Mucor* and *Rhizopus* belong to the *Phycomycetes* and they do not have a septate mycelium.

343. *Clostridium tetani* produces its clinical picture due to the production of a neurotoxin.

344. *Bacteroides fragilis* is the most common organism in the intestinal tract.

345. Gas gangrene may be caused by a mixture of clostridia species.

346. The most common isolate from nonepidemic meningitis is *Neisseria meningitidis*.

347. The carrier state (e.g., typhoid, diphtheria) may persist for long periods and serve as reservoir of infection.

348. *Clostridium botulinum* has been associated only with food-borne disease.

349. Skin ulcers may be caused by both *Bacillus anthracis* and *Corynebacterium diphtheriae*.

350. Syphilis is characterized by the disease occurring in three stages.

351. The beta hemolysis of group A streptococci on blood agar is due to the production of streptolysin O.

352. A pathogen is an organism which is capable of producing a disease in a susceptible host.

353. Injection of tetanus toxoid results in acquired passive active immunity.

354. During an outbreak, persons who are Schick test positive do not need immunization.

355. Saccharolytic species of clostridia obtain energy from fermentation of amino acids.

356. Isolation of *Campylobacter jejuni* requires increased CO_2 and temperature as well as selective media.

357. Penicillin may be destroyed by beta-lactamase produced by certain organisms.

358. Zone sizes in the Kirby-Bauer antibiotic susceptibility test are not affected by the inoculum size.

359. Some sera, when tested for agglutinating antibodies, produce positive reactions

only when diluted several hundred or thousand fold. This is known as prozone phenomenon.

360. Sulfonamides interfere with the synthesis of para-amino-benzoic acid by bacteria.

361. Antibiotics when used in combination may enhance the emergence of resistant strains.

362. Chromatic aberration in microscopy refers to the bending of light rays passing from one medium to the other.

363. In the absence of a carbon dioxide incubator, a candle jar may be used to give an atmosphere of 5 - 10 per cent CO_2.

364. Identification of dermatophytes is dependant on the presence of spiral hyphae and chlamydospores.

365. *Shigella sonnei* may be differentiated from other shigellae in that it is ONPG positive.

366. *Salmonella typhi* may be differentiated from other salmonellae in that it is a weak hydrogen sulphide producer.

367. Normal human flora may contain all of the following: *Actinomyces israelii*, *Clostridium perfringens*, *Haemophilus influenzae* and *Bacteroides fragilis*.

368. Gentamicin and tobramycin are examples of polypeptide antibiotics.

369. The enzyme tryptophanase breaks down tryptic soy to produce tryptophane.

370. Incubation of blood plates under anaerobic conditions for the isolation of *Streptococcus pyogenes* may be useful because streptolysin O is oxygen labile.

SECTION D: SPECIAL QUESTIONS

371. A young man helped his father clean up an old mill and farm yard prior to establishing a country inn and restaurant. He received a small cut on his thumb which was healed over by the next day. Approximately twelve days later, he visited his dentist complaining of some difficulty in opening his mouth which he thought was due to emerging wisdom teeth.

The probable etiologic agent is:
(a)   invasive
(b)   a virulent virus
(c)   a toxin producer
(d)   a gram negative bacillus

Assuming the organism to be *Clostridium tetani*, the microscopic appearance may be described as:
(e)   pleomorphic
(f)   drumstick
(g)   serpentine
(h)   bipolar

The source of the organism in the farm yard was most probably:
(i)   horse manure
(j)   rusty wagon
(k)   water wheel
(l)   old hay

Treatment of the patient should be with which of the following:
(m)   tetanus antitoxin
(n)   debridment of the port of entry
(o)   penicillin
(p)   all of the above

372. A school teacher returns after visiting several countries in the Orient. Three days later she has a sudden onset of nausea, vomiting and profuse watery diarrhea. The diarrhea is intense, producing watery stools. Culture reveals an almost pure growth in alkaline peptone broth in 6 - 8 hours.

The most probable diagnosis is:
(a)   typhoid fever
(b)   cholera
(c)   amebiasis
(d)   shigellosis

Assume the organism isolated is a gram negative nonmotile bacillus, then the probable diagnosis would be:
(e)   cholera
(f)   shigellosis
(g)   salmonellosis
(h)   none of the above

Assume the teacher had consumed an eggnog for breakfast. Which one of the following organisms would be the most likely causative agent?
(i)   *Staphylococcus aureus*
(j)   *Vibrio comma*
(k)   *Salmonella* species
(l)   *Shigella sonnei*

If the causative agent is *Vibrio cholerae*, which of the following may be observed:
(m)   the organism ferments sucrose
(n)   the organism is oxidase positive
(o)   the organism does not grow at 7 per cent NaCl
(p)   all of the above

373. The hospital night nursing supervisor received several reports from wards that some patients and staff members had been experiencing cramping, nausea and vomiting and diarrhea. A few had been taken ill in the afternoon approximately four to five hours after lunch, but more were sick two to three hours after dinner.

The foods consumed at lunch and dinner included the following. Which is the most likely source?
(a)   baked ham
(b)   ice cream
(c)   chicken salad sandwich
(d)   vegetable soup

All patients recovered by the following morning - this would indicate the organism to have been:
(e)   *Staphylococcus aureus*
(f)   *Shigella flexneri*
(g)   *Giardia lamblia*
(h)   *Salmonella typhimurium*

What is the usual source of this organism in contaminated food?
  (i) cutting board in the kitchen
  (j) butter used in sandwich
  (k) mayonnaise used in making chicken salad
  (l) hands of person making chicken salad

374. A foul smelling sample of pleural pus was sent to the laboratory. Gram stain showed the presence of pleomorphic gram negative bacilli, gram positive cocci in chains and gram negative bacilli with pointed ends.

Cultures should be set up on which of the following combinations:
  (a) laked blood plate containing kanamycin and vancomycin (anaerobic), blood agar (CO_2)
  (b) blood agar (CO_2) chocolate agar (CO_2)
  (c) blood agar (CO_2) MacConkey agar (O_2)
  (d) Thayer-Martin (CO_2) blood agar (anaerobic)

The specimen most likely contains:
  (e) viridans streptococci, *Bacteroides* species and *Escherichia coli*
  (f) viridans streptococci, *Bacteroides* species and *Fusobacterium*
  (g) *Staphylococcus epidermidis*, *Klebsiella pneumoniae*, *Bacteroides* species
  (h) *Streptococcus pyogenes*, *Escherichia coli* and *Bacteroides* species

Colonies present on the laked

kanamycin-vancomycin plate show a brick red fluorescence at 18 hours. The most likely organism is:
  (i) *Serratia marcescens*
  (j) Group B beta-hemolytic streptococcus
  (k) *Bacteroides melaninogenicus*
  (l) none of the above

Culture of specimens for anaerobes can be expensive and is time consuming. Which of the following specimens should not be cultured anaerobically?
  (m) pus
  (n) sputum
  (o) blood
  (p) transtracheal aspirate

375. A mother brings her eight year old boy into the hospital emergency room. He has a fever of 39.5°C, is sleepy and complains of having a stiff neck. A spinal tap reveals a cloudy fluid which on gram stain shows many polymorphonuclear leukocytes and gram negative diplococci.

The most likely organism is:
  (a) *Klebsiella pneumoniae*
  (b) *Neisseria meningitidis*
  (c) *Haemophilus influenzae*
  (d) *Streptococcus pneumoniae*

The organism will be isolated on:
  (e) blood agar, chocolate agar
  (f) blood agar, MacConkey agar
  (g) blood agar only
  (h) nutrient agar

The organism will be identified by:
  (i) acid production from
       glucose, maltose and
       sucrose
  (j) acid production from
       glucose, maltose and
       lactose
  (k) acid production from
       glucose only
  (l) acid production from
       glucose and maltose

SECTION E: QUESTIONS AND ANSWERS

*Answer the following questions in
the space provided.*

376. Salmonella disease may be
      seen in many forms, but
      the two most common are
      enteric fever and gastro-
      enteritis; with which is
      Salmonella typhi associated?
      ANSWER: _____

377. An oxidase negative, glucose
      nonfermenting bacillus was
      isolated. After 18 hours
      incubation, glucose was nega-
      tive and maltose was oxidized.
      What is this organism?
      ANSWER: _____

378. An organism causing respira-
      tory disease with character-
      istic paroxysms requires
      Bordet-Gengou medium for
      growth. What is the organism?
      ANSWER: _____

379. What single test could be
      done to differentiate
      Listeria monocytogenes from
      other aerobic nonsporeforming
      gram positive bacilli?
      ANSWER: _____

380. The scolex of *Taenia saginata*
      has a characteristic mechanism
      for attachment. What is it
      called?
      ANSWER: _____

381. Common tapeworms require one
      or more hosts in which the
      larval form develops. Name
      the host for *Taenia solium*.
      ANSWER: _____

382. India ink is useful for
      demonstrating what feature
      of certain bacteria and
      Cryptococcus?
      ANSWER: _____

383. What can be done to make a
      diagnosis of syphilis when
      the causative organism
      cannot be grown?
      ANSWER: _____

384. In order to be toxigenic,
      Corynebacterium diphtheriae
      must have one characteristic.
      What is this?
      ANSWER: _____

385. What is the term given to
      the ability of an organism
      to spread through tissue?
      ANSWER: _____

386. When two antibiotics act
      together to achieve an effect
      greater than either acting
      alone, what is the effect
      called?
      ANSWER: _____

387. Chronic infection of the
      valves of the heart is
      caused by several genera
      of bacteria. What is the
      clinical name of this con-
      dition?
      ANSWER: _____

388. A colony of *Clostridium per-fringens* has a characteristic effect on the blood agar plate. What is the term used for this appearance?
ANSWER: _____

389. A useful primary differentia-tion can be made between pathogenic and nonpathogenic enteric bacilli using one medium. What is the name of the medium?
ANSWER: _____

390. A number of organisms per ml of urine is accepted as the baseline for indicating a urinary tract infection. What is that number?
ANSWER: _____

391. Ova that are characteristically flattened on one side belong to which worm?
ANSWER: _____

392. Gram positive bacilli that are frequently isolated from vaginal specimens and are able to exist under acid con-ditions belong to which genus?
ANSWER: _____

393. The viridans group of strepto-cocci are normal inhabitants of the body's mucous membranes and are a frequent isolate in cases of endocarditis. What specimen should be sent to the laboratory for isolation of this group?
ANSWER: _____

394. Flagellar or H antigens may mask the O or somatic antigen when performing slide agglu-tinations. How can this be overcome?
ANSWER: _____

395. Cultures for isolation of *Mycobacterium tuberculosis* must be incubated for 6 - 8 weeks before discarding as negative. Why is this?
ANSWER: _____

396. Scarlet fever is caused by strains of streptococci which must have one charac-teristic. What is it?
ANSWER: _____

397. The capsules of pneumococci enable us to classify the organisms into more than 85 specific antigenic types. What other function does the capsule have?
ANSWER: _____

398. Food poisoning due to staphy-lococci characteristically has a sudden onset of nausea occurring a few hours after ingestion of contaminated food. Would you expect to isolate the causative organ-ism from vomitus?
ANSWER: _____

399. Why do mycobacteria species resist the gram stain?
ANSWER: _____

400. Shigellae unlike salmonellae are seldom isolated from blood cultures. Is this because they are nonmotile?
ANSWER: _____

401. The organisms causing per-tussis have been placed in a separate genus (*Bordetella*) from *Haemophilus*. Why has this been done?
ANSWER: _____

402. How can you make a presumptive diagnosis of gonorrhoea in

smears of pus from the male urethra?
ANSWER: _____

403. Gram positive pleomorphic nonsporeforming bacilli are frequently referred to as "diphtheroid" bacilli. Why is this term used?
ANSWER: _____

404. Following tooth extraction, a patient developed a cervico-facial abscess. What organism which may be part of the normal flora of the mouth is the most likely infecting organism?
ANSWER: _____

405. Spores are commonly seen in the various members of the *Clostridium* genus except for one organism. What is the name of the organism?
ANSWER: _____

406. What is the name given to the engulfment of micro-organisms or other particles by leukocytes?
ANSWER: _____

407. Although more than 90 per cent of infected people may be asymptomatic, severe disease may result from hepatic abscesses due to invasion with this protozoan.
ANSWER: _____

408. Specimens for isolation of *Francisella tularensis* are best handled by reference centers. Why is this?
ANSWER: _____

409. *Brucella abortus* has one requirement for isolation that differentiates it from the other *Brucella* species.

What is that requirement?
ANSWER: _____

410. Performing acid fast stains of gastric fluid and urines is not a good practice. Why?
ANSWER: _____

411. What is the organism that is the cause of "wool-sorters" disease?
ANSWER: _____

412. Several severe sequelae may result from infection with *Streptococcus pyogenes*. What are two?
ANSWER: _____

413. Why does infection with *Clostridium tetani* occur although the organism rarely invades past the point of entry?
ANSWER: _____

414. Resistance of *Staphylococcus aureus* and many gram nega-tive organisms to penicillin is due to the production of an enzyme. What is its action?
ANSWER: _____

415. Sporadic cases of typhoid fever may result from asymptomatic individuals. What do we call such people?
ANSWER: _____

416. Most of the bacterial RNA is found in what structures in the cell?
ANSWER: _____

417. When the term "g-c ratio" is used, what do the letters "g" and "c" refer to?
ANSWER: _____

418. *Edwardsiella tarda* may be con-
      fused biochemically with what
      genus?
      ANSWER: _____

419. Optochin discs are used to
      differentiate pneumococci
      from the viridans group of
      streptococci. What is the
      compound present in the disc?
      ANSWER: _____

420. How do *Mycoplasma* species
      differ from bacteria?
      ANSWER: _____

421. Tetrazolium salts are used
      in various bacterial media
      to detect what?
      ANSWER: _____

422. What test may be used to
      differentiate *Mycobacterium
      tuberculosis* from other acid
      fast pathogens?
      ANSWER: _____

423. False negative coagulase
      tests may result from lysis
      of the coagulase-produced
      clot by what enzyme?
      ANSWER: _____

424. When fecal specimens must be
      held for some time before
      plating, what solution may
      be used as a preservative?
      ANSWER: _____

425. An organism that fails to
      grow on MacConkey agar al-
      though good growth occurs
      on nutrient agar may be
      sensitive to what ingred-
      ient in the MacConkey agar?
      ANSWER: _____

ANSWERS

SECTION A: MULTIPLE CHOICE

1. (c) Viable bacteria are count-
         ed by production of colo-
         nies on solid media.

2. (a) Cell walls of gram posi-
         tive bacteria contain
         polysaccharides such as
         teichoic acids and pro-
         teins. Thin sections
         reveal it to be relatively
         thick compact layer.

3. (d) Identification of enteric
         bacilli is done using
         their cultural appearance
         on selective media, their
         reactions in biochemical
         tests and in some in-
         stances (*Salmonella*,
         Shigella) serological
         characteristics.

4. (c) *Staphylococcus aureus*
         elaborates enterotoxin
         into the food.

5. (d) *Neisseria gonorrhoeae* may
         be isolated from blood,
         synovial fluids, eyes and
         other specimens.

6. (b) A common character of
         Klebsiella, *Enterobacter*
         and *Serratia* is a posi-
         tive reaction in the
         V.P. test. Some species
         in each group may fer-
         ment lactose; *Serratia*
         and *Enterobacter* are
         motile and *Klebsiella*
         are not pigmented.

7. (d) Clumping of staphylococci
         when emulsified in saline
         is autoagglutination and
         a slide coagulase cannot
         be done on such a strain.

8. (c) Red blood cells in the
         medium produce catalase
         causing breakdown of
         hydrogen peroxide.

9. (d) Enteric streptococci

are resistant to peni-
cillin.

10. (c) Precipitin lines formed
by combination of toxin
and antitoxin are the
basis of the Elek test.

11. (b) *Haemophilus influenzae*
requires nicotinamide
adenine dinucleotides
for growth (V factor).

12. (d) Alcohol and formalin
would kill any fungal
elements present in
the skin scraping so
that isolation of the
dermatophyte could not
be made. Small scrap-
ings could easily be
lost in a transport
medium.

13. (d) Sterilization in an
autoclave can be achieved
at temperatures in excess
of 100°C; for most bac-
teriological media, the
combination of 121°C at
15 lbs/sq. inch and
15 minutes is satisfactory.

14. (a) The usual means of acquir-
ing *Salmonella* is by eating a contaminated food
source.

15. (d) A thermolabile substance
is destroyed or inactiva-
ted by heat.

16. (b) Most bacteria grow between 10°C and 45°C and
are termed mesophiles.

17. (c) Hot air sterilization
requires a higher tem-
perature when moisture
and pressure are not
present and articles

should be held for one
hour or longer.

18. (c) The heat resistance of
bacterial spores can
be used to isolate a
sporeforming organism
from a bacterial mix-
ture by heating the
mixture at 100°C for
15 - 20 minutes.

19. (a) Bacteria do not begin
to multiply immediately
after inoculation; they
are in a period of
stationary population.

20. (c) The process introduced
by Tyndall makes use
of flowing steam on 3
successive days and
therefore lower tem-
peratures than usually
used in autoclaves.
Incubation of the mate-
rial between exposure
allows spores to ger-
minate which are de-
stroyed by the next
steam process.

21. (a) Diameter of a staphylococcus is 0.8 - 1
micron.

22. (c) Following infection
with group A streptococci,
a patient develops anti-
bodies to streptolysin
O; in the ASO test, this
antibody combines with
and neutralizes strepto-
lysin O thus inhibiting
its hemolytic activity
on red blood cells.

23. (b) The intermediate host
of *Taenia solium* is
the pig; man acquires
the infection by eating

undercooked infected pork which may contain encysted parasites.

24. (d) Bacterial endocarditis is colonization of the valves of the heart by various bacteria usually streptococcal species. It may present as "sub-acute" or "acute" endo-carditis.

25. (d) Resazurin turns pink in the presence of oxygen.

26. (b) To adjust the pH of 1 liter of medium with N/10 NaOH, one would have to add a considerable volume of fluid (35 ml in this instance) which would dilute the medium. Using a more concentrated solution, there is less dilution.

27. (b) The purpose of the sub-stage condenser on the microscope is to condense or focus the light source on the object you wish to observe.

28. (b) The fish tapeworm (Diphyllo-bothrium latum) egg is non-embryonated, the walls are thinner than eggs of the Taenia species and are operculate.

29. (b) Temperatures of 100°C, 45°C apply to commercially available agars; other agars are known which have widely different tempera-ture characteristics which make them unsuitable for usual microbiological pur-poses.

30. (c) The viridans streptococci are the usual isolates from cases of bacterial endocarditis. They reach the heart valves via the blood stream from the mouth.

31. (b) Botulism is caused by the ingestion of toxin elaborated by Clostridium botulinum, an anaerobic sporeforming bacillus.

32. (a) Triple sugar iron agar commonly used in bac-teriology for enteric bacilli incorporates ferrous ammonium sul-phate for H_2S detection.

33. (b) Sterilization by steam is accomplished by coagulation of the bacterial protein.

34. (a) Mistakes and difficul-ties in identification of bacteria frequently result from a mixed culture, although in-appropriate media, abbreviated schemata and insensitive tests will also result in misidentifications.

35. (c) Tetrazolium compounds are reduced to red salts by bacterial growth.

36. (c) The media commonly described as O/F media were originally described by Hugh and Leifson to determine the method of carbohydrate utilization.

37. (c) An increasing titer of

antistreptolysin O indi-
cates a patient has had
infection with group A
streptococcal infection
in the past and is diag-
nostic of acute rheumatic
fever.

38. (d) *Nocardia asteroides* is
a gram positive, aerobic
bacillus which is also
partially acid - fast.

39. (b) *Enterobacter aerogenes*
produces acetoin (acetyl-
methyl carbinol) in the
V.P. test and its pres-
ence is determined by
the addition of alpha
naphthol and KOH -
creatine to a 48-hour
dextrose broth culture
and formation of a red
color.

40. (c) The mode of antibacterial action of alcohols
is probably a denatura-
tion of proteins. In
the absence of water,
this denaturation does
not occur and a 70 per
cent aqueous solution
alcohol has been found
to be the most effective.

41. (c) The addition of a small
amount of agar (usually
0.07 per cent) to thio-
glycollate slows the
diffusion of oxygen into
the medium, making it
suitable for anaerobic
organisms.

42. (b) A positive methyl red
test is detected by the
addition of a methyl red
solution to a 24 - 48-
hour glucose broth cul-
ture resulting in a red

color.

43. (c) Beta lactamase is an
enzyme produced by
penicillin-resistant
Staphylococcus aureus
and other bacteria
which split the beta
lactam ring.

44. (b) One of the identifying
tests for the enteric
streptococci is their
ability to grow in
the presence of 4 per
cent bile salts; other
characteristics are
hydrolysis of esculin,
growth in the presence
of 6.5 per cent sodium
chloride and belonging
to Lancefield group D.

45. (d) The enzyme tryptophanase
splits tryptophan to form
indole; this is the basis
of the indole test com-
monly used in identifi-
cation of the *Entero-
bacteriaceae*.

46. (c) Lactose fermentation
is dependent on two
enzymes - permease and
beta-galactosidase.
Slow lactose fermenters
are deficient in permease
which enables lactose to
enter the bacterial cell.
The ONPG test detects
the presence of beta-
galactosidase and a
positive ONPG test indi-
cates the organism con-
tains lactose-fermenting
enzymes.

47. (c) Only toxigenic strains of
C. diphtheriae can pro-
duce disease.

48. (c) A culture suspected of being *Listeria monocytogenes* may be rapidly identified by demonstrating characteristic "tumbling" motility in a wet mount made from a 2 - 4 hour room temperature broth culture.

49. (d) A broad spectrum antibiotic affects both gram positive and gram negative bacteria.

50. (a) Media that are allowed
    (b) to dry out lose the
    (c) correct concentration of ingredients for bacterial growth; excessive heating will cause breakdown of some materials and excessive condensation could lead to contamination.

51. (c) The cell wall constitutes a significant portion of the total dry weight of a cell; depending on the species, the amount may vary from 10 - 40 per cent.

52. (b) Many factors influence heat resistance of spores - their complex structure, suspending medium, age of the spore, etc. Moist heat under pressure has the best effect.

53. (b) Tissue taken from one portion of the body to another for grafting is referred to as an "autograft." A tissue from another body of the same species may be termed a "homograft."

54. (d) Food poisoning due to *Salmonella* may be caused by *S. typhimurium*, *S. enteriditis* as well as many other *Salmonella* species.

55. (b) Infection with *Bacillus anthracis* was frequently associated with handlers of sheep wool, various animal hides and cattle workers. It is rarely seen in North America but a few cases occur each year.

56. (c) Colonies of *Mycobacterium tuberculosis* growing on a solid medium such as Lowenstein-Jensen are typically dry and heaped, resembling bread crumbs in appearance.

57. (c) There are more than 80 serologically distinct types of *Streptococcus pneumoniae* based on capsular antigens. In practice a polyvalent serum containing a pool of antibodies is used in a quellung reaction. It is of use primarily in epidemiologic studies.

58. (d) The meningococcus requires added CO_2, is gram negative and does not ferment sucrose.

59. (c) Tetanus spores are terminal and distend the bacterial cell.

60. (c) *Haemophilus influenzae* is a fastidious organism that requires a medium

containing X and V factors. Luxuriant growth occurs on chocolate agar whereas a streak of *Staphylococcus* is required on a blood agar plate.

61. (a) *Brucella abortus* requires 3 - 10 per cent CO_2 on primary isolation but this requirement may be lost on subculture.

62. (c) Anaerobic bacteria lack the enzyme superoxide dismutase and some species are highly sensitive to even traces of oxygen.

63. (a) Many bacteria, particularily the gram negative bacilli, produce endotoxins which are not liberated until the bacterial cell disintegrates. Endotoxins are complex in nature, being composed of carbohydrates, protein and phospholipids.

64. (d) Ribosomes are an integral part of a bacterial cell and are not media dependent.

65. (c) Penicillin acts on synthesis of cell wall so is most effective during period of maximum cell division.

66. (c) An agar thickness of 4 mm is recommended for the K-B test. Too thick a layer results in a three dimensional effect and resulting smaller zone of inhibition. Too thin an agar layer allows greater outward diffusion of antibiotic with a resulting large zone of inhibition.

67. (c) *Enterobius vermicularis* is one of the smaller round worms infecting man and is commonly referred to as the "pinworm."

68. (b) Glucose is the one sugar characteristically fermented by all members of the family *Enterobacteriaceae* with or without the production of gas.

69. (c) *Epidermophyton floccosum* characteristically produces clusters of 3 club-shaped smooth-walled macroconidia and no microconidia.

70. (b) The enzyme phenylalanine deaminase produced by various members of the *Enterobacteriaceae* deaminates phenylalanine to pyruvic acid.

71. (b) The bacitracin disk for identifying group A streptococci contains 0.04 units of bacitracin, zone size may be affected by an old dry plate and a sensitivity disc is 10 units.

72. (a) N-acetyl-1-cysteine is a mucolytic agent used to break up sputum samples for routine culture and in combination with NaOH for tuberculosis isolation.

73. (a) Dermatophytes characteristically invade

the superficial skin lay-
ers as they possess kera-
tinolytic enzymes enabling
them to use keratin as a
nitrogen source.

74. (c) Hydrogen is explosive when
present in concentrations
of more than 4 per cent.

75. (b) Trophozoites of *Entamoeba
histolytica* contain one
nucleus with chromatoidal
bars present only in the
cyst stage. The presence
of ingested red blood
cells is considered diag-
nostic of *E. histolytica*.

76. (d) *Proteus*, *Providencia* and
Morganella are all phenylalanine deaminase pro-
ducers thus giving a
positive phenylalanine
test.

77. (c) Most strains of *Staphylococcus aureus* isolated
in hospitals are resis-
tant to penicillin.

78. (c) The key phrase "foul
smelling" is one of the
useful clinical clues
of a possible anaerobic
infection and the pres-
ence of small gram posi-
tive cocci in chains would
suggest *Peptostreptococcus*
species.

79. (c) Phosphates in bacteriological media act as
buffers preventing wide
changes in pH.

80. (c) *Trichomonas* may be recog-
nized in gram stains by
its size and presence of
axostyle.

81. (b) The yeast, *Cryptococcus
neoformans*, produces
only yeast-like colonies
in culture. No mycelial
phase has been described
for this organism and
most saprophytic strains
do not grow at 35°C.

82. (a) Synergism is when the
combined effect of two
(or more) agents is
greater than the sum
of their individual
effects.

83. (d) Meningitis in infants
under two months of
age is most frequently
due to *Haemophilus
influenzae*. The organism
enters via the respiratory
tract where it may enter
the blood stream and be
carried to the meninges.

84. (a) Cells of *Streptococcus
pneumoniae* are susceptible
to lysis by surface active
agents such as bile or
bile salts. This is the
basis of the bile solu-
bility test which may be
performed on broth cul-
tures or directly on
colonies on blood agar.

85. (c) Identification of *Staphylococcus aureus* is most
reliably done by the
coagulase test, either
by tube (detecting free
coagulase) or slide
(detecting bound coagu-
lase) tests. A negative
slide test should always
be checked by a tube
test.

86. (b) Statistics have shown

that asymptomatic carriers
of *Salmonella typhi* are
most likely to be middle-
aged females. The organ-
ism is frequently present
in the gallbladder, which
can be removed surgically
to clear up the carrier
state.

87. (d) Complement is present in
most sera, but the usual
source for testing pur-
poses is guinea pig
serum.

88. (b) Aerogenic is defined as
production of gas, usually
from carbohydrate fermen-
tation.

89. (c) Metachromatic granules
are characteristically
produced on Loeffler's
serum slants or Pai's
egg medium.

90. (b) Lecithinase splits lecithin, resulting in opaci-
ty in the medium.

91. (c) Lancefield grouping is
based on the cell wall
polysaccharides of beta
hemolytic streptococci.

92. (d) Presumptive identification of *Salmonella typhi*
may be easily made when
a TSI with minimal amount
of H_2S is seen and a small
amount of gas in the butt.

93. (b) A red color which develops
after the addition of zinc
dust to a nitrate test
indicates that unreduced
nitrates were present in
the broth. Zinc reduces
nitrate to nitrite.

94. (c) Many disinfectants are
inactivated by organic
material.

95. (c) *Citrobacter freundii*
is ONPG positive,
Salmonella enteritidis
is negative. Citrate
and methyl red are
positive for both
organisms.

96. (b) Iodine belongs to the
halogen group of chem-
icals which also in-
cludes bromine and
chlorine.

97. (d) Excretion of ova is
not consistent so
several samples should
be examined.

98. (b) The exact mode of
chlorine action on
bacteria is not
thoroughly understood
but is probably oxi-
dation. It is thought,
however, that the un-
dissociated chloramine
molecule acts directly
on bacteria and that
the hypochlorus acid
formed in a chlorine -
water mixture is the
killing agent.

99. (d) A double zone of beta
hemolysis on anaerobic
blood plates by *Clos-
tridium perfringens* is
frequently referred to
as "target hemolysis."

100. (a) A CAMP test is performed on blood plates
using a central streak
of *Staphylococcus* and
streaks at right angles
to it of beta hemolytic

streptococci. Group B
streptococci will show
a broad arrow-shaped
zone of hemolysis adja-
cent to the staphylo-
coccus after overnight
incubation.

101. (d) All members of the genus
Klebsiella and the genus
Shigella are nonmotile.

102. (c) The presence of oxygen
is essential to the
proper final reaction
of a TSI test. After
the initial utilization
of glucose, a non-lactose,
non-sucrose fermenting
organism will proceed to
oxidation of the peptones
resulting in a reversion
to alkalinity of the
slope.

103. (b) *Klebsiella pneumoniae*
is by definition an
oxidase negative, non-
motile fermentative
organism which usually
produces large amounts
of gas from carbohydrate
fermentation.

104. (b) Strong alkali solutions
are used to eliminate
other bacteria from
specimens for mycobac-
terial isolation, as *M.
tuberculosis* is rela-
tively resistant to
short exposures of
alkaline solutions.

105. (c) Diseases capable of being
transmitted to man from
animals are described
as "zoonoses."

106. (b) A yeast isolated in the
laboratory which pro-

duces germ tubes in
serum and/or chlamy-
dospores on corn meal
agar may be identified
as *Candida albicans*
without further testing.

107. (a) Both the Ziehl-Neelsen
and modified Kinyoun
stains use basic fuchsin
and phenol as ingredients
of the stain for mycobac-
teria.

108. (d) Safety shields should be
used in centrifuges;
rubber stoppers opened
in a safety hood and ex-
cess material removed
from loops before flam-
ing.

109. (d) *Brucella* are most usually
isolated from blood, but
are occasionally isolated
from bone marrow or lymph
node biopsies.

110. (a) Lecithinase C is only
one of the many toxins
which enable *Clostridium
perfringens* to produce
disease in tissues. It
is also called alpha
toxin and will attack
lecithin and sphingo-
myelin and red blood
cells.

111. (a) Phagocytosis of pneumococci is prevented by
presence of capsules.

112. (a) Infections with either
Clostridium tetani or
*Corynebacterium diph-
theriae* may be prevented
by conferring passive
immunity using the spe-
cific antitoxin.

113. (d) The 3 genera, *Proteus*, *Pseudomonas* and *Serratia*, are all gram negative bacilli which are commonly present in many hosptial reservoirs or fomites and may become resistant to many antibiotics.

114. (b) *Neisseria* species are all oxidase positive.

115. (d) *Shigella* species are non-motile, are not isolated from animal reservoirs and with the exception of *Shigella sonnei*, which is ONPG positive, are non-lactose fermenting.

116. (b) Sabouraud's dextrose agar has a low pH which inhibits most bacteria allowing fungi to grow.

117. (b) In typhoid fever, a blood culture may be positive before stool cultures become positive. During the first week about 90 per cent of blood cultures will be positive and stool cultures only about 10 per cent.

118. (b) Most of nonpathogenic mycobacteria are niacin negative.

119. (d) The *Bacteroides fragilis* group of gram negative bacilli are the most frequently isolated anaerobes in the clinical laboratory and are also the predominant organisms in the human intestinal tract.

120. (b) *Actinomyces israelii* is nonacid-fast, is anaerobic and will not grow on Sabouraud's agar.

121. (c) *Pasteurella multocida* is frequently isolated from animal bites.

122. (c) Chocolate agar would support the growth of all spinal fluid pathogens and brain heart infusion broth is a good all purpose broth.

123. (b) Selenite broth is an example of an enrichment medium; it should be subcultured 6 - 8 hours after inoculation.

124. (d) The tube coagulase test for staphylococci detects the presence of free coagulase and a positive reaction identifies *Staphylococcus aureus*.

125. (d) Two serum samples should enable detection of a rising titre.

126. (c) Disks of ethylhydrocupreine HCl are the basis of the optochin susceptibility test for differentiation of *Streptococcus pneumoniae* from viridans streptococci. Pneumococci must exhibit a zone of inhibition of at least 14 - 16 mm with a 10 mm disk.

127. (b) Some bacteria such as citrate-utilizing enter-ococci or gram negative bacilli may coagulate citrated plasma as well as staphylococci so that use of oxalated plasma or EDTA will prevent a false positive.

128. (a) Variable reactions in V.P. and M.R. tests when incubated at 22°C or 35°C are useful in the identification of *Hafnia alvei*.

129. (b) Methylene blue, when reduced, becomes colorless so that it may be used to indicate presence of oxygen in an anaerobic jar.

130. (c) Production of staphy-lokinase may cause lysis of the coagulase induced clot, resulting in an apparently negative result. Tube coagulase tests should be checked at 2 and 4 hour intervals after inoculation.

131. (a) By definition, *Haemophilus* species require blood or blood factors for growth whereas the members of the *Bordetella* genus can be isolated without these additions.

132. (d) *Corynebacterium diphtheriae* usually ferment glucose and maltose only; a rare sucrose fermenting strain has been reported.

133. (a) The gel strength of an agar will be adversely affected by heat, pH and concentration. Container

size is irrelevant.

134. (d) Sodium hydroxide, NAC and trisodium phosphate are all mucolytic agents.

135. (b) Thayer-Martin is a selective medium for isolation of *Neisseria gonorrhoeae* from clinical specimens.

136. (b) Phage type is particu-larly used in epide-miological studies of *Staphylococcus aureus*.

137. (c) The palladium catalyst must be heated after each use to remove water.

138. (a) The enteric strepto-cocci belong to Lance-field group D.

139. (c) Tumbling motility of
     (d) a two hour room tem-perature broth culture and a rapidly positive bile esculin reaction are excellent rapid presumptive tests for *Listeria* cultures.

140. (d) *Bacteroides melanino-genicus* produces black colonies on laked blood agar; the colonies also fluoresce with a brick red fluorescence.

141. (a) *Alcaligenes* produces an alkaline reaction in O/F media.

142. (a) Ringworm in schoolage children is commonly due to *Microsporum audouini* and it spreads rapidly throughout a

school population.

143. (c) Capsules of *Cryptococcus*, *Klebsiella*, *Streptococcus pneumoniae*, *Haemophilus influenzae* may be seen in India ink preparations.

144. (a) Eggs of *Enterobius vermicularis* are deposited on the skin of the anal region during the night. Use of Scotch ® tape will enable the diagnosis of pinworm infection to be made. Eggs are seldom seen in feces.

145. (a) Sheep cell agglutinating antibodies will still be present in the guinea pig absorbed titration row making the differential diagnosis of infectious mononucleosis.

146. (b) The complement present in human serum can be readily inactivated by 30 minutes exposure to 56°C.

147. (d) Lowenstein-Jensen medium for the isolation of *Mycobacterium tuberculosis* is made with the addition of fresh eggs.

148. (c) Ribosomes are composed of rRNA and proteins and are small granules which fill the cytoplasm of bacterial cells. They synthesize protein; the type depends on mRNA supplied.

149. (a) Membrane filters of which the Millipore ® filter is

an example are made of cellulose acetate and can be made with specific pore sizes.

150. (a) The higher lipid content of gram negative cells is removed by the alcohol used in the decolorization step. This increases cell permeability and the crystal violet-iodine complex is removed.

151. (b) Tetramethylparaphenylene diamine hydrochloride is the commonly used oxidase test reagent for *Neisseria* and *Pseudomonas*.

152. (a) To achieve saturated steam and a resulting 121°C, all air must be removed from the autoclave.

153. (c) Yeast extract is an excellent source of vitamin B and is added to many media to enhance bacterial growth.

154. (c) The Elek test for detecting toxin-producing strains of *Corynebacterium diphtheriae* uses anti-toxin-soaked filter paper strip and precipitation lines are formed in agar between the toxin and the antitoxin.

155. (a) Gentamicin is an aminoglycoside antibiotic as are tobramycin, amikacin and netilmycin.

156. (b) Durham tubes are small

glass tubes closed at one end which when inverted in a fluid medium permit the detection of gas production.

157. (c) A good transport medium preserves the initial proportions of organisms present in the specimen without allowing growth or inhibition.

158. (d) SPS is an effective anticoagulant in blood cultures and in addition it appears also to neutralize bactericidal effects of human serum and prevent phagocytosis.

159. (a) The gram positive lactobacilli are commensals of the mucous membranes and are frequently isolated from genital specimens.

160. (c) Immersion oil with its refractive index close to that of glass allows light to pass directly from the condenser to the objective.

161. (b) Antitoxin to *Clostridium perfringens* will inhibit the opacity produced by this organism on a lecithin containing medium (e.g., egg yolk agar).

162. (c) *Neisseria gonorrhoeae*, a human pathogen, produces acid from glucose only, is a gram negative, catalase positive bean-shaped diplococcus.

163. (d) *Shigella sonnei* does

not produce hydrogen sulphide, is nonmotile, does not produce gas from glucose and is ONPG positive.

164. (c) Inhibition of growth by a 0.04 unit disk of bacitracin is a presumptive identification of group A streptococci.

165. (b) *Klebsiella pneumoniae* utilizes citrate as sole carbon source, is nonmotile, is usually lactose fermenting and does not decarboxylate ornithine.

166. (a) *Entamoeba coli* and *Giardia lamblia* are protozoa; *Enterobius vermicularis* and *Trichuris trichiura* are round worms.

167. (d) Blood may contain hepatitis B surface antigen which can be inactivated by chlorine.

168. (c) Tetramethylparaphenylene diamine dihydrochloride is the oxidase reagent and a positive test is indicated by colonies turning blue-black.

169. (a) The pH range of phenol red is 6.8 - 8.4 and the color change is yellow to red.

170. (b) *Streptococcus agalactiae* belongs to Lancefield group B and is commonly present on mucous membranes such

as the respiratory and genital tracts.

171. (a) The cellular response in bacterial meningitis other than due to *Mycobacterium tuberculosis* is predominantly polymorphonuclear.

172. (b) Concentrations of blood used in plates for the clinical laboratory are usually 3 - 5 per cent.

173. (b) Maximum growth is over; the nutrients are becoming exhausted.

174. (c) Thermostable substances are unaffected by heat as opposed to thermolabile, adversely affected by heat.

175. (c) Chromatographic profiles of volatile acids produced by anaerobic fermentation of carbohydrates are used in identification of anaerobic bacteria.

176. (d) A eugonic organism grows luxuriantly as opposed to dysgonic organisms - poor growth.

177. (d) Some organisms require increased amounts of carbon dioxide; they are termed "capneic."

178. (d) Gram stains of *Corynebacterium diphtheriae* show pleomorphic gram positive bacilli, some of which are club shaped.

179. (d) *Citrobacter freundii* is VP negative and *Enterobacter cloacae* is VP positive.

180. (c) The enteric gram negative bacilli look very similar in gram stain and you cannot tell *E. coli* from *S. typhi* on this stain.

181. (c) The breakdown of hydrogen peroxide is the catalase test. *Staphylococcus epidermidis* is positive while *Streptococcus* species and *Clostridium* species are negative.

182. (d) MacFarland standards are prepared using solutions of barium chloride and sulphuric acid. They should be stored in the dark and prepared fresh each month.

183. (b) Plastic Petri plates are sterilized for use by ethylene oxide. Gamma radiation may also be used.

184. (c) *Pasteurella multocida* is a small gram negative coccobacillus which grows readily on most laboratory media.

185. (d) *Pseudomonas aeruginosa* and other pseudomonads attack carbohydrates oxidatively.

186. (d) *Campylobacter* species may be identified in the laboratory by their characteristic curved morphology, positive oxidase reaction and

temperature requirements.

187. (d) Lowenstein-Jensen medium is made with glycerol, potato flour, eggs, malachite green and is sterilized in flowing steam without pressure.

188. (c) *Acinetobacter* are aerobic gram negative coccoid shaped bacilli which are oxidase negative and attack carbohydrates oxidatively.

189. (a) The addition of vancomycin, colistin and nystatin to Thayer-Martin medium inhibits bacteria and yeasts to enhance the isolation of *N. gonorrhoeae*.

190. (d) Articles packed too tightly prevent steam access to all parts of the load. Superheated steam condenses on items thus lowering their temperature. Timing does not begin until the temperature gauge reads the correct temperature.

191. (c) In transformation, DNA is transferred from one strain to another. An example of this is the R-S transformation in pneumococci described by Griffith in 1928.

192. (c) A facultative anaerobe is an organism which will grow in the absence or presence of oxygen.

193. (b) Bacterial spores may be termed as a "resting"

stage; they do not have metabolic activity.

194. (a) Bacteria which require molecular oxygen for metabolism are obligate aerobes.

195. (d) Antibiotics act on bacterial cells by a variety of methods - disruption of the cell wall, denaturation of protein, competition for metabolic substances, damage the cell membrane or inhibit nucleic acid metabolism.

196. (b) A bacterial cell surrounded by flagella is said to be peritrichate.

197. (c) By definition, a disinfectant is usually a chemical agent which destroys micro-organisms but not usually spores. An antiseptic on the other hand is a substance that arrests the growth or action of micro-organisms either by inhibiting or destroying.

198. (c) A symbiotic relationship is beneficial to both members.

199. (d) The number of organisms per ml of urine may be calculated by counting the number of colonies produced by plating a known volume of the urine.

200. (b) Chromatic aberration occurs when white light

is split into its com-
ponent colors by the
lens to form a spectrum.
The result will be a
hazy outline and a fringe
of various colors.

201. (a) *Bacillus stearothermophilus*
          is used for testing routine
          autoclave conditions of
          121°C, 15 minutes.

202. (d) A 10^3 dilution is 1 in a
          thousand.

203. (b) Most oil immersion objec-
          tives are 90X.

204. (c) *Shigella* species are not
          motile.

205. (d) Fluorescent staining of
          mycobacteria is accom-
          plished by use of fluo-
          rescent dyes; no antibody
          labelling is used.

206. (a) Trophozoites may be dem-
          onstrated better by hemo-
          toxylin staining than by
          wet mounts. The inter-
          nal structure is more
          readily examined.

207. (d) *Clostridium perfringens*
          can cause both gas gan-
          grene and food poison-
          ing.

208. (b) *Neisseria meningitidis*
          is carried in the naso-
          pharynx so a throat
          swab or a swab of the
          nasopharyngeal wall
          would be the best sam-
          ples for carrier detec-
          tion.

209. (b) *Moraxella*, like *Neisseria*,

are oxidase positive
and are also present
on mucous membranes.

210. (a) Man is infected by
          Leptospira transmitted
          in urine and tissues
          of infected animals
          such as rats.

211. (c) Chickens are colonized
          by *Salmonella* with
          the result that dried
          egg preparations were
          frequently contaminated.

212. (b) *Enterobacter agglomerans*
          has been implicated in
          contamination of I.V.
          solutions.

213. (d) *Pseudomonas aeruginosa*
          is motile by means of
          a single polar flagellum.

214. (a) A positive indole test
          for *Escherichia coli*
          results from the break-
          down of tryptophan in
          the medium by the enzyme
          tryptophanase.

215. (c) *Vibrio parahemolyticus*
          requires at least 2
          per cent NaCl for
          growth.

216. (a) If the crystal violet-
          iodine complex is not
          formed in the gram
          stain the cells would
          only take up the count-
          erstain.

217. (d) Bacteria do not have
          lipopolysaccharides
          in their cell envelopes
          and *Mycoplasma* cause
          pneumonia among other

diseases.

218. (c) Beta hemolytic streptococci, *Staphylococcus
aureus* and *Corynebacterium diphtheriae* all pro-
duce exotoxins which are
responsible for the
disease states. *Bacillus
subtilis* is rarely asso-
ciated with disease.

219. (a) *C. diphtheriae* phage
provides genetic mater-
ial for toxin synthesis
by the bacterium.

220. (b) *Arizona* are malonate
positive, *Salmonella*
are malonate negative.

221. (d) *Bordetella* pertussis
is not normally car-
ried; its presence
in the nasopharynx
usually is associated
with disease.

222. (a) Drug addicts are frequent victims of hepa-
titis due to the hepa-
titis B antigen.

223. (b) Phase microscopy enables
the observation of liv-
ing organisms and con-
sequently their internal
structures.

224. (b) B.C.G. is a bovine strain
of *Mycobacterium tuberculosis* and is used as a
vaccine to confer immunity
to *M. tuberculosis* var.
hominis.

225. (c) Some fungi have two growth
forms which are tempera-
ture related.

226. (c) Two types of bacterial

viruses are known:
lytic or virulent and
temperate (lysogenic)
or avirulent. When
cells are infected
by lytic phage, a
large number of new
virions may be pro-
duced, resulting in
bursting of the host
cell. In temperate
phage infection, no
such replication
takes place and the
phage is simply passed
on to cells of the
next generation.

227. (d) *Herpesvirus hominis*
is a DNA virus; it
is not the cause of
smallpox and is
responsible for one
of the sexually trans-
mitted diseases.

228. (b) Use of bovine heart
tissue for detecting
antibodies to *Treponema
pallidum* is an example
of a nontreponemal
test and thus is not
specific for syphilis
and not the most sen-
sitive test.

229. (c) Quellung is the capsular swelling test
for pneumococci and
other encapsulated
bacteria.

230. (b) *Escherichieae* is the
tribe name and includes
two genera - *Escherichia*
and *Shigella*.

231. (a) Chemolithotrops are
bacteria that can
utilize inorganic com-
pounds such as elemen-

tal sulphur and nitrites for energy.

232. (d) V factor is a heat labile substance required by some species of *Haemophilus* and is coenzyme I, nicotinamide adenine dinucleotide.

233. (b) The presence of a capsule in *S. pneumoniae* is associated with virulence.

234. (d) Phosphates for bacterial cell use are best supplied as free inorganic phosphates.

235. (a) The cell walls of gram positive and gram negative bacteria both contain muramic acid.

236. (c) *Proteus* species possess the enzyme phenylalanine deaminase which breaks phenylalanine to phenylpyruvic acid.

237. (d) Cysteine, resazurin and thioglycollic acid may all be used in anaerobic fluid media but ascorbic acid is a preserving agent used in food.

238. (b) *Staphylococcus epidermidis* is coagulase negative whereas *Staph. aureus* is coagulase positive.

239. (b) Knowing the gram reaction, the presence of a spore and its shape and position in a bacterial cell can assist you in determining which

species of *Clostridium* you are dealing with.

240. (a) Mycobacteria belonging to the Group II scotochromogens produce a deep yellow to orange pigment when grown in the dark. Some of the group, *M. scrofulaceum*, *M. szulgai* and *M. xenopi* are potential human pathogens.

241. (d) A potential lactose fermenter may be identified by the ONPG test to detect the enzyme beta galactosidase.

242. (a) Conjugation is a mating process characterized by the temporary fusion of mating partners; it occurs particularly in unicellular organisms.

243. (b) Bacterial cell walls maintain the shape of a bacterium.

244. (b) Media for obligate anaerobes should be of the low oxidation-reduction type, as many of these organisms are sensitive to even trace amounts of oxygen.

245. (b) A positive Schick test indicates a lack of immunity to diphtheria. The test material is diluted diphtheria toxin; 0.1 ml is injected intradermally and a positive result is red-

dening and edema.

246. (a)   Detection and identifi-
            cation of an unknown
            antigen using a fluores-
            cent labelled known
            antibody is an example
            of direct immunofluores-
            cence.

247. (d)   The skin infection termed
            tinea versicolor is caused
            by the fungus *Pityrosporon*
            (Malassezia) *furfur* and in
            KOH preparations the skin
            scrapings contain the
            characteristic "spaghetti
            and meatballs" morphology.

248. (b)   The limit of the light
            microscope is usually
            0.2 micron. The electron
            microscope has allowed
            us to see ultrastructures
            within the bacterial cell.

249. (b)   Serological identifica-
            tion of the various
            Salmonella species is
            based on their O (somatic)
            and H (flagella) antigens.

250. (d)   Mycobacteria are all acid
            fast, but like other
            bacteria, the species
            differ in growth rate,
            pathogenicity for guinea
            pigs and humans as well
            as having varying bio-
            chemical reactions.

254. (e)   *Corynebacterium
            diphtheriae*

255. (d)   *Treponema pallidum*

(2)
256. (d)   *Staphylococcus aureus*

257. (a)   *Neisseria meningitidis*

258. (e)   *Staphylococcus epider-
            midis*

259. (b)   *Neisseria gonorrhoeae*

260. (c)   *Branhamella catarrhalis*

(3)
261. (e)   *Clostridium tetani*

262. (d)   *Bacteroides fragilis*

263. (a)   *Streptococcus pyogenes*

264. (b)   *Streptococcus faecalis*

265. (c)   *Clostridium perfringens*

(4)
266. (c)   *Yersinia enterocolitica*

267. (d)   *Borrelia vincentii*

268. (b)   *Trichophyton mentagro-
            phytes*

269. (e)   *Yersinia pestis*

270. (a)   *Epidermophyton flocco-
            sum*

SECTION B: HEADINGS

(1)
251. (b)   *Bordetella pertussis*

252. (c)   *Haemophilus influenzae*

253. (a)   *Mycobacterium tuberculo-
            sis*

SECTION C: TRUE OR FALSE

271. True

272. True

273. False   Steam at 121°C for
              15 minutes is most
              effective method.

274. False   Penicillin is effec-
             tive only against
             organisms with cell
             walls.

275. False   Gram positive bacteria
             have teichoic acid.

276. True

277. True

278. False   Most clinical speci-
             mens contain aerobes
             and anaerobes.

279. True

280. True

281. False   Viridans streptococci
             are most frequently
             isolated in cases of
             SBE.

282. True

283. False   The cold catalyst ab-
             sorbs water and gases
             and must be regenerated
             after each use.

284. True

285. False   *Clostridium tetani*
             has the "drumstick"
             appearance.

286. True

287. False   Some pathogenic fungi
             may take three weeks
             to grow on primary
             culture.

288. False   Scotch ® tape prepar-
             ations are useful for
             Enterobius vermicularis.

289. True

290. False   Streptolysin O
             is a product of
             Lancefield group
             A streptococci.

291. False   Some *Serratia* strains
             are non-pigmented.

292. False   *Listeria* is catalase
             positive.

293. True

294. False   Its pH range (8.3 -
             10.0) is useful
             only in urease
             test.

295. True

296. True

297. True

298. False   Exotoxins are pro-
             duced by intact
             cells.

299. False   The only time one
             may see spores in
             *Clostridium per-
             fringens* is in
             tissue, seldom in
             culture.

300. False   Many strains of
             *Staphylococcus
             aureus* are beta
             lactamase producers.

301. True

302. True

303. True

304. False   The dimple results
             from autolysis of
             cells in the center
             of the colony.

305. False Rarely do *Shigella* invade the blood stream.

306. True

307. False Pathogenicity is determined by presence of toxin in the Elek test.

308. False *Haemophilus influenzae* is usually pleomorphic and frequently coccobacillary.

309. True

310. False Infants have passive immunity from their mothers.

311. False Some bacterial spores require long boiling times.

312. True

313. False BCG is a vaccine containing live attenuated organisms.

314. False PEA inhibits the swarming of *Proteus* and the growth of most other enteric bacilli.

315. True

316. True

317. True

318. False *Shigella* are nonmotile and do not possess H antigens.

319. True

320. False Steam is more effective.

321. True

322. True

323. False The reaction on egg yolk agar (Nagler reaction) is due to lecithinase.

324. True

325. True

326. True

327. False A positive reaction is a pH of less than 4.5.

328. False *Neisseria* are bean-shaped diplococci.

329. True

330. False The solution is 10 per cent potassium hydroxide.

331. True

332. True

333. False *Plasmodium falciparum* shows multiple infections of erythrocytes.

334. False The acid resulting from carbohydrate fermentation is lactic.

335. True

336. True

337. False Vaccines have proven of little value in preventing staphylococcus

infections; prevention
is predominantly by
good hygiene and good
health.

338. True

339. False   *Brucella* does not cause
             pneumonia.

340. False   *Neisseria meningitidis*
             is sensitive to low
             temperatures and dry-
             ing.

341. False   Low temperature organ-
             isms are called psych-
             rophiles.

342. True

343. True

344. False   Anaerobes are the most
             numerous organisms in
             the gut, but *Bacter-
             oides fragilis* is only
             a small per cent.

345. True   Frequently a mixture
             of clostridia will be
             present - *perfringens*,
             novyi and *septicum*.

346. False   The most frequent
             isolate is *Haemophilus
             influenzae*.

347. True

348. False   *Clostridium botulinum*
             is being reported
             from infected wounds.

349. True

350. True

351. False   Streptolysin S is also
             active in production

of hemolysis.

352. True

353. False   The result is ac-
             quired artificial
             active immunity.

354. False   Schick positive
             persons are suscepti-
             ble to diphtheria and
             need immunization.

355. False   Amino acid fermentation
             is characteristic of
             the proteolytic clos-
             tridia; saccharolytic
             clostridia ferment
             sugars.

356. True

357. True

358. False   Inoculum concentra-
             tion is an important
             factor in K-B testing.

359. True

360. True

361. False   Antibiotic combinations
             may be synergistic, re-
             sulting in rapid kill-
             ing of the infecting
             organism.

362. False   It refers to the break
             up of light into its
             component parts giving
             a hazy image fringed
             with color.

363. True

364. False   Dermatophytes are
             identified by their
             characteristic mac-
             roconidia and/or

microconidia.

365. True

366. True

367. True All these organisms may be present either in the respiratory, genital or intestinal tracts.

368. False They belong to the group of antibiotics called aminoglycosides.

369. False Tryptophanase breaks down tryptophane to produce indole.

370. True

SECTION D: SPECIAL QUESTIONS

371. (c) A toxin producer - *Clostridium tetani* is not invasive.

    (f) Drumstick - the characteristic spore of *Clostridium tetani* is terminal and distends the cell.

    (i) Horse manure - spores of *Clostridium tetani* are commonly present in horse manure.

    (p) All of the above.

372. (b) Cholera - it is characterized by "rice water" diarrhea and rapid onset.

    (f) Shigellosis

    (k) *Salmonella* species -

many chickens carry *Salmonella* and raw eggs may be infected.

    (p) All of the above.

373. (c) Chicken salad sandwich.

    (e) *Staphylococcus aureus*.

    (l) Hands

374. (a) Laked blood (kanamycin and vancomycin) (anaerobic), blood agar (CO_2).

    (f) Viridans streptococci, *Bacteroides* species and *Fusobacterium*.

    (k) *Bacteroides melaninogenicus*.

    (n) Sputum

375. (b) *Neisseria meningitidis*.

    (e) Blood agar, chocolate agar.

    (l) Acid production from glucose and maltose.

SECTION E: QUESTIONS AND ANSWERS

376. Enteric fever

377. *Pseudomonas maltophilia*

378. *Bordetella pertussis*

379. Motility at room temperature.

380. Sucking discs

381. Hog

382. Capsules

383. Dark field microscopy of
      lesions.

384. Organism must carry phage
      to be toxigenic.

385. Invasiveness

386. Synergy

387. Subacute bacterial endocar-
      ditis.

388. Double zone, target hemo-
      lysis.

389. MacConkey agar

390. 10^5

391. *Enterobius vermicularis*

392. Lactobacilli

393. Blood

394. Boiling a suspension of
      the organism for 15 minutes.

395. *M. tuberculosis* is character-
      istically slow growing.

396. They produce erythrogenic
      toxin.

397. The capsule protects the
      pneumococcus from phago-
      cytosis.

398. No, the infection is due to
      production of enterotoxin
      before the food is eaten.

399. The cell walls have a high
      lipid content (up to 60 per
      cent).

400. No, shigellae are much less
      invasive than salmonellae.

401. Unlike *Haemophilus*, they
      do not require X and V
      factors for isolation.

402. Gram negative intracellular
      diplococci; in other samples
      this is less reliable.

403. Largely because of their
      morphologic resemblance
      to *Corynebacterium diph-
      theriae*.

404. *Actinomyces israelii*

405. *Clostridium perfringens*

406. Phagocytosis

407. *Entamoeba histolytica*

408. The organism has a high
      infectivity and requires
      enriched media contain-
      ing cysteine.

409. The presence of 3 - 10
      per cent carbon dioxide.

410. Many acid fast saprophytes
      are present in urines and
      gastric fluids.

411. *Bacillus anthracis*

412. Rheumatic fever and acute
      glomerular nephritis.

413. The infection is due to
      production and spread of
      a potent neurotoxin.

414. The enzyme betalactamase
      splits the beta lactam
      ring.

415. Carriers

416. Ribosomes

417. Guanine and cytosine, two
      of the base pairs of the
      DNA molecule.

418. *Salmonella*

419. Ethylhydrocupreine hydro-
      chloride.

420. *Mycoplasma* lack a cell
      wall.

421. Bacterial growth.

422. Niacin

423. Staphylokinase

424. Buffered glycerol saline.

425. Bile salts

HEMATOLOGY

J. BARRY ATKINSON
A.R.T.,F.I.M.L.S.
Chief Technologist
Hematology – Oncology
THE HOSPITAL FOR SICK CHILDREN
TORONTO, ONTARIO, CANADA

QUESTIONS

Select the phrase, sentence or symbol which completes the statement or answers the question. More than one answer may be correct in each case.

1. Which of the following hemoglobins is present in a normal
   adult?
   (a) C
   (b) D
   (c) A_2
   (d) S

2. The alkaline denaturation test
   measures:
   (a) hemoglobin A
   (b) hemoglobin A_2
   (c) hemoglobin S
   (d) hemoglobin F

3. *Plasmodium vivax* differs from
   Plasmodium falciparum by:
   (a) presence of a large ring
        form
   (b) enlargement of the red
        cell

   (c) presence of Schuffner's
        dots
   (d) all of the above

4. As a safety measure in
   chemical storage, water
   must always be added to
   stocks of:
   (a) thymol
   (b) phenol
   (c) trichloroacetic acid
   (d) picric acid

5. In a preparation that is
   positive for lupus erythematosus which of the following tests could be done
   to confirm the disease?
   (a) Incubate patient's
        buffy coat with
        normal serum
   (b) Incubate patient's
        buffy coat with
        normal plasma
   (c) Incubate normal
        buffy coat with
        patient's serum
   (d) None of the above

146

6. Sites for bone marrow aspiration may be:
   (a) iliac crest
   (b) sternum
   (c) lumbar vertebrae
   (d) tibia

7. In normal bone marrow there
   are:
   (a) many plasma cells
   (b) many pronormoblasts
   (c) a myelo-erythroid ratio
        of 3:1
   (d) approximately 10 mega-
        karyocytes per oil-
        immersion field

8. Which of the following statements is/are true about platelet counting methods?
   (a) E.D.T.A. (ethylene-
        diaminetetra acetic acid)
        in concentration greater
        than 2 mg/ml of blood
        gives a falsely increased
        platelet count
   (b) E.D.T.A. prevents plate-
        let clumping
   (c) The normal range is 150 -
        400 x 10^9/liter
   (d) All of the above

9. The ideal capillary blood
   collection site in a 6 week
   old child is:
   (a) thumb
   (b) earlobe
   (c) plantar surface of the
        heel
   (d) the back of the heel

10. An electronic impedence cell
    counter depends on:
    (a) the cell being less con-
         ductive than the isotonic
         diluent
    (b) the cell being more con-
         ductive than the isotonic
         diluent
    (c) the cell interrupting a
         light source as it passes

through a flow cell
(d) none of the above

11. Which of the following is
    a leukocyte inclusion body?
    (a) Heinz body
    (b) Maurer's dots
    (c) Dohle body
    (d) Pappenheimer body

12. In vitamin B_{12} deficiency
    anemia which of the follow-
    ing is a typical finding?
    (a) Hypersegmented neu-
         trophils
    (b) Thrombocytopenia
    (c) Oval macrocytes
    (d) None of the above

13. A blood sample preparation
    giving a positive reaction
    for Heinz bodies may indi-
    cate which of the following?
    (a) Unstable hemoglobins
    (b) Hereditary hemolytic
         anemia
    (c) Ingestion of aspirin
    (d) None of the above

14. In beta thalassemia major
    which of the following is
    usually increased?
    (a) Hemoglobin H
    (b) Hemoglobin F and A_2
    (c) Hemoglobin A_2
    (d) Hemoglobin A

15. A nanometer is which part
    of a meter?
    (a) 10^{-9}
    (b) 10^{-12}
    (c) 10^{-15}
    (d) 10^{-3}

16. "Shift to the left" refers
    to:
    (a) increase in the number
         of segments in a neu-
         trophil
    (b) increase in band and
         juvenile forms in the

granulocyte series
(c) decrease in band and
juvenile forms in the
granulocyte series
(d) (a) and (b) are correct

17. Basophilic stippling can be
differentiated from reticulocytes in the fact that:
(a) they both stain by any
Romanowsky stain
(b) basophilic stippling
is stained by any
Romanowsky stain and
reticulocytes by new
methylene blue
(c) basophilic stippling
is stained by brilliant
cresyl blue and reticu-
locytes are stained by
any Romanowsky stain
(d) both are stained with
methylene blue

18. Auer rods may be found in
which of the following?
(a) Proerythroblasts
(b) Lymphoblasts
(c) Myeloblasts
(d) Pelger-Huet anomaly

19. In chronic granulocytic leukemia which of the following is often seen?
(a) An increased basophil
count
(b) Decrease in leukocyte
alkaline phosphatase
activity
(c) Philadelphia chromosome
(d) Only (b) and (c) are
correct

20. Which of the following cells
give a positive staining reaction for nonspecific esterase?
(a) Myeloblast
(b) Lymphoblasts
(c) Monoblast

(d) Proerythroblast

21. The normal adult hemoglobin
contains which of the following?
(a) Two alpha and two
beta chains
(b) Two alpha and two
gamma chains
(c) Two alpha and two
delta chains
(d) Four beta chains

22. When doing an Ivy method
bleeding time the blood
pressure cuff is inflated
to:
(a) 10 mm. Hg
(b) 40 mm. Hg
(c) 60 mm. Hg
(d) 80 mm. Hg

23. Which of the following is
not a Romanowsky type dye?
(a) Wright's
(b) Leishman
(c) Methylene blue
(d) Jenner-Giemsa

24. Which of the following
would be most useful in
distinguishing hereditary
from acquired hemolytic
anemia?
(a) Bilirubin estimation
(b) Direct anti-globulin
test
(c) Osmotic fragility
(d) Reticulocyte count

25. Two standard deviations
from the mean in a normal
distribution curve would
include?
(a) 95 per cent of all
values
(b) 99 per cent of all
values
(c) 68 per cent of all
values

(d) 75 per cent of all
     values

26. A nanogram is which decimal
    part of a gram?
    (a) 10^{-3}
    (b) 10^{-6}
    (c) 10^{-9}
    (d) 10^{-12}

27. The leukocyte alkaline phos-
    phatase is helpful in dis-
    tinguishing:
    (a) leukemoid reactions
         from chronic myelogenous
         leukemia
    (b) chronic myelogenous leu-
         kemia from acute myelo-
         genous leukemia
    (c) chronic myelogenous leu-
         kemia from acute lympha-
         tic leukemia
    (d) acute myelogenous leu-
         kemia from acute lympha-
         tic leukemia

28. In erythroblastosis of the new-
    born caused by ABO incompata-
    bility there is typically a
    considerable:
    (a) anisocytosis
    (b) macrocytosis
    (c) spherocytosis
    (d) poikilocytosis

29. Which of the following is not
    associated with hemolytic
    anemias?
    (a) Decreased red cell sur-
         vival
    (b) Increase in reticulo-
         cytes
    (c) Decreased erythrocyte
         count
    (d) Increase in haptoglobins

30. Typically in which of the fol-
    lowing are hypersegmented neu-
    trophils found?
    (a) May-Hegglin anomaly
    (b) Pelger-Huet Neubauer

(c) Megaloblastic anemia
(d) Myeloproliferative
     diseases

31. The process of cell multi-
    plication occurs by:
    (a) amitosis
    (b) meiosis
    (c) mitosis
    (d) karyokinesis

32. In a normal adult body the
    iron content is:
    (a) 300 mgm - 500 mgm
    (b) 1 - 2 grams
    (c) 3 - 5 grams
    (d) 6 - 8 grams

33. The ruled area of the Fuchs-
    Rosenthal hemocytometer
    differs from the ruled area
    of the improved Neubauer
    hemocytometer in which of
    the following?
    (a) Area
    (b) Depth
    (c) Width
    (d) All of the above

34. Coefficient of variation
    refers to which of the
    following?
    (a) Plus or minus 1
         standard deviation
    (b) Plus or minus 2
         standard deviations
    (c) Error of the method
         in per cent
    (d) Reliability

35. Nuclear remnants in the
    erythrocyte are called?
    (a) Pappenheimer bodies
    (b) Dohle bodies
    (c) Reticulocytes
    (d) Howell-Jolly bodies

36. Chronic granulocytic leu-
    kemia is characterized by
    which of the following?
    (a) Increased total white

cell count
(b) White cell population
    shows a "left shift"
(c) Less than 10 per cent
    blasts
(d) Decreased leukocyte
    alkaline phosphatase

37. Hypochromic microcytic anemia
    is seen in all of the follow-
    ing *except:*
    (a) iron deficiency anemia
    (b) chronic G.I. bleeding
    (c) beta-thalassemia minor
    (d) multiple myeloma

38. Splenic functions in the nor-
    mal adult are thought to be:
    (a) red cell reservoir
    (b) red cell production
    (c) regulates release of
        cells from the bone
        marrow
    (d) removes nuclear frag-
        ments

39. In the maturation process of
    red blood cells the youngest
    cell is called?
    (a) Basophilic normoblast
    (b) Polychromatophilic
        normoblast
    (c) Promormoblast
    (d) Orthochromic normoblast

40. In normal reticulocytes when
    stained with new methylene
    blue demonstrates the follow-
    ing features:
    (a) basophilic stippling
    (b) inclusion bodies
    (c) reticulitis
    (d) network of granular
        filaments

41. If in the Westergren method
    for erythrocyte sedimentation
    the tube is not placed exactly
    in a vertical position the
    rate will be:
    (a) increased

(b) decreased
(c) nonaffected
(d) not affected unless
    it is more than 10°
    from the vertical

42. In the maturation process
    of the lymphocytes the
    youngest cell is called:
    (a) prolymphocyte
    (b) lymphoblast
    (c) large lymphocyte
    (d) plasmablast

43. The precursor cell of the
    reticulocyte is:
    (a) myeloblast
    (b) megakaryoblast
    (c) pronormoblast
    (d) plasmablast

44. Which of the following is
    not demonstrated by Wright's
    stain?
    (a) Pappenheimer bodies
    (b) Howell-Jolly bodies
    (c) Heinz bodies
    (d) Auer rods

45. Thrombocytopenia may occur in?
    (a) Von-Willebrand's disease
    (b) Megaloblastic anemia
    (c) Lupus erythematosus
    (d) Thalassemia

46. Hemophilia A is?
    (a) A sex-link recessive
        characteristic
    (b) An acquired disease
    (c) Thrombocytopenic
    (d) Has a prolonged
        prothrombin time

47. An abnormally prolonged
    activated partial throm-
    boplastin time may indicate:
    (a) circulating anticoag-
        ulent
    (b) afibrinogenemia
    (c) Factor VIII deficiency
    (d) none of the above

48. The conversion of fibrinogen
    to fibrin requires:
    (a) calcium chloride
    (b) normal plasma
    (c) thrombin
    (d) prothrombin

49. Aspirin ingestion has the
    following hemostatic effect:
    (a) no effect
    (b) prolongs the bleeding
         time
    (c) interferes with plate-
         let aggregation
    (d) prolongs the prothrom-
         bin time

50. Which of the following anti-
    coagulants neutralizes throm-
    bin?
    (a) Ammonium and potassium
         oxalate
    (b) Dipotassium E.D.T.A.
    (c) Heparin
    (d) Sodium citrate

51. A diluent for erythrocyte
    enumeration should have as
    one of its properties:
    (a) hypotonicity
    (b) high viscosity
    (c) high specific gravity
    (d) isotonicity

52. The total blood volume of a
    healthy adult is?
    (a) 70 ± 10 ml/kg of body
         weight
    (b) 70 ± 5 ml/kg of body
         weight
    (c) 60 ± 10 ml/kg of body
         weight
    (d) 45 ± 5 ml/kg of body
         weight

53. Utilizing the following data,
    Hgb. 12.9 gm/dl, RBC 4.1 x
    10^{12}/1 Hct. 0.39(1/1)
    what is the mean cell volume
    in femtoliters?
    (a) 89

    (b) 94
    (c) 108
    (d) 92

54. Utilizing the following data,
    Hgb. 8.0 g/dl, RBC 3.2 x
    10^{12}/1 Hct. 0.26(1/1)
    what is the mean cell hemo-
    globin in picograms (pg)?
    (a) 25
    (b) 23
    (c) 29
    (d) 31

55. Utilizing the following data,
    Hgb. 15 g/dl, Hct. 0.45(1/1)
    what is the M.C.H.C. in g/dl?
    (a) 30.5
    (b) 35.0
    (c) 33.3
    (d) 29.5

56. Heterophile antibodies are
    increased in?
    (a) Neutrophilia
    (b) Acute lymphoblastic
         leukemia
    (c) Infectious mononeu-
         cleosis
    (d) Polycythemia vera

57. Hemoglobin S and hemoglobin C
    are usually found in persons
    having the following ancestry?
    (a) Mediterranean
    (b) Oriental
    (c) American Indian
    (d) Negro

58. The Donath-Landsteiner anti-
    body test is positive when
    a blood sample shows hemo-
    lysis:
    (a) at 4°C
    (b) at 37°C
    (c) after cooling to 4°C
         and rewarming to 37°C
    (d) after cooling to 4°C
         and rewarming to 56°C

59. With a prolonged prothrombin

time of 17 seconds which of
the following possibilities
could you eliminate as the
probable cause?
(a) Ingestion of salicylates
(b) Liver disease
(c) Mild Factor VIII deficiency
(d) Vitamin K deficiency

60. The source of phospholipid
for the intrinsic pathway of
coagulation is:
(a) tissue thromboplastin
(b) thrombin
(c) serotonin
(d) platelet factor 3

61. A disease characterized by
growth of one or more tumor
masses in the bone marrow,
bone pain and abnormal plasma
proteins is most consistent
with:
(a) multiple myeloma
(b) Hodgkin's disease
(c) Histiocytosis
(d) Erythroleukemia

62. Sudan black B stains?
(a) Peroxidase granules
(b) Lipids
(c) D.N.A.
(d) R.N.A.

63. The Periodic acid-Schiff reaction stains:
(a) polysaccharides
(b) mucopolysaccharides
(c) glycoproteins
(d) mucoproteins

64. The peroxidase reaction
stains:
(a) myeloblasts
(b) lymphoblasts
(c) Auer rods
(d) lymphocytes

65. A positive acid phosphatase
reaction in a peripheral

blood film identifies:
(a) lymphoblastic leukemia
(b) T-cell acute lympho-
blastic leukemia
(c) chronic lymphocytic
leukemia
(d) erythroblastosis
fetalis

66. Platelets in Von Willebrand's
disease give an abnormal
aggregation result when reacted with:
(a) adenosine diphosphate
(b) epinephrine
(c) ristocetin
(d) collagen

67. Vitamin B_{12} is chiefly absorbed in:
(a) terminal ileum
(b) stomach
(c) colon
(d) duodenum

68. Which of the following
should be used in a good
routine quality program?
(a) Instrument calibration
(b) Control specimens
(c) Statistical analysis
(d) Correlation assess-
ment

69. A milligram expressed in
System International (S.I.)
units is which of the following?
(a) $x\ 10^{-1}$
(b) $x\ 10^{-6}$
(c) $x\ 10^{-12}$
(d) $x\ 10^{-3}$

70. A microliter expressed in
System International (S.I.)
units is which of the following?
(a) 10^{-3}
(b) 10^{-6}
(c) 10^{-12}
(d) 10^{-15}

71. A femtoliter expressed in
    System International (S.I.)
    units is which of the follow-
    ing?
    (a) 10^{-3}
    (b) 10^{-6}
    (c) 10^{-12}
    (d) 10^{-15}

72. To calculate the relative
    centrifugal force of the
    centrifuge which of the
    following is required?
    (a) Speed of rotation
    (b) Radius of the rotor
    (c) Number of centrifuge
         tube holders
    (d) Weight of the centri-
         fuge tube holders

73. In the Duke method for bleed-
    ing time which of the fol-
    lowing is the usual puncture
    site?
    (a) Forearm
    (b) Thumb
    (c) Heel
    (d) Earlobe

74. Which cell best fits the fol-
    lowing description? The nu-
    cleus is eccentrically placed,
    with a clear perinuclear halo
    and clumped nuclear chromatin:
    (a) intermediate megaloblast
    (b) monoblast
    (c) plasma cell
    (d) pronormoblast

75. In the Schilling test, the
    excretion of radioactive B_{12}
    is measured in:
    (a) urine
    (b) blood
    (c) gastric fluid
    (d) feces

76. The optimum stain for demon-
    strating malarial parasites
    is?
    (a) Pappenheim's stain

(b) Giemsa stain
(c) Wright's stain
(d) Leishman stain

77. Cabot's rings are seen in
    which of the following?
    (a) Non-nucleated erythro-
         cyte
    (b) Monoblast
    (c) Myeloblast
    (d) Promegaloblast

78. Macrocytic erythrocytes
    may be seen in all except:
    (a) after gastrectomy
    (b) pernicious anemia
    (c) sprue
    (d) thalassemia

79. Schumm's test is used to
    detect the presence of:
    (a) methemoglobin
    (b) methemalbumin
    (c) sulfhemoglobin
    (d) carboxyhemoglobin

80. Ham's test (acidified-
    serum) is used in the
    diagnosis of:
    (a) paroxysmal nocturnal
         hemoglobinuria
    (b) paroxysmal cold hemo-
         globinuria
    (c) pernicious anemia
    (d) DiGuglielmo's disease

81. Transferrin is which of the
    following?
    (a) Apoferritin
    (b) Alpha globulin
    (c) Ferric-beta$_1$ globulin
         complex
    (d) Gamma-globulin

82. In megaloblastic anemia the
    characteristic white cell
    changes are:
    (a) toxic granulation
    (b) hypersegmented neutro-
         phils
    (c) a "left shift"

(d) vaculated lymphocytes

83. To differentiate between homozygous and heterozygous sickle
cell anemia which of the following tests would be pertinent?
(a) Wet preparation using
sodium metabisulphite
(b) Blood smear examination
(c) Hemoglobin electrophoresis
(d) Alkali resistant hemoglobin determination

84. Which of the following terms
refers to sickle cells?
(a) Acanthocytes
(b) Schistocytes
(c) Elliptocytes
(d) Drepanocytes

85. The test used to detect the
presence of hemoglobin F in
a suspected fetal-maternal
bleed is called:
(a) alkali denaturation
test
(b) Kleihauer-Betke test
(c) Schumm's test
(d) Ham's test

86. The cause of idiopathic thrombocytopenic purpura (I.T.P.)
is:
(a) acute leukemia
(b) radiation
(c) drug toxicity
(d) unknown

87. Which of the following coagulation factors is *not* vitamin
K dependent?
(a) Factor VII
(b) Factor VIII
(c) Factor IX
(d) Factor X

88. Which of the following coagulation factors is a contact
factor?
(a) Prothrombin

(b) Prekallikrein
(c) Factor V
(d) Factor XIII

89. The Philadelphia chromosome is most commonly
seen in:
(a) acute myeloblastic
leukemia
(b) acute lymphoblastic
leukemia
(c) chronic lymphatic
leukemia
(d) chronic myelogenous
leukemia

90. The Sahli hemoglobin method
converts hemoglobin to:
(a) acid hematin
(b) cyanmethemoglobin
(c) carboxyhemoglobin
(d) oxyhemoglobin

91. In lead poisoning, punctate
basophilia is found in:
(a) neutrophils
(b) lymphocytes
(c) eosinophils
(d) erythrocytes

92. Which of the following stains
is used to demonstrate siderocytes?
(a) Perl's Prussian blue
reaction
(b) Brilliant cresyl blue
(c) Methyl violet
(d) Methyl green

93. Aplastic anemia may be caused
by which of the following?
(a) Chloramphenicol
(b) Radiation
(c) Benzene poisoning
(d) All of the above

94. To correct a total white cell
count for the number of nucleated erythrocytes one has
to:
(a) do both a red cell

count and a white cell
count
(b) use a special stain
(c) determine the number
of nucleated erythro-
cytes per 100 white
cells
(d) differentiate between
white cells and nucleated
erythrocytes in the hemo-
cytometer

95. The synonym for coagulation
Factor X is?
(a) Hageman factor
(b) Stuart-Prower factor
(c) Proconvertin
(d) Proaccelerin

96. The Roman numerical nomenclature for fibrin stabilizing factor is:
(a) II
(b) V
(c) VII
(d) XIII

97. The synonym for coagulation
Factor XI is?
(a) Plasma thromboplastin
antecedent
(b) Anti-hemophilic factor
(c) Hageman factor
(d) Christmas factor

98. Gaucher cells have:
(a) abundant pale staining
cytoplasm
(b) fibrillae in the cytoplasm
(c) usually do not have
nucleoli
(d) all of the above

99. Which of the following coagulation factors is present in
serum?
(a) Factor I
(b) Factor V
(c) Factor VII
(d) Factor VIII

100. Which of the following
coagulation factors is
not adsorbed by adsorbing
agents?
(a) Factor II
(b) Factor VII
(c) Factor VIII
(d) Factor IX

101. The normal range of white
cells in the adult is:
(a) $7.5 \pm 3.5 \times 10^9/l$
(b) $5.5 \pm 3.5 \times 10^9/l$
(c) $6.5 \pm 3.5 \times 10^9/l$
(d) $6.0 \pm 4.5 \times 10^9/l$

102. The normal range of mean
cell volume in the adult
is:
(a) 80 ± 8 fl
(b) 85 ± 8 fl
(c) 70 ± 10 fl
(d) 75 ± 10 fl

103. The normal range for hemoglobin in the adult male
is:
(a) 13.5 ± 2.5 g/dl
(b) 15.5 ± 2.5 g/dl
(c) 14.5 ± 1.5 g/dl
(d) 14.0 ± 2.5 g/dl

104. The normal range for hemoglobin in the adult female
is:
(a) 13.5 ± 2.5 g/dl
(b) 15.5 ± 2.5 g/dl
(c) 14.5 ± 1.5 g/dl
(d) 14.0 ± 2.5 g/dl

105. The normal range for plasma
fibrinogen in the adult is:
(a) 1.3 - 4.5 g/l
(b) 1.25 - 4.25 g/l
(c) 1.5 - 4.0 g/l
(d) 1.75 - 4.0 g/l

106. The range for serum iron in
a normal adult is:
(a) 13 - 32 µmol/l
(b) 10 - 45 µmol/l

(c)   17 - 50 μmol/l
(d)   20 - 35 μmol/l

107. The normal range for total
      iron binding capacity is
      2.5 - 4.0 mg/l. What is
      this value when expressed
      in μmol/l?
      (a)   45 - 70
      (b)   30 - 65
      (c)   50 - 85
      (d)   75 - 100

108. The normal range for the
      Westergren method for ESR
      in the normal adult male
      is:
      (a)   0 - 5 mm
      (b)   5 - 10 mm
      (c)   0 - 7 mm
      (d)   0 - 10 mm

109. The normal range for Wester-
      gren method for ESR in the
      normal adult female is:
      (a)   0 - 5 mm
      (b)   0 - 7 mm
      (c)   5 - 10 mm
      (d)   0 - 10 mm

110. The accuracy of a 20 μl blood
      pipet may be checked by:
      (a)   filling with water and
            then weighing the water
      (b)   filling with blood and
            then weighing the blood
      (c)   filling with mercury
            and then weighing the
            mercury
      (d)   filling with buffer
            and then weighing the
            buffer

111. The presence of hemosiderin
      in urine may be demonstrated
      by?
      (a)   Perl's Prussian blue
            reaction
      (b)   Sudan black B
      (c)   P.A.S. reaction
      (d)   L.A.P. reaction

112. Which of the following
      porphyrins is/are present
      in the normal adult?
      (a)   Protoporphyrin
      (b)   Uroporphyrin
      (c)   Corproporphyrin
      (d)   All of the above

113. Which of the following
      electrophoretic techniques
      is used in the demonstration
      and estimation of hemoglobin
      A_2?
      (a)   Starch gel at pH 8.6
      (b)   Starch block at pH
            8.9
      (c)   Agar gel at pH 5.9
      (d)   Cellulose acetate
            at pH 6.5

114. Hemoglobin S can be sepa-
      rated from hemoglobin D
      by which of the following
      methods?
      (a)   Agar gel pH 5.9
      (b)   Cellulose acetate
            pH 6.5
      (c)   Starch gel pH 8.6
      (d)   Starch block pH 7.0

115. In auto-immune hemolytic
      anemia the commonest type
      of warm autoantibody is?
      (a)   IgA
      (b)   IgM
      (c)   IgG
      (d)   None of the above

116. In auto-immune hemolytic
      anemia the commonest type
      of cold autoantibody is?
      (a)   IgA
      (b)   IgM
      (c)   IgG
      (d)   None of the above

117. Which of the following
      tests would be done for
      diagnosis of disseminated
      intravascular coagulation?
      (a)   P.T. and A.P.T.T.

(b) Thrombin time
(c) Platelet count and
     blood smear
(d) All of the above

118. In the microbiological assay
      for serum and red cell folate
      which of the following organ-
      isms is used?
      (a) *S. faecalis*
      (b) *L. casei*
      (c) *L. leichmanii*
      (d) *Euglena gracilis*

119. Which of the following terms
      refers to a normal red blood
      cell?
      (a) Drepanocyte
      (b) Discocyte
      (c) Codocyte
      (d) Echinocyte

120. Which of the following terms
      refers to a burr cell?
      (a) Drepanocyte
      (b) Discocyte
      (c) Codocyte
      (d) Echinocyte

121. Which of the following terms
      refers to a target cell?
      (a) Shizocyte
      (b) Acanthocyte
      (c) Codocyte
      (d) Stomatocyte

122. The chloroacetate esterase
      stain is useful in differen-
      tiating which of the follow-
      ing cells?
      (a) Myeloblast
      (b) Lymphocyte
      (c) Monocyte
      (d) Lymphoclast

123. The Ph chromosome may be found
      in:
      (a) chronic lymphatic leu-
           kemia
      (b) Down's syndrome
      (c) chronic myelogenous

           leukemia
      (d) acute monocytic leukemia

124. The precursor cell of plate-
      lets found in the bone mar-
      row is:
      (a) profibroblast
      (b) thrombocyte
      (c) megakaryocyte
      (d) myeloblast

125. The etiology of idiopathic
      thrombocytopenic purpura
      is:
      (a) bacterial infection
      (b) viral infection
      (c) radiation
      (d) unknown

126. In which of the following
      pathologies would reticu-
      locytosis not be a feature?
      (a) Hereditary sphero-
           cytosis
      (b) Auto-immune hemolytic
           anemia
      (c) Post-hemorrhagic
           anemia
      (d) Aplastic anemia

127. A vital stain is used for
      staining which of the fol-
      lowing?
      (a) Reticulocytes
      (b) Malarial parasites
      (c) Nucleoli in lympho-
           blasts
      (d) D.N.A.

128. The normal number of reti-
      culocytes in an adult does
      not commonly exceed:
      (a) 0.2 per cent
      (b) 2.0 per cent
      (c) 3.0 per cent
      (d) 5.0 per cent

129. Reticulocytosis is an in-
      dication of:
      (a) erythrocyte regen-
           eration

  (b) erythrocyte degenera-
       tion
  (c) erythrocyte aplasia
  (d) Vitamin B_{12} deficiency

130. Drabkin's reagent for the
     estimation of hemoglobin by
     the cyanmethemoglobin has
     which of the following?
     (a) Potassium ferrocyanide
     (b) Potassium ferricyanide
     (c) Potassium dichromate
     (d) Potassium cyanide

131. The cyanmethemoglobin method
     for hemoglobin measures all
     of the following except:
     (a) sulfhemoglobin
     (b) methemoglobin
     (c) carboxyhemoglobin
     (d) oxyhemoglobin

132. Which of the following hemo-
     globins is insoluble when
     reduced?
     (a) Hemoglobin C
     (b) Hemoglobin A
     (c) Hemoglobin S
     (d) Hemoglobin D

133. All of the following hemo-
     globins are denatured by
     alkaline solutions except:
     (a) hemoglobin A
     (b) hemoglobin C
     (c) hemoglobin S
     (d) hemoglobin F

134. Which of the following factors
     affects the result of the ery-
     throcyte sedimentation rate?
     (a) Anemia
     (b) Diameter of the tube
     (c) Sunlight
     (d) All of the above

135. Which of the following anti-
     coagulants cannot be used
     for routine coagulation and
     factor assay studies?
     (a) Sodium oxalate

  (b) Tri-sodium citrate
  (c) Di-potassium E.D.T.A.
  (d) All of the above

136. Which of the following
     anticoagulants is un-
     suitable for coagulation
     studies?
     (a) Tri-sodium citrate
     (b) Sodium oxalate
     (c) Sodium heparin
     (d) All of the above

137. In lupus erythematosus
     the nucleoprotein acquires
     chemotactic properties and
     and attracts phagocytes
     usually:
     (a) myelocytes
     (b) monocytes
     (c) segmented neutrophils
     (d) lymphocytes

138. Leukopenia is a decrease
     in the total white cells
     below:
     (a) $4.0 \times 10^9/1$
     (b) $5.0 \times 10^9/1$
     (c) $3.0 \times 10^9/1$
     (d) $2.0 \times 10^9/1$

139. Neutropenia in adults is
     a decrease in neutrophilic
     granulocytes below:
     (a) $4.0 \times 10^9/1$
     (b) $5.0 \times 10^9/1$
     (c) $3.0 \times 10^9/1$
     (d) $2.0 \times 10^9/1$

140. Neutropenia in children
     is a decrease in neutro-
     philic granulocytes below:
     (a) $2.0 \times 10^9/1$
     (b) $3.0 \times 10^9/1$
     (c) $1.5 \times 10^9/1$
     (d) $4.0 \times 10^9/1$

141. A marked lymphatic leuko-
     cytosis is usually seen
     in:
     (a) acute myeloblastic
          leukemia

(b) acute appendicitis
(c) pertussis
(d) none of the above

142. Cerebrospinal fluid that
     is yellow in color is
     termed:
     (a) icteric
     (b) xanthochromic
     (c) achromic
     (d) polychromatic

143. Which of the following
     solutions is a lysing
     agent?
     (a) E.D.T.A.
     (b) Saponin
     (c) Mercuric chloride
     (d) Mercuric oxide

144. Anemia due to acute blood
     loss is typically:
     (a) microcytic
     (b) hypochromic
     (c) normochromic
     (d) megaloblastic

145. The synonym for polycythemia
     is:
     (a) eosinophilia
     (b) thrombocytopenia
     (c) leukopenia
     (d) erythremia

146. In ABO erythroblastosis of
     the newborn there is con-
     siderable:
     (a) macrocytosis
     (b) spherocytosis
     (c) poikilocytosis
     (d) ovalocytosis

147. Sickle cell anemia is:
     (a) a deficiency anemia
     (b) a hemolytic anemia
     (c) a hemorrhagic anemia
     (d) an aplastic anemia

148. Elevated values for erythro-
     cyte count, hematocrit, hemo-

globin and leukocyte count
would indicate further in-
vestigations for:
     (a) polycythemia
     (b) leukemia
     (c) Hodgkin's disease
     (d) anemia

149. A vitamin B_6 deficiency
     blood smear may resemble
     that of:
     (a) megaloblastic anemia
     (b) iron deficiency
          anemia
     (c) auto-immune hemolytic
          anemia
     (d) pyruvate-kinase de-
          ficiency

150. Di Guglielmo's syndrome is
     a disorder involving the
     precursors of:
     (a) thrombocytes
     (b) granulocytes
     (c) lymphocytes
     (d) erythrocytes

151. A decreased erythrocyte
     osmotic fragility is
     usually associated with:
     (a) polycythemia vera
     (b) multiple myeloma
     (c) microcytic hypochromic
          anemia
     (d) hereditary sphero-
          cytosis

152. Punctate basophilia is:
     (a) seen only in basophils
     (b) a manifestation of
          lead poisoning
     (c) Prussian-blue posi-
          tive
     (d) not stained by Roman-
          owsky dyes

153. The hereditary disorder
     characterized by the in-
     complete segmentation of
     nuclei of granulocytes is:

(a) May-Hegglin anomaly
(b) Chediak-Higashi anomaly
(c) Alder-Reilly anomaly
(d) none of the above

154. Aleukemic leukemia differs from other leukemias in that it has:
(a) more mature cell forms
(b) a normal or less than normal peripheral blood leukocyte count
(c) a higher than normal peripheral blood leukocyte count
(d) no granules in the cells

155. Drug induced hemolysis in G-6-PD- deficient red blood cells is generally accompanied by the formation of?
(a) Pappenheimer bodies
(b) Dohle bodies
(c) Heinz bodies
(d) Hgb. H bodies

156. In a patient with post-splenectomy pyruvate-kinase deficiency the peripheral blood shows:
(a) reticulocytosis
(b) target cells
(c) siderocytes
(d) Howell-Jolly bodies

157. The oral anticoagulant Coumadin acts by:
(a) interference with the fibrinogen-fibrin reaction
(b) interference with liver synthesis of vitamin K dependent factors
(c) inducing hypocoagulability by the removal of fibrinogen
(d) none of the above

158. Which of the following HL-A antigens are predominantly characteristic of Caucasians?
(a) HL-A1
(b) HL-A8
(c) HL-A3 and HL-A7
(d) HL-A2

159. Which of the following factors affect the osmotic fragility test?
(a) Hydrogen ion concentration
(b) Temperature
(c) Venous blood
(d) Maximally aerated blood

160. The isopropanol test for unstable hemoglobin is unsuitable when:
(a) Hemoglobin A is present
(b) Hemoglobin H is present
(c) Hemoglobin F is present
(d) Hemoglobin Barts is present

161. Hemophilia A:
(a) results in a prolonged activated partial thromboplastin time
(b) is inherited as a sex-linked recessive
(c) shows variable expression in females
(d) all of the above

162. The bone marrow in chronic idiopathic thrombocytopenic purpura has an increase in:
(a) plasma cells
(b) promyelocytes
(c) megakaryocytes
(d) Gaucher's cells

163. Megaloblastic erythropoiesis may be due to a deficiency of:
(a) pyridoxine
(b) Vitamin B_{12}
(c) folic acid

(d) iron

164. A patient with an M.C.V. of
      122 fl, an M.C.H.C. of 35 per
      cent and a white cell count
      of 3.0 x 10^9/l and a platelet
      count of 95.0 x 10^9/l which
      of the following tests would
      contribute towards diagnosis?
      (a) Reticulocyte count
      (b) Platelet factor 3
      (c) Schilling test
      (d) Leukocyte alkaline
           phosphatase

165. Hemophilia A or B may be sus-
      pected in patients with a:
      (a) prolonged prothrombin
           time
      (b) prolonged partial throm-
           boplastin time and pro-
           longed prothrombin time
      (c) prolonged partial throm-
           boplastin time
      (d) low fibrinogen

166. The area of the smallest
      square in the Neubauer hemo-
      cytometer is:
      (a) 0.025 mm^2
      (b) 0.0025 mm^2
      (c) 0.00025 mm^2
      (d) 0.02 mm^2

167. What is the volume counted
      for platelets in the improved
      Neubauer hemocytometer ex-
      pressed in cmm?
      (a) 0.4 cmm
      (b) 0.02 cmm
      (c) 0.1 cmm
      (d) 0.2 cmm

168. The thymus is important in
      the development of:
      (a) B lymphocytes
      (b) T lymphocytes
      (c) basophils
      (d) eosinophils

169. Megaloblastic erythropoiesis

may be due to a deficiency
of:
      (a) Vitamin B_6
      (b) iron
      (c) pyridoxine
      (d) none of the above

170. In sickle cell anemia the
      abnormality in the hemo-
      globin molecule is located
      on which polypeptide chain?
      (a) Alpha
      (b) Beta
      (c) Gamma
      (d) Delta

171. The type of acute leukemia
      most commonly seen in chil-
      dren is:
      (a) acute monocytic
      (b) acute myeloblastic
      (c) acute myelomonocytic
      (d) acute lymphocytic

172. The type of acute leukemia
      most commonly seen in adults
      is:
      (a) acute monocytic
      (b) acute myeloblastic
      (c) acute myelomonocytic
      (d) acute lymphoblastic

173. Which of the following is
      not present in serum?
      (a) Alpha globulin
      (b) Beta globulin
      (c) Albumin
      (d) Fibrinogen

174. In which of the following
      would the "sugar-water"
      test be appropriate?
      (a) Hereditary spherocy-
           tosis
      (b) Erythroblastosis
           fetalis
      (c) Paroxysmal nocturnal
           hemoglobinuria
      (d) Paroxysmal cold hemo-
           globinuria

175. Perl's Prussian-blue reaction demonstrates:
     (a) ferric iron
     (b) ferrous iron
     (c) pyridoxine
     (d) Howell-Jolly bodies

176. A total nucleated cell count of $11.0 \times 10^9/l$ and having 100 nucleated RBC's/100 WBC's has a corrected white cell count of:
     (a) $11.0 \times 10^9/l$
     (b) $10.0 \times 10^9/l$
     (c) $9.0 \times 10^9/l$
     (d) $10.5 \times 10^9/l$

177. When handling a blood sample that is positive for Australia antigen:
     (a) the sample must be centrifuged in closed tubes
     (b) rubber gloves must be worn when handling the sample
     (c) report at once any mishaps with the sample to the Infection Control Committee
     (d) all of the above

178. If a blood sample is spilled on the work bench or floor area:
     (a) clean with a 1 per cent available chlorine solution
     (b) wash with water
     (c) wash with 70 per cent isopropanol
     (d) use a concentrated soap solution

179. Pipeting of a blood sample for hemoglobin determination is:
     (a) by mouth suction
     (b) by automatic pipet
     (c) manual suction device
     (d) all of the above

180. A pressurized water fire extinguisher must not be used on:
     (a) ignited xylol
     (b) ignited paper
     (c) burning lab coat
     (d) none of the above

181. A Gaussian curve shows:
     (a) standard deviation
     (b) coefficient of variation
     (c) the variance curve
     (d) curve of normal distribution

182. Acceptable limits of a value are:
     (a) within plus or minus 1 S.D.
     (b) not within plus or minus 1 S.D. but within plus or minus 2 S.D.
     (c) not within plus or minus 2 S.D. but within plus or minus 3 S.D.
     (d) all of the above

183. The molecular weight of hemoglobin is:
     (a) 55,000
     (b) 40,000
     (c) 65,000
     (d) 75,000

184. The number of amino acids present in the alpha chain of hemoglobin is:
     (a) 98
     (b) 115
     (c) 231
     (d) 141

185. Hemoglobin S may be associated with:
     (a) thalassemia
     (b) hemoglobin C
     (c) hemoglobin D
     (d) all of the above

186. Which of the following give

a similar peripheral blood picture?
  (a) Hereditary spherocytosis and pyridoxine deficiency
  (b) Beta-thalassemia minor and iron deficiency anemia
  (c) Vitamin B_{12} deficiency and vitamin B_6 deficiency
  (d) All of the above

187. Using starch gel electrophoresis at pH 8.6, hemoglobin E has the same mobility as:
  (a) hemoglobin S
  (b) hemoglobin F
  (c) hemoglobin A_2
  (d) hemoglobin H

188. Hemolytic crisis may be precipitated in glucose 6-phosphate dehydrogenase deficient individuals by?
  (a) Chloramphenicol
  (b) Primaquine
  (c) Fava beans
  (d) All of the above

189. Drug induced hemolysis in G-6-PD cells is generally accompanied by the formation of?
  (a) Howell-Jolly bodies
  (b) Heinz bodies
  (c) Dohle bodies
  (d) Reilly bodies

190. Acanthocytes are typically present in the peripheral blood smear of an individual with:
  (a) congenital absence of beta-lipoprotein
  (b) hereditary elliptocytosis
  (c) sickle cell disease
  (d) hepatocellular disease

191. Pyruvate kinase deficiency is:
  (a) inherited as an autosomal dominant
  (b) inherited as an autosomal recessive
  (c) is not an inherited disease
  (d) has a marked autohemolysis

192. An example of a congenital platelet defect is in:
  (a) Glanzmann's disease
  (b) uremia
  (c) scurvy
  (d) glycogen storage disease

193. Which of the following show little physiological variation?
  (a) Hemoglobin
  (b) Red blood cells
  (c) White blood cells
  (d) Thrombocytes

194. Stomatocytes in blood smears:
  (a) may be present as an artefact
  (b) may be associated with a mild or severe anemia
  (c) are present as an inherited disorder
  (d) all of the above

195. A 1 per cent solution of potassium ferricyanide is used in:
  (a) staining siderocytes
  (b) the Prussian-blue reaction
  (c) staining hemosiderin
  (d) none of the above

196. The substance which will hasten the sickling of erythrocytes is:

(a)   sodium sulphate
(b)   sodium metabisulphite
(c)   sodium citrate
(d)   sodium oxalate

197. The highest hemoglobin value
      is found in:
      (a)   children aged one year
      (b)   newborn infants
      (c)   adolescents
      (d)   adult males

198. The macrocytes typically
      seen in vitamin B_{12} defi-
      ciency are:
      (a)   hypochromic
      (b)   pyknotic
      (c)   oval in shape
      (d)   tear drop shape

199. Microspherocytes in the
      peripheral blood indicate:
      (a)   thalassemia
      (b)   siderosis
      (c)   hemolytic process
      (d)   megaloblastosis

200. Contain pipets:
      (a)   deliver a specific
            volume
      (b)   must be rinsed out
            after they have drained
      (c)   contain a specific
            volume
      (d)   none of the above

201. Using the following data
      Hemoglobin 8.2 g/dl
      Red cell count 2.78 x 10^{12}/l
      Hematocrit 0.26 L/L
      Which of the following is the
      correct value for mean cell
      volume in femtoliters (fl)?
      (a)   90
      (b)   92
      (c)   94
      (d)   96

202. Using the following data
      Hemoglobin 8.2 g/dl
      Red cell count 2.78 x 10^{12}/l

Hematocrit 0.26 L/L
Which of the following
is the correct value for
mean cell hemoglobin in
picograms (pg)?
      (a)   29.5
      (b)   31.5
      (c)   33.5
      (d)   35.5

203. Using the following data
      Hemoglobin 8.2 g/dl
      Red cell count 2.78 x 10^{12}/l
      Hematocrit 0.26 L/L
      Which of the following is the
      correct value for mean cell
      hemoglobin concentration in
      grams per deciliter?
      (a)   27.5 g/dl
      (b)   27.9 g/dl
      (c)   29.9 g/dl
      (d)   31.9 g/dl

204. If in the central square
      millimeter of an improved
      Neubauer counting chamber
      there are 200 platelets,
      what is the total number
      present per liter of blood?
      (a)   200 X 10^9/L
      (b)   400 X 10^9/L
      (c)   350 X 10^9/L
      (d)   375 X 10^9/L

205. The protein that binds
      with free hemoglobin is?
      (a)   Ferritin
      (b)   Haptoglobin
      (c)   Pyridoxine
      (d)   None of the above

206. When staining with Giemsa
      stain, the blood smear
      must first be:
      (a)   immersed in concen-
            trated stain
      (b)   immersed in stain
            prediluted with buffer
      (c)   fixed with methanol
      (d)   none of the above

207. A congenital non-spherocytic hemolytic anemia characterized by sensitivity to primaquine and the formation of Heinz bodies is:
    (a) pyruvate kinase deficiency
    (b) glucose-6-phosphate dehydrogenase deficiency
    (c) auto-immune hemolytic anemia
    (d) microangiopathic anemia

208. The characteristic abnormality in the 21 - 22 chromosome group may occur in:
    (a) acute myeloblastic leukemia
    (b) chronic lymphatic leukemia
    (c) chronic myelogenous leukemia
    (d) acute myelo-monocytic leukemia

209. Salicylate ingestion gives:
    (a) prolonged prothrombin time
    (b) prolonged bleeding time
    (c) prolonged activated partial thromboplastin time
    (d) all of the above

210. Protamine sulphate neutralizes the effect of:
    (a) heparin
    (b) coumadin
    (c) anti-thrombin III
    (d) platelet Factor III

211. The bone marrow in vitamin B_{12} or folic acid deficiency typically shows:
    (a) megaloblastic changes
    (b) erythroid hyperplasia
    (c) giant metamyelocytes
    (d) nuclear-cytoplasmic asynchrony

212. The specific stain for demon-

stration of Howell-Jolly bodies is?
    (a) Wright's stain
    (b) May-Grunwald Giemsa
    (c) Feulgen reaction
    (d) Jenner-Giemsa

213. Field's stain demonstrates which of the following?
    (a) Heinz bodies
    (b) Malarial parasites
    (c) Chromosomes
    (d) White cell inclusion bodies

214. A blood sample for coagulation studies is contaminated with tissue fluid; the effect will be:
    (a) no effect
    (b) good only for prothrombin time
    (c) unsuitable
    (d) good for factor assays only

215. Erythrocytes that form in chains in a peripheral blood film is/are:
    (a) agglutination
    (b) rouleaux formation
    (c) agglutinates
    (d) none of the above

216. Aspirin ingestion has the following effect:
    (a) decreases fibrinogen levels
    (b) prolongs A.P.T.T.
    (c) interferes with platelet aggregation
    (d) has no effect

217. Adsorbed plasma can be prepared by using:
    (a) aluminum sulphate
    (b) barium hydroxide
    (c) barium sulphate
    (d) aluminum hydroxide

218. The prothrombin time is

useful in the diagnosis of
which of the following?
(a) Vitamin K deficiency
(b) Liver damage
(c) Reduced Factor VII
     concentration
(d) All of the above

219. The platelet count would be
      useful as an aid for diagnosis
      of:
(a) acute leukemias
(b) cirrhosis of the liver
(c) polycythemia vera
(d) chronic myelogenous
     leukemia

220. Precision is:
(a) to be within ± 1SD of
     the correct value
(b) to be within ± 2SD of
     the correct value
(c) to be within ± 3SD of
     the correct value
(d) reproducibility

221. Thrombasthenia refers to:
(a) an increased platelet
     count
(b) a decreased platelet
     count
(c) a defect in the coagu-
     lation mechanism of
     the blood
(d) functional defect in
     blood platelets

222. In a citrated blood sample,
      with a hematocrit of 55 per
      cent or more, that is re-
      quired for coagulation
      studies, should the volume
      of anticoagulant used:
(a) remain the same as
     usual
(b) be reduced in volume
(c) be increased in volume
(d) be collected into oxa-
     late

223. Inspection of quality con-

trol data may reveal:
(a) a loss of precision
(b) the method is out of
     control
(c) the method is in con-
     trol
(d) all of the above

224. Which of the following is
      not a factor in hereditary
      spherocytosis?
(a) There is an increase
     in osmotic fragility
(b) Erythrocytes are
     thicker than normal
(c) Erythrocytes are
     larger than normal
(d) Is transmitted by
     either parent

225. The prothrombin time and
      partial thromboplastin time
      are increased in all except:
(a) thrombocytopenia
(b) afibrinogenemia
(c) Factor VII deficiency
(d) Factor X deficiency

226. A post-splenectomy blood
      smear would show all of
      the following, except?
(a) Howell-Jolly bodies
(b) Thrombocytopenia
(c) Thrombocytosis
(d) Target cells

227. A prolonged bleeding time
      would indicate further
      testing is necessary.
      Which of the following would
      be most useful?
(a) Thromboplastin gener-
     ation test
(b) Platelet count
(c) Thrombin time
(d) Prothrombin time

228. Which of the following would
      be a suitable diluent for
      manual platelet counts?
(a) 0.85 per cent sodium

chloride
- (b) 1 per cent ammonium oxalate
- (c) Eagle's solution (modified)
- (d) 1 per cent formalin in 3 per cent sodium citrate

229. The normal range for the absolute lymphocyte count in a normal adult expressed in SI units is:
- (a) $0.5 - 2.5 \times 10^9/l$
- (b) $0.3 - 0.8 \times 10^9/l$
- (c) $1.5 - 3.5 \times 10^9/l$
- (d) $2.5 - 6.5 \times 10^9/l$

230. A relative neutrophilic granulocytosis is when the granulocyte percentage is elevated above:
- (a) 90 per cent
- (b) 80 per cent
- (c) 75 per cent
- (d) 70 per cent

231. Leukopenia is when the total white cell count is depressed below:
- (a) $5.0 \times 10^9/l$
- (b) $4.0 \times 10^9/l$
- (c) $3.5 \times 10^9/l$
- (d) $3.0 \times 10^9/l$

232. When rouleaux formation is identified in a blood smear which of the following tests would be appropriate for further studies?
- (a) E.S.R.
- (b) Total protein
- (c) Protein electrophoresis
- (d) None of the above

233. The normal absolute eosinophil count in the adult is:
- (a) $0.04 - 0.4 \times 10^9/l$
- (b) $0 - 1.0 \times 10^9/l$
- (c) $0.5 - 1.5 \times 10^9/l$
- (d) $1.0 - 1.7 \times 10^9/l$

234. What is the unit of electrical resistance?
- (a) Volt
- (b) Ampere
- (c) Ohm
- (d) Watt

235. Which of the following syringe needles has the smallest bore?
- (a) 18 gauge
- (b) 19 gauge
- (c) 20 gauge
- (d) 21 gauge

236. The process of cell division in the myeloid series is called:
- (a) meiosis
- (b) oogenesis
- (c) mitosis
- (d) regeneration

237. An Angstrom unit is:
- (a) a unit for measurement of wavelength of light
- (b) 1/10,000 of an inch
- (c) 1/1,000 of an millimeter
- (d) none of the above

238. A chemical is said to be deliquescent when:
- (a) it is only soluble in alcohol
- (b) it absorbs water from the air
- (c) it is in powder form
- (d) none of the above

239. The end product of the Embden-Meyerhoff pathway of glucose metabolism is:
- (a) pyruvate
- (b) lactate
- (c) G-6-PD
- (d) 2-P-glycerate

240. Chromosomes with a terminal centromere are termed:

(a) acrocentric
(b) metacentric
(c) centric
(d) none of the above

241. Which of the following are sex-linked disorders?
(a) Hemophilia A
(b) G-6-PD deficiency
(c) Christmas disease
(d) All of the above

242. Erythrocyte production is directly related to the hormone erythropoietin which is mainly produced in:
(a) pituitary
(b) spleen
(c) kidney
(d) thymus

243. Pancytopenia refers to:
(a) hypoplasia of the bone marrow
(b) leukemoid reaction
(c) decrease in platelets
(d) decrease in all formed blood elements

244. The center square millimeter of an improved Neubauer hemacytometer is subdivided into:
(a) 400 squares
(b) 320 squares
(c) 500 squares
(d) 425 squares

245. A rod-shaped body in the cytoplasm of blasts that is peroxidase positive is?
(a) Barr body
(b) Auer body
(c) Howell-Jolly body
(d) Pappenheimer body

246. The following description is of which cell? Usually large but can vary widely in size. Irregular cytoplasmic margin with blunt pseudopods. Cytoplasm very basophilic and quite often more intense at the edge of the cytoplasmic margin. Nucleus shows irregularly distributed chromatin:
(a) plasma cell
(b) large lymphocyte
(c) monocyte
(d) atypical lymphocyte

247. Neutropenia is present in:
(a) megaloblastic anemia
(b) acute hemorrhage
(c) acute hemolysis
(d) all of the above

248. Lymphocytosis is present in:
(a) lymphatic leukemia
(b) acute viral infection
(c) infectious hepatitis
(d) none of the above

249. A femtoliter is which part of a liter?
(a) 10^{-3}
(b) 10^{-9}
(c) 10^{-12}
(d) 10^{-15}

250. In the adult, extra medullary hematopoiesis is usually in the:
(a) kidney
(b) sternum
(c) spleen
(d) iliac crest

SECTION B: HEADINGS

For each numbered word or phrase, select one heading that is most closely related to it.

(1) (a) Lymphoblast
     (b) Myeloblast
     (c) Myelocyte
     (d) Giant metamyelocyte

251. May show Auer rods.
     ANSWER: _____

252. Is present in pernicious
     anemia.
     ANSWER: _____

253. May contain P.A.S. positive
     material.
     ANSWER: _____

254. Are present in large numbers
     in chronic leukemia.
     ANSWER: _____

(2) (a) Maurer's dots
     (b) Punctate basophilia
     (c) Schuffner's dots
     (d) Dohle bodies
     (e) Pappenheimer bodies
     (f) Heinz bodies

255. Is Prussian-blue positive.
     ANSWER: _____

256. Is present in P. falciparum.
     ANSWER: _____

257. May be present in neutrophils.
     ANSWER: _____

258. Is present in P. vivax.
     ANSWER: _____

259. Is present in lead poisoning.
     ANSWER: _____

260. Is present in glucose-6-
     phosphate dehydrogenase
     deficiency.
     ANSWER: _____

(3) (a) Hemophilia A
     (b) Von-Willebrand's disease
     (c) Christmas disease
     (d) Factor XII
     (e) Factor X

261. Platelets do not aggregate
     with ristocetin.
     ANSWER: _____

262. Is present in aged serum.
     ANSWER: _____

263. Is not present in adsorbed
     plasma.
     ANSWER: _____

264. Is Factor IX deficient.
     ANSWER: _____

265. Is Factor VIII deficient.
     ANSWER: _____

(4) (a) Hemoglobin A
     (b) Hemoglobin F
     (c) Hemoglobin S
     (d) Hemoglobin A_2
     (e) Hemoglobin D

266. Has 2 alpha and 2 gamma
     chains.
     ANSWER: _____

267. Has 2 alpha and 2 beta
     chains.
     ANSWER: _____

268. Migrates with Hgb. S on
     cellulose acetate at pH
     8.6.
     ANSWER: _____

269. Is increased in beta thal-
     assemia minor.
     ANSWER: _____

270. Glutamic acid is replaced
     by valine.
     ANSWER: _____

SECTION C: TRUE OR FALSE

*Mark the following statements
either TRUE (T) or FALSE (F).*

271. Pyruvate kinase deficiency
     is a congenital non-spherocytic
     hemolytic anemia characterized
     by a sensitivity to primaquine

and the formation of Heinz bodies.

272. Plasmin is a proteolytic enzyme that can break down fibrin and fibrinogen.

273. Protamine sulphate neutralizes the effect of heparin.

274. Aspirin ingestion interferes with platelet aggregation.

275. In aleukemic leukemia there is a leukopenia.

276. The Philadelphia chromosome is present in acute lymphoblastic leukemia.

277. The thrombin time is abnormal in afibrinogenemia.

278. Factor V is preserved when a blood sample is mixed with sodium oxalate.

279. Fibrinogen is present in blood at the highest concentration of any of the clotting factors.

280. Blood contaminated with tissue fluid will have no effect on the coagulation times using capillary methods.

281. Ethylenediaminetetraacetic acid is the anticoagulant of choice for routine hematological work.

282. E.D.T.A. in excess of 2 mg/ml of blood may result in a decrease in packed cell volume.

283. The improved Neubauer hemacytometer is 0.1 mm deep.

284. The Fuchs-Rosenthal hemacytometer is 0.1 mm deep.

285. Drabkin's reagent contains potassium cyanide and potassium ferricyanide.

286. Drepanocytes are never present in the peripheral blood.

287. Dohle bodies may be found in the cytoplasm of neutrophils.

288. May-Hegglin anomaly characteristically has Dohle bodies and giant platelets.

289. Auer rods are present in the cytoplasm of lymphoblasts.

290. Erythrocyte osmotic fragility is decreased in liver disease.

291. Tear-drop shaped erythrocytes are frequently seen in myelofibrosis and are indicative of extramedullary hematopoiesis.

292. One per cent ammonium oxalate may be used as a diluent for manual platelet counts.

293. A "shift to the left" is a common consequence of severe sepsis.

294. Hypersegmented neutrophils are characteristic of vitamin B_6 deficiency.

295. Most of the iron destined for hemoglobin biosynthesis is taken into the cell at the pronormoblast stage.

296. A Fuchs-Rosenthal hemacytometer is used for manual

eosinophil counts.

297. Howell-Jolly bodies are Feulgen positive.

298. Schuffner's dots are seen in *Plasmodium falciparum*.

299. Paroxysmal nocturnal hemoglobinuria is an acquired red cell defect.

300. Iron deficiency anemia presents with a microcytic-hypochromic blood smear.

301. *Diphyllobothrium latum* infestation causes an iron deficiency anemia.

302. The alkali denaturation test measures hemoglobin F.

303. Reticulocytes can be stained supravitally.

304. The osmotic fragility is decreased in thalassemia.

305. Basophilia may be seen in chronic myelogenous leukemia.

306. The leukocyte alkaline phosphatase stain helps in differentiating leukemoid reactions from leukemia.

307. Chronic lymphatic leukemia occurs mainly in children.

308. Auer rods are diagnostic in chronic myelogenous leukemia.

309. Sternberg-Reed cells are found in the lymph node in Hodgkin's disease.

310. The periodic acid-Schiff reaction demonstrates glycogen in white blood cells.

311. The Giemsa stain is not suitable to use in hot climates.

312. In a normal bone marrow the myelo-erythroid ratio is 3:1.

313. The nonspecific esterase in monoblasts can still be demonstrated after sodium fluoride exposure.

314. Hemoglobin A_2 is increased in beta thalassemia minor.

315. Hemoglobin D can be separated from hemoglobin S by agar-gel electrophoresis at pH 5.9.

316. The Donath-Landsteiner antibody is present in paroxysmal cold hemoglobinuria.

317. Inheritance of Factor X is autosomal recessive.

318. Siderocytic granules are Prussian-blue positive.

319. Malarial parasites are demonstrated by Giemsa stain.

320. Hemophilia A is Factor VIII deficient.

321. The S.I. unit for expression of mean cell volume is cu. microns.

322. Electrical resistance is measured in amperes.

323. The first stage in cell mitosis is called the prophase.

324. The APTT is increased in afibrinogenemia.

325. Erythropoietin is mainly produced in the spleen.

326. Sickle cell disease is a beta chain abnormality.

327. Normal adult hemoglobin has 2 alpha and 2 delta chains.

328. Oval macrocytes are associated with pyridoxine deficiency.

329. Factor VII is vitamin K dependent.

330. Factor VIII has a half life of 12 hours.

331. Factor V is the most labile of the coagulation factors.

332. Heinz bodies are best demonstrated by a Romanowsky stain.

333. Platelets from a case of Von Willebrand's disease do not aggregate with epinephine.

334. The erythrocyte sedimentation rate is not increased in polycythemia vera.

335. The di-sodium salt of E.D.T.A. has greater solubility.

336. Infected erythrocytes of *P. vivax* may contain Maurer's dots.

337. Numerous nucleated red cells are present in the peripheral blood in hemolytic disease of the newborn.

338. In an A.B.O. incompatability of the newborn there are many spherocytes present in the peripheral blood.

339. The resolving power of a

microscope is its ability to correct spherical abberation.

340. A soda-acid fire extinguisher is suitable for paper fires.

341. The Ortho ELT-8 cell counter detects cells by using a laser beam.

342. The thymus is important in the development of B-lymphocytes.

343. The Coulter 'S' cell counter uses an optical cell detection system.

344. The "millimicron" is being replaced by the S.I. unit "nanometer" and it is 10^{-12} of a meter.

345. Hb. F. and Hb. A_2 are increased in beta thalassemia major.

346. A decreased erythrocyte life span would be indicative of hemolytic anemia.

347. There would be a prolonged one-stage prothrombin time in severe liver disease.

348. The Pelger-Huet anomaly is seen in monocytes.

349. Heinz bodies are associated with G-6-PD deficiency.

350. The clot retraction test may be used as an indicator of platelet function.

351. Increased numbers of atypical lymphocytes occur in infectious mononucleosis.

352. Target cells are a prominent

feature in hemoglobin C
disease.

353. Myeloblasts may contain
Dohle bodies.

354. In thrombocytopenic purpura
the platelet count is normal
but platelet function is
impaired.

355. Red cell energy is derived
from glucose metabolism.

356. The plasma cell is not normally
found in the peripheral blood.

357. Megaloblastic erythropoiesis
may be due to a deficiency
of folic acid.

358. Reticulocytosis is an indica-
tion of erythrocyte regeneration.

359. The bleeding time is a screening test for platelet numbers
and function.

360. The thrombin time is a screening test for circulating anticoagulants.

361. The activated partial thromboplastin time is prolonged
when there is a factor deficiency in the extrinsic
system.

362. Serum does not contain fibrinogen.

363. Adsorbed plasma contains
Factor XII.

364. Aged serum contains Factor
VII.

365. In a leukemoid reaction there
is a high alkaline phosphatase
activity.

366. The enzyme peroxidase is
contained within the granules
of cells in the myeloid
series.

367. A cerebrospinal fluid that
is xanthochromic is yellow
in color.

368. The xanthochromia of C.S.F.
is due to hemoglobin breakdown products.

369. A increased lymphocyte count
in the C.S.F. may be due to
T.B. meningitis.

370. The L.E. factor is present
in serum.

SECTION D: MISSING WORDS

*Fill in the blanks with a word
or phrase to complete the statement.*

371. Aged serum is deficient in
_____.(name one only)

372. Adsorbed plasma is deficient
in _____.(name one
only)

373. The Schilling test is usual
in the diagnosis of _____.

374. Aggregation of erythrocytes
in chains is called _____.

375. A measure of the variable
about the mean is called
_____.

376. The depth of a Fuchs-Rosenthal
hemacytometer is _____.

377. Myeloblasts may contain _____.

378. Dohle bodies may be present in _____.

379. Heinz bodies may be present in _____.

380. Reticulocytes appear in a Wright stained smear as _____.

381. The depth of an improved Neubauer hemacytometer is _____.

382. The normal lymphocyte count in cerebrospinal fluid is _____.

383. A decrease in granulocytes is called _____.

384. The substance stimulating erythrocyte production is _____.

385. Hematopoiesis that takes place in the liver and spleen is _____.

386. The presence of free hemoglobin in the plasma is _____.

387. Nuclear remnants that consist of D.N.A. and are in the erythrocyte are _____.

388. Erythrocytes that are primaquine sensitive are _____.

389. A mononuclear leukocyte capable of synthesizing antibodies is _____.

390. 10^{-12} gram is called a _____.

391. 10^{-15} liters is called a _____.

392. The erythrocyte inclusions seen in sideroblastic anemias are _____.

393. The best anticoagulant for routine coagulation studies is _____.

394. The coagulation factor that is very labile in sodium oxalate is _____.

395. Glycogen is stained in leukocytes with _____.

396. Hemosiderin is stained by _____.

397. Favism is seen in _____.

398. The action of heparin is neutralized by _____.

399. The osmotic fragility is increased in _____.

400. Fish tapeworm may cause a _____.

401. Chronic alcoholism may give a _____.

402. The largest normal cell in a normal bone marrow is _____.

403. Target cells are characteristic of _____.

404. A non-sickling hemoglobin that migrates with hemoglobin S is _____.

405. The bone marrow myeloid-erythroid ratio is _____.

406. Agranulocytosis includes which cells _____.

407. The Philadelphia chromosome occurs in _____.

408. The characteristic cell in the peripheral blood in multiple myeloma is _____.

409. The ideal anticoagulant for routine hematology testing is _____.

410. A predominance of lymphocytes is normally present in _____.

411. Lymphocytosis occurs in _____.(name one only)

412. Heterophile antibodies are present in _____.

413. Heterophile antibodies are absorbed by _____.

414. Aspirin ingestion affects the function of _____.

415. Aspirin ingestion will prolong the _____.

416. The normal adult platelet count in S.I. units is _____.

417. A functional defect of blood platelets is called _____.

418. Beta thalassemia minor is characterized by an increase in _____.

419. One per cent ammonium oxalate is used as a diluent for _____.

420. Reticulocytes can be stained with brilliant cresyl blue and _____.

SECTION E: SPECIAL QUESTIONS

421. A 49 year old male admitted to hospital with malaise. A routine hematology screen revealed.

Hgb. 9.7 g/dl
RBC 3.1 x 10^{12}/l
WBC 170 x 10^9/l
Platelets 34 x 10^9/l

White cell differential

Neutrophils	33%
Bands	7%
Metamyelocytes	9%
Myelocytes	21%
Promyelocytes	3%
Blasts	1%
Eosinophils	2%
Basophils	10%
Lymphocytes	4%
Monocytes	10%

The erythrocytes showed microcytes and hypochromasia.

(a) What is a possible diagnosis?

(b) Give two confirmatory tests with their expected results.

422. A 5 year old boy of Mediterranean descent was admitted to
hospital for tonsillectomy. A pre-operative hematology
screen revealed.

Hgb. 10.0 g/dl   White cell differential
RBC 5.85 x 10^{12}/l   Neutrophils   50%
WBC 5.3 x 10^9/l   Eosinophils   3%
MCV 59 fl   Basophils   1%
Platelets 170 x 10^9/l   Lymphocytes   44%
                                  Monocytes   2%

The erythrocytes show a hypochromic-microcytic picture.

(a) What is the probable diagnosis?

(b) Name one confirmatory test with expected values.

423. Fill in the spaces of the following chart.

(+ denotes present)   (0 denotes absent)

DISTRIBUTION OF COAGULATION FACTORS

	I	II	V	VII	VIII	IX	X	XI	XII
Fresh Normal Plasma	+	+	+	+	+	+	+	+	+
Stored Plasma	+		+			+		+	+
Adsorbed Plasma	+	0				0		+	
Aged Serum		0				+	+		+

424. Fill in the missing factors in this simplified cascade chart of
the coagulation mechanism.

/continued...

COAGULATION MECHANISM

Intrinsic System

contact with foreign surface; platelets (PF3)

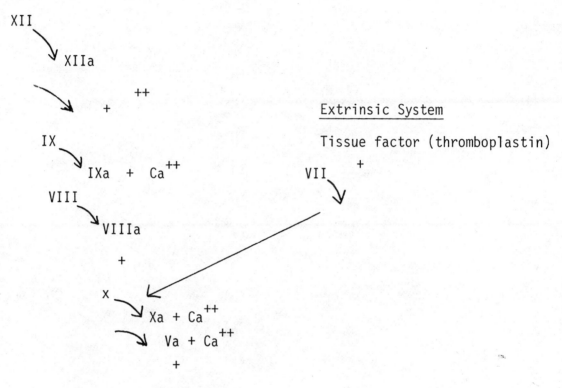

XII

XIIa

+ $^{++}$

Extrinsic System

Tissue factor (thromboplastin)

IX

IXa + Ca^{++} VII   +

VIII

VIIIa

+

X

Xa + Ca^{++}

Va + Ca^{++}

+

Phospholipid

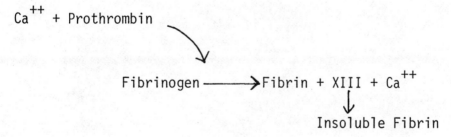

Ca^{++} + Prothrombin

Fibrinogen ———→ Fibrin + XIII + Ca^{++}

Insoluble Fibrin

425.   Give the numerical values of the following metric prefixes.

THE METRIC SYSTEM PREFIXES

		Value
tera	(T)	
giga	(G)	
mega	(M)	
kilo	(K)	
hecto	(H)	
deca	(da)	
deci	(d)	
centi	(c)	
milli	(m)	
micro	(u)	
nano	(n)	
pico	(p)	
femto	(f)	
atto	(a)	

ANSWERS

SECTION A: MULTIPLE CHOICE

1. (c) A_2 is the only normal adult hemoglobin, all the others are beta chain variants.

2. (d) A blood hemolysate is prepared by treating 1 volume of anticoagulated washed packed red cells with 2 volumes of distilled water. The red cells are lysed and hemoglobin is released into solution. If this resulting hemolysate is treated with dilute sodium hydroxide the hemolysate will remain red in color. If either hemoglobin A, hemoglobin A_2 or hemoglobin S is present the hemolysate will turn green (denaturation). This principle of denaturation is the basis for a quantitative method for hemoglobin F.

3. (d) A large ring form, en-largement of the red cell and Schuffner's dots are all present in *Plasmodium vivax*.

4. (d) Picric acid in its dry state is unstable and has explosive properties so it must always be kept moist with water.

5. (c) The lupus erythematosus phenomenon is present in serum. If neutrophils from a normal donor are incubated with the serum from a lupus erythematosus patient, lupus erythematosus (L.E.) cells will form in the normal neutrophils.

6. (a) The iliac crest, sternum,
   (b) lumbar vertebrae and tibia
   (c) are all potential sites
   (d) for bone marrow aspiration. The preferred sites are the sternum in adults and

179

the iliac crest in chil-
dren.

7. (c) Plasma cells, pronormoblasts and megakaryocytes
are present in normal bone
marrow but not in large
numbers.

8. (d) The normal range for platelets is 150 - 400 x 10^9/
liter. Ethylenediamine
tetra acetic acid is the
ideal anticoagulant for
platelet counting because
it prevents clumping of
platelets. If it is used
in concentrations of >2
mg/ml of blood it causes
swelling and rupture of
the platelets with a sub-
sequent false high plate-
let count.

9. (c) The ideal capillary blood
collection site in a 6
week old infant is the
plantar surface of the
heel. The heel bone is
usually well below the
skin surface in these
areas to be protected
from damage by the
puncturing lancet. Never-
theless, the puncture
should not be more than
2.5 mm in depth. The
thumbs and earlobes are
generally too small for
a satisfactory blood col-
lection and at the back
of the heel there is the
danger of puncturing the
heel bone.

10. (a) The electronic impedence
counter depends on the
cell being less conduc-
tive than the isotonic
diluent. If an electric
current is passed between

two electrodes through
a good conductor (normal
saline) and a cell in-
terrupts this electric
current, then it is de-
tected by the cell coun-
ter because it is a poor
conductor of electricity
and it causes a change
in resistance between
the two electrodes.

11. (c) A Dohle body is present
in neutrophils in chronic
infections and the May-
Hegglin anomaly.
Heinz bodies, Maurer's
dots and Pappenheimer
bodies are all red cell
inclusions.

12. (a) Hypersegmented neutrophils,
    (b) thrombocytopenia and oval
    (c) macrocytes are all typical
findings in vitamin B_{12}
deficiency.

13. (a) The ingestion of aspirin
    (b) is known to affect plate-
let function and not
cause the formation of
Heinz bodies.

14. (b) Hemoglobin H is present
in alpha thalassemia
and hemoglobin A_2 is
increased in beta thal-
assemia minor.

15. (a) A nanometer is 10^{-9}
meters.

16. (b) An increase in the
number of segments in
a neutrophil is termed
"shift to the right."
An increase in band
and juvenile forms in
the granulocyte series
is termed "shift to
the left."

17. (b) Basophilic stippling is
        stained by any Romanowsky
        stain and reticulocytes
        are stained supravitally
        using new methylene blue
        or brilliant cresyl blue.

18. (c) Auer rods may be present
        in myeloblasts.
        Proerythroblasts and
        lymphoblasts do not show
        Auer rods.
        Pelger-Huet anomaly is
        a congenital defect in
        the neutrophils.

19. (a) An increased basophil
    (b) count, decrease in
    (c) leukocyte alkaline phos-
        phatase activity and the
        Philadelphia chromosome
        are usually seen in chronic
        granulocytic leukemia.

20. (a) Both myeloblasts and mono-
    (c) blasts give a positive
        staining reaction for
        nonspecific esterase.
        Differentiation between
        myeloblasts and mono-
        blasts may be made by
        treating them with sodium
        fluoride. After sodium
        fluoride treatment, mye-
        loblasts give a positive
        staining reaction and
        monoblasts give a negative
        staining reaction for non-
        specific esterase.

21. (a) Two alpha and two beta
        chains are present in
        hemoglobin A. Two alpha
        and two gamma chains are
        present in hemoglobin F.
        Two alpha and two delta
        chains are present in
        hemoglobin A_2. Four beta
        chains are present in
        hemoglobin H.

22. (b) In the Ivy method for
        bleeding time, the
        blood pressure cuff is
        inflated to 40 mm of
        mercury.

23. (c) Wright's stain, Leish-
        man stain and Jenner-
        Giemsa stain are all
        Romanowsky stains;
        methylene blue is not.

24. (b) The direct anti-globulin
        test will distinguish
        hereditary from acquired
        hemolytic anemia.
        The bilirubin estimation
        measures red cell des-
        truction.
        The reticulocyte count
        indicates the rate of
        red cell regeneration.
        The osmotic fragility
        measures the fragility
        of red cells in vary-
        ing hypotonic strengths
        of sodium chloride.

25. (a) Two standard deviations
        from the mean in a nor-
        mal distribution curve
        would include 95 per
        cent of all values.

26. (c) A nanogram is 10^{-9}
        gram.

27. (a) The leukocyte alkaline
        phosphatase is high in
        leukemoid reactions
        and low in chronic mye-
        logenous leukemia.

28. (c) The most prominent
        feature in a blood
        smear of erythroblas-
        tosis of the newborn
        caused by ABO incom-
        patability would be a
        marked spherocytosis.

29. (d) In hemolytic anemias haptoglobin binds with free hemoglobin; there-fore, the haptoglobin level would decrease below normal.

30. (c) Neutrophils with hyper-segmented nuclei are found in vitamin B_{12} and folate deficiencies. The diagnosis can be confirmed by finding giant metamyelocytes in the bone marrow, as well as megaloblasts.

31. (c) Mitosis has four stages of cell division, pro-phase, metaphase, ana-phase, telophase.

32. (c) There are between 3 and 5 gm of iron present in the human body, represent-ing approximately only 0.006 - 0.007 per cent of total body weight.

33. (d) The Fuchs-Rosenthal hemacytometer measures 4 mm x 4 mm and is 0.2 mm deep compared to the improved Neubauer which is 3 mm x 3 mm x 0.1 mm deep.

34. (c) The formula for calcula-tion of the coefficient of variation is
$$\frac{\text{standard deviation}}{\text{mean}} \times 100$$

35. (d) Nuclear remnants in the erythrocyte are called Howell-Jolly bodies and are regularly seen in post-splenectomy blood smears.

36. (a) All are typical findings

(b) in chronic granulo-
(c) cytic leukemia.
(d)

37. (d) Hypochromic microcy-tic anemia is seen in iron deficiency anemia, chronic G.I. bleeding and beta-thalassemia minor. Multiple mye-loma usually shows a moderate normocytic anemia.

38. (c) The spleen removes
(d) aging cells and imper-fect cells from the circulation and regu-lates release of young cells from the bone marrow.

39. (c) The sequence of ery-throcyte maturation is Pronormoblast (proerythroblast or rubriblast) Basophilic normoblast (early erythroblast or prorubricyte) Polychromatophilic normoblast (late ery-throblast or rubricyte) Orthochromic normoblast (normoblast or metaru-bricyte) Polychromatophilic ery-throcyte (reticulocyte) Mature erythrocyte.

40. (d) Reticulocytes contain remnants of the ribo-somes and ribonucleic acids from their nucl-eated precursors which appear as granular fil-aments when supravi-tally stained.

41. (a) If the ESR tube is not in an exact vertical

position, the second
phase of erythrocyte
sedimentation will be
increased.

42. (b) The maturation sequence
of the lymphocyte series
is:
lymphoblast
prolymphocyte
large lymphocyte
intermediate lymphocyte
small lymphocyte

43. (c) The pronormoblast is the
youngest cell in the
erythrocyte maturation
process.

44. (c) Heinz bodies are stained
with 0.5 g per cent methyl
violet in 0.9 per cent
NaCl and they stain an
intense purple. Auer
rods, Howell-Jolly bodies
and Pappenheimer bodies
are stained by Wright's
stain.

45. (b) Megaloblastic anemia
(c) and lupus erythematosus
may present with a throm-
bocytopenia. Von
Willebrand's disease and
the thalassemia syndromes
have normal platelet
counts.

46. (a) Hemophilia A is a sex-
linked recessive charac-
teristic.

47. (a) An abnormally prolonged
(b) activated partial throm-
(c) boplastin time may indicate the presence of a
circulating anticoagu-
lant, afibrinogenemia
or Factor VIII deficiency.

48. (c) Thrombin converts fibri-

nogen to fibrin in the
presence of calcium ions.

49. (b) Aspirin ingestion pro-
(c) longs the bleeding time
and interferes with
platelet aggregation.
The aspirin effect can
last from 4 - 7 days
after ingestion.

50. (c) Heparin is thought to
have the power of neu-
tralizing thrombin in
the presence of a co-
factor located in the
albumin fraction of
plasma.

51. (d) A diluent for erythrocyte enumeration must
be isotonic to main-
tain the integrity of
the cell.

52. (a) The total blood volume
in a healthy adult is
70 ± 10 ml/kg of body
weight. The blood
volume is the same
for male and female
but there are differ-
ences in red cell
volume.

53. (b) The formula for calculation of MCV =
$\dfrac{\text{Hematocrit}}{\text{RBC in millions}}$ x 1000

MCV is expressed as
femtoliters (fl).

54. (a) The formula for calculation of M.C.H. =
$\dfrac{\text{Hb. in grams/liter}}{\text{RBC counts/liter}}$

e.g. Hgb = 15.0 g/dl
RBC = $5.0 \times 10^{12}/1$
= $\dfrac{150}{5 \times 10^{12}}$ = $\dfrac{3}{10^{11}}$ = 30 picograms
(pg)

55. (c) The formula for calculation of MCHC is

$$\frac{Hgb\ g/dl}{Hct\ (1/1)} = MCHC\ g/dl$$

56. (c) Infectious mononucleosis, also known as "glandular fever," typically gives a WBC count of 10.0 x $10^9/1$ - 20.0 x $10^9/1$ with Downey cells in large numbers. Heterophil agglutinins (absorbed by beef erythrocyte antigen, but not completely by guinea pig antigen, which absorbs Forssman antibodies) appears from the first week of the disease. The highest titer usually occurs during the second to third week. The positive heterophil (Paul-Bunnell) test in typical clinical hematologic cases is diagnostic from 1:56 to 1:224 titer as minimum levels.

57. (d) Homogygous hemoglobin S anemia occurs in one in 600 American Negroes while homoxygous hemoglobin C anemia occurs in one out of 6000.

58. (c) The highest temperature at which D-L antibodies are usually adsorbed to red cells is about 18°C. Little or no lysis can be expected unless the cell-serum suspension is cooled below this temperature. Chilling in crushed ice results in maximum adsorption of the antibody and leads to fixation of complement which brings about lysis

when the cell suspension is subsequently warmed to 37°C.

59. (c) Factor VIII deficiency will give a normal prothrombin time and a prolonged activated partial thromboplastin time.

60. (d) Activated Factor XII activates Factor XI to form a contact product. The contact product in the presence of calcium, platelets, phospholipid, Factor IX and Factor VIII activates Factor X.

61. (a) In multiple myeloma the blood smear shows a slight to moderate normochromic-normocytic anemia, becoming progressively more severe where there is an associated uremic or hemolytic pattern. Blood films take a greyish blue underlying color presumably because of an associated dysproteinemia. The leukocyte count varies from slightly decreased to slightly increased levels occasionally with myelocytes, metamyelocytes, eosinophils and foci of plasma cells.

62. (b) Sudan black B is used to stain the granules of leukocytes, many of which appear to contain phospholipids. There is a close parallel between sudanophilia and a positive peroxidase reaction.

63. (a) The P.A.S. reaction de-
    (b) pends on the liberation
    (c) of carbohydrate radicals
    (d) from combination with
        protein and their oxida-
        tion to aldehydes by the
        Schiff reagent. In blood
        cells a positive reaction
        usually denotes the pres-
        ence of glycogen. This
        can be confirmed by de-
        monstrating that the
        positive reaction disap-
        pears when the blood
        film is treated with
        diastase before it is
        stained.

64. (a) Myeloperoxidase is a
    (c) lysomol enzyme localized
        in the azurophilic gran-
        ules of neutrophils and
        monocytes. Peroxidase
        activity can also be
        demonstrated in basophils
        and eosinophils. Devel-
        oping granulocytes give
        a positive peroxidase
        reaction but the earliest
        myeloblasts are usually
        negative. Auer rods in
        leukemic blasts are near-
        ly always positive. The
        main practical value of
        the reaction is in the
        distinction between mye-
        loblastic and lympho-
        blastic leukemias.

65. (b) Acute lymphoblastic
        leukemia and chronic
        lymphocytic leukemia
        give a typically nega-
        tive or very weak acid
        phosphatase reaction.
        T-cell acute lympho-
        blastic leukemia is
        moderately to strongly
        positive.

66. (c) In most cases of
        classic Von Willebrand's
        disease there is a total
        lack of platelet aggre-
        gation when low concen-
        trations (1 mg/ml) of
        ristocetin are added to
        platelet-rich plasma.

67. (a) In order for vitamin B_{12}
        to be absorbed from the
        diet (extrinsic factor),
        it must combine with a
        mucoid substance (in-
        trinsic factor) secreted
        by the mucosal cells of
        the gastric fundus.
        Intrinsic factor is a
        thermolabile glyco-
        protein that binds
        strongly with ingested
        vitamin B_{12}, facilitating
        its absorption by ileal
        mucosal cell receptors.

68. (a) Instrument calibration
    (b) should be done at in-
    (c) tervals, some daily,
    (d) some weekly. Control
        specimens should be
        checked daily by re-
        testing samples from
        a previous batch and
        checking with reference
        preparations.
        Statistical analysis
        should be done daily
        and should include mean
        and standard deviation.
        Frequency distribution
        pattern, cusum on daily
        means and cusum on ref-
        erence preparations.
        Correlation assessment
        is done at all times
        using a cumulative
        report form.

69. (b) A milligram expressed

in System International
(S.I.) units is 10^{-6}
gram.

70. (b) A microliter expressed
in System International
(S.I.) units is 10^{-6}
liter.

71. (d) A femtoliter expressed
in System International
(S.I.) units is 10^{-15}
liters.

72. (a) Relative centrifugal
     (b) force is calculated
with the following
formula:

RCF - 0.0000118 x r x N^2,
where r = radius (c.m.)
and N = speed of rotation
(rpm).

73. (d) The Duke method for bleeding time is not the method
of choice but may be used
when the patient is a
small infant. The punc-
ture site is the earlobe.

74. (c) A plasma cell (plasmocyte)
is egg shaped; narrower
on one end than the other.
The nucleus is ovoid,
eccentrically placed,
usually in the small end
of the cell. Chromatin
is purplish, extremely
coarse and clumped with
distinct sparse para-
chromatin. The nucleus-
cytoplasm ratio is ap-
proximately 1:2. The
cytoplasm is deep blue
with a pale perinuclear
halo near one side of
the nucleus.

75. (a) In the Schilling test at
the same time as 1.0
microgram of radioactive
B_{12} is given by mouth,
1000 micrograms of non-
radioactive cyanocobal-
amin are given intra-
muscularly. Urine is
collected over a 24-
hour period. The radio-
activity of the urine
and a standard are
measured.
Percentage excreted =
total CPM in 24

$$\frac{\text{hours urine}}{\text{CPM in standard}} \times 100$$

Normal values $>$10 per
cent excreted in the
first 24 hours.
B_{12} deficient patient
$<$5 per cent excreted
in the first 24 hours.

76. (b) Although malarial parasites can be demonstra-
ted using other Romanowsky
dyes, Giemsa is one of
choice.

77. (a) Cabot's rings are seen
in non-nucleated erythro-
cytes and are red or
reddish purple, loop
shaped or form figures
of eight. These struc-
tures most likely indi-
cate regenerative acti-
vity and are seen in
Romanowsky stained blood
smears.

78. (d) Macrocytic erythrocytes
may be seen in the peri-
pheral blood after gas-
trectomy, in pernicious
anemia and sprue.
Thalassemia typically
presents as a hypochromic-
microcytic anemia.

79. (b) Schumm's test demonstrates the presence of methem-albumin and it is found in the plasma when hapto-globins are absent in hemolytic anemia when the lysis is predominant-ly intra-vascular.

80. (a) Paroxysmal nocturnal hemo-globinuria (PNH) is an acquired disorder in which the patient's ery-throcytes are abnormally sensitive to lysis by normal constituents of plasma. In its classic form PNH is characterized by nocturnal hemoglobin-uria, jaundice and hemo-siderinuria.

81. (c) Ferric iron combines with $beta_1$ globulin to form a ferric compound termed transferrin, siderophilin or iron binding protein.

82. (b) In megaloblastic anemia the peripheral blood shows hypersegmented neutrophils and bone marrow smears would show giant metamyelocytes.

83. (c) In heterozygous sickle cell anemia, electro-phoresis would show the presence of hemoglobin A and hemoglobin S Homozygous sickle cell disease would not have any hemoglobin A, only hemoglobin S.

84. (d) Sickle cells are also called drepanocytes.

85. (b) The identification of cells containing Hgb-F depends on the fact that they resist acid elution to a greater extent than do normal cells. After stain-ing, the cells contain-ing Hgb-F appear as isolated darkly stained cells amongst a back-ground of pale stained ghost cells.

86. (d) The word idiopathic means of unknown origin.

87. (b) Vitamin K dependent factors include Pro-thrombin, Factors VII, IX, X and protein C.

88. (b) The contact factors include Factors XI and XII, prekallikrein and high molecular weight kininogen.

89. (d) In chronic myelo-genous leukemia (C.M.L.) a characteristic feature is deletion of one arm, of one of the small acrocentric chro-mosomes; the result is an abnormally small chromosome now referred to as the Philadelphia (Ph[1]) chromosome.

90. (a) Hemoglobin is converted to acid-hematin by addition of N/10 HCl in the Sahli method for hemoglobin deter-mination.

91. (d) "Classical" punctate basophilia is found as a variant of diffuse basophilia, in many blood diseases, as well

as in infections and in-
toxications such as lead
poisoning.

92. (a) Siderocytes contain granules of hemosiderin and
give a positive Prussian
blue reaction. When
these granules are stain-
ed by Wright's stain they
are referred to as
"Pappenheimer bodies."

93. (d) Chloramphenicol, radiation
and benzene poisoning are
all causative agents of
aplastic anemia.

94. (c) To correct a total white
cell count for the number
of nucleated erythrocytes,
the number of nucleated
erythrocytes per 100 WBC's
must be determined. Cor-
rection is made by the
following formula:

$$\frac{\text{Total Nucleated Count}}{100\ \text{WBC} + \dfrac{\text{NUCRBC}}{100\ \text{WBC}}} \times 100$$

95. (b) Coagulation Factor X is
also called Stuart-Prower
factor.

96. (d) The fibrin stabilizing
factor is Factor XIII.

97. (a) The synonym for coagulation Factor XI is plasma
thromboplastin antecedent.

98. (d) Gaucher cells have abundant pale staining cyto-
plasm, fibrillae in the
cytoplasm and usually
do not have nucleoli.

99. (c) Factors present in serum
include VII, IX, X, XI,

XII; Factor XIII
is present in a re-
duced amount.

100. (c) Factors adsorbed by
adsorbing agents in-
clude II, VII, IX
and X.

101. (a) The normal range for
white blood cells in
the normal adult is
7.5 ± 3.5 x 10^9/liter.

102. (b) The normal range of
mean cell volume in
the adult is 85 ±
8 femtoliters (fl).

103. (b) The normal range for
hemoglobin in the
adult male is 15.5 ±
2.5 g/deciliter.

104. (d) The normal range for
hemoglobin in the
adult female is 14.0 ±
2.5 g/deciliter.

105. (c) The normal range for
plasma fibrinogen in
the adult is 1.5 -
4.0 g/l.

106. (a) The normal range for
serum iron in the
adult is 0.7 - 1.8
mg/l and this is
equivalent to 13-32
umol/l.

107. (a) The normal range for
total iron binding
capacity is 2.5 -
4.0 mg/l and this is
equivalent to 45 -
70 umol/l.

108. (a) The normal range for
the Westergren sedi-
mentation rate in the

adult male is 0 - 5 mm/hr.

109. (b) The normal range for the
Westergren sedimentation
rate in the adult female
is 0 - 7 mm/hr.

110. (c) A 20 μl blood pipet should
be filled to the gradua-
tion line with mercury.
The mercury is expelled
into a suitable container
and weighed, 20 μl of
mercury weighs 272 mg.
Mercury is used because
it will not wet the
glass surface of the
pipet so all of it is
expelled for weighing.

111. (a) Hemosiderin in urine
can be demonstrated
with Perl's Prussian
blue reaction. Deposits
of iron stain a blue-
black color.

112. (d) Protoporphyrin is a
precursor of heme in
hemoglobin and myoglobin
and a precursor of cyto-
chromes and catalse.
Uroporphyrin and copro-
porphyrin are precursors
of protoporphyrin.

113. (b) Hemoglobin A_2 is demonstrated in starch block
with barbitone buffer
at pH 8.9.

114. (a) Hemoglobin S and hemoglobin D migrate to the
same position as cellulose
acetate at pH 8.6.
These two hemoglobins
migrate to separate posi-
tions when run on agar
gel at pH 5.9.

115. (c) IgG is the commonest
type of warm auto-
antibody present in
auto-immune hemolytic
anemia. Rarely are
warm autoantibodies
of either IgM or IgA
present.

116. (b) In vivo IgM antibody
causes chronic intra-
vascular hemolysis,
the intensity of which
is characteristically
influenced by the
ambient temperature.

117. (d) In intravascular
coagulation the P.T.
and A.P.T.T. are
prolonged due to con-
sumption of coagula-
tion factors. The
thrombin time is pro-
longed from fibrinogen
deficiency and the
presence of fibrin
split products. Throm-
bocytopenia is present
and the blood smear
may show evidence of
microangiopathic hemo-
lytic anemia.

118. (b) The folate activity
of serum is due mainly
to the presence of a
folic acid co-enzyme,
5-methyl-tetrahydrofolic
acid. Because this
compound is microbio-
logically active for
L. casei and not *S.
faecalis*, the former
organism is used for the
assay of naturally occur-
ring folates in serum
and red cells.

119. (b) The normal red blood

cell is also referred to as a discocyte. The word originates from the Greek *diskos* disk or platter and *kytos* hollow vessel.

120. (d) A burr cell is also referred to as an echinocyte and comes from the Greek *echinos* spiny, prickly and *kytos* hollow vessel.

121. (c) A target cell is also referred to as a codocyte.

122. (a) Mature and immature granulocytes including late myeloblasts have a positive reaction for chloroacetate esterase. Little or no activity is found in cells of the monocytic or lymphocytic series.

123. (c) The Philadelphia (Ph^1) chromosome is present in chronic myelogenous leukemia. The characteristic feature is deletion of one of the small acrocentric chromosomes; the result is an abnormally small chromosome now referred to as the Philadelphia chromosome (Ph^1).

124. (c) The precursor cell of the platelet is the megakaryocyte found in the bone marrow. The megakaryocyte measures approximately 100 microns. This stage of development in the platelet system is the last which still constitutes a com-

plete cell. It is formed from the promegakaryocyte after it has lost the power of karyokinesis.

125. (d) Idiopathic means from unknown origins.

126. (d) In aplastic anemia there may be reduction of all formed elements in the peripheral blood. Hereditary spherocytosis and auto-immune hemolytic anemia would both show reticulocytosis because of the ongoing hemolytic process. Post-hemorrhagic anemia would also show reticulocytosis due to erythrocyte regeneration.

127. (a) Reticulocytes are stained with toxin free dyes in unfixed preparations using either new methylene blue or billiant cresyl blue.

128. (b) The normal range for reticulocytes in the adult is 0.2 - 2.0 per cent.

129. (a) Reticulocytes are juvenile red cells and an increase in numbers is evidence of red cell regeneration.

130. (b) Drabkin's reagent con-
     (d) tains a mixture of potassium ferricyanide and potassium cyanide. Carboxyhemoglobin, methemoglobin and oxyhemoglobin are all converted to cyanmeth-

emoglobin.

131. (a) The cyanmethemoglobin method (Drabkin's method) converts carboxy-hemoglobin, methemoglobin, and oxyhemoglobin to cyanmethemoglobin with the exception of sulf-hemoglobin.

132. (c) Tests to detect the presence of hemoglobin S depend on the decreased solubility at low oxygen tensions.

133. (d) The basis of the test for the estimation of hemoglobin F is that it is not denatured by alkali solutions (NaOH).

134. (d) Anemia, sunlight and variation in the internal diameter of the sedimentation tube will all affect the result of the erythrocyte sedimentation rate.

135. (c) Di-potassium ethylene-diamine tetra acetic acid (E.D.T.A.) is unsuitable as an anticoagulant for hemostosis studies because Factor V is very labile in this anticoagulant. E.D.T.A. may also inhibit the thrombin-fibrinogen reaction.

136. (c) Sodium heparin is unsuitable for coagulation studies because it functions as an antithrombin and it also inhibits many of the coagulation factors.

137. (c) In Romanowsky stained preparations the L.E. cell appears as a neutrophil in the cytoplasm of which is a large spherical body which stains shades of pale purple. The L.E. body, although derived from nuclear material, usually shows no evidence of nuclear structure and appears as an opaque homogenous mass.

138. (a) Leukopenia may be defined as a reduction of the total number of leukocytes below $4.0 \times 10^9/l$. In most situations the decrease is due to a marked decrease in the number of cells of the granulocyte series.

139. (d) Specific reduction of neutrophilic granulocytes below $2.0 \times 10^9/l$ in adults and $1.5 \times 10^9/l$ in children is caused by the peripheral distribution of abnormally large numbers of polymorphonuclear cells as seen in infections by the salmonellae, in which there is mild early leukocytosis followed by neutropenia with relative and absolute lymphocytosis and occasionally monocytosis.

140. (c) Childhood neutropenia is characterized by a decrease in neutrophilic

granulocytes below 1.5
x 10^9/l.

141. (c) Pertussis is characterized by a marked lympho-
cytosis. Acute appendi-
citis is characterized
by a neutrophilia and
in acute myeloblastic
leukemia the predominant
cell is the myeloblast
which may contain Auer
rods.

142. (b) The yellow or xanthochromic color of cerebro-
spinal fluid (C.S.F.) is
usually associated with
cerebral hemorrhage.

143. (b) Saponin may be used to
lyse erythrocytes when
enumerating white cells.

144. (c) Anemia due to acute blood
loss is typically normo-
chromic.

145. (d) The synonym for polycythemia is erythremia

146. (d) Spherocytosis is a typical finding in ABO incom-
patability of the newborn.

147. (b) Sickle cell anemia is a
hemolytic anemia and is
a beta chain variant.

148. (a) Elevated values for RBC,
WBC, Hct and Hgb are
typical findings in
polycythemia.

149. (b) Vitamin B_6 (pyridoxine)
deficiency has been des-
cribed as being associa-
ted with certain hypo-
chromic microcytic ane-
mias.

150. (d) Di Guglielmo's syndrome
is the erythrocytic
counterpart of acute
leukemia characterized
by progressive and
irreversible prolifera-
tion of neoplastic
developing red cells.

151. (d) Hypochromic erythrocytes are more resis-
tant to lysis in hypto-
tonic solutions than
are normal erythrocytes.

152. (b) Punctate basophilia is
a classic   finding in
lead poisoning.

153. (d) Incomplete segmentation
of the nuclei of granu-
locytes is typical of
Pelger-Huet anomaly.

154. (b) Aleukemic leukemia is
defined as a state in
which the leukocyte
count is less than
normal and the periph-
eral blood supposedly
contains no abnormal
immature cells of the
myeloid or lymphoid
series.

155. (c) Drug induced hemolysis
of glucose-6-phosphate
dehydrogenase (G-6PD)
deficient red cells
often shows the forma-
tion of Heinz bodies.
Heinz bodies are par-
ticles of denatured
hemoglobin and stromal
protein which form
only in the presence
of oxygen.

156. (a) Reticulocytosis, target
(b) cells, siderocytes and

(c) Howell-Jolly bodies are
(d) typical findings in a
post-splenectomy blood
picture.

157. (b) Coumadin interferes with
the liver synthesis of
vitamin K dependent
Factors II, VII, IX and
X.

158. (a) HL-A1 and HL-A8 are pre-
(b) dominantly Caucasian
whilst the Caucasoid
antigens HL-A3 and HL-
A7 are also found in
Negroid and Oriental
populations. HL-A2
antigen is spread
throughout all popula-
tions but has the high-
est frequency in American
Indians.

159. (a) There are small differ-
(b) ences between strictly
(c) venous blood and maxi-
(d) mally aerated blood
and for the most accur-
ate results blood should
be mixed until it is
bright red. Testing
should always be carried
out at the same temper-
ature, a rise of 5°C is
equivalent to an altera-
tion in saline concen-
tration of about 0.1 g/l.
The effect of pH is also
important, the fragility
of the red cells being
increased by a fall in
pH. A shift of 0.1 in
pH is equivalent to
altering the saline
concentration by 0.1 g/l.

160. (c) The isopropanol test
for unstable hemoglobin
may give a false posi-
tive result if there is

an increased amount
of hemoglobin F.

161. (d) Hemophilia A gives
a prolonged activated
partial thromboplastin
time. It is inherited
as a sex-linked reces-
sive and shows variable
expression in females.

162. (c) In chronic idiopathic
thrombocytopenic pur-
pura (ITP) there are
increased numbers of
megakaryocytes; they
are normal in size,
mature in construction,
but have reduced granu-
larity and fewer plate-
lets are formed.

163. (b) Deficiences of pyri-
(c) doxine and iron give
rise to a hypochromic-
microcytic picture
and vitamin B_{12} and
folic acid give a
megaloblastic picture.

164. (c) A patient with a mean
cell volume of 122 fl.,
a mean cell hemoglobin
concentration of 35
per cent, a reduced
total white cell count
and platelet count.
These results are sus-
picious of megaloblastic
anemia. The most appro-
priate test would be
the Schilling test for
vitamin B_{12} uptake.

165. (c) Both hemophilia A
(Factor VIII deficiency)
and hemophilia B (Factor
IX deficiency) give a
prolonged P.T.T.

166. (b) The area of the smallest

square in the Neubauer
hemacytometer is .05 mm
x .05 mm = .0025 mm^2.

167. (c) The central square of
          the improved Neubauer
          hemacytometer is used
          for platelet counting
          and this is subdivided
          into 25 smaller squares,
          each of an area of 0.04
          mm^2; the hemocytometer
          has a depth of 0.1 mm.
          Therefore, the total
          area counted is 25 x
          0.04 x 0.1 = 0.1 cmm.

168. (b) Marrow produced lymphoid
          cells which eventually
          participate in cellular
          immunity have been sub-
          jected to thymus-induc-
          tive influences and
          therefore are referred
          to as T-lymphocytes.

169. (d) Megaloblastic erythro-
          poiesis is due to a de-
          ficiency of vitamin B$_{12}$
          or folic acid.

170. (b) In sickle cell anemia
          the abnormality in the
          hemoglobin molecule is
          located on the beta
          chain. There is replace-
          ment of glutamic acid by
          valine at the sixth amino
          acid locus from the N-
          terminal end of the beta
          chain.

171. (d) Acute lymphocytic leu-
          kemia is most commonly
          seen in children.

172. (b) Acute lymphoblastic
          leukemia is most commonly
          seen in children. A
          disease of similar

appearance occurs
in adults but is un-
common. Acute granu-
locytic, myelogenous
or myeloblastic leu-
kemia (A.M.L.) occurs
most commonly in adults
and less frequently in
children.

173. (d) Fibrinogen is consumed
          in the formation of
          the fibrin clot and
          would not be present
          in serum.

174. (c) The sugar-water test
          shows marked hemolysis
          in patients with par-
          oxysmal nocturnal hemo-
          globinuria and is speci-
          fic for the disorder.

175. (a) The Prussian blue
          reaction shows the
          presence of ferric
          iron. The ferrocyanide
          reacts with ferric
          iron forming a blue-
          black ferric-ferro-
          cyanide complex.

$$4Fe^{+3} + (K_4Fe(CN)_6)_3 =$$
$$Fe_4(Fe(CN)_6)_3 + 12K^+$$

176. (b) The corrected white
          cell count is cal-
          culated from the formula.

$$100xWBC(11.0x10^9/l) = \frac{}{100+NRBC/100WBC}$$

$$\frac{100x11}{110} = 10x10^9/l$$

177. (d) When handling Australia
          antigen positive material
          it is imperative that the
          greatest care be taken.

178. (a) All blood samples should be treated as potentially hazardous. The World Health Organization (W.H.O.) advisory committee recommends the use of "strong chlorine" solutions containing 10,000 parts/million of available chlorine for clean up of blood spills and for work bench cleaning.

179. (b) Pipetting of any clinical
     (c) material by mouth suction must be strictly forbidden.

180. (a) A pressurized water fire extinguisher may be used for an ignited paper or burning laboratory coat fire. This type of extinguisher is unsuitable for an ignited xylol fire because water and xylol are not miscible.

181. (d) Gaussian curve is a symmetrical bell-shaped curve representative of many types of numerical distributions.

182. (b) A laboratory result that falls within ± 2 standard deviations of the mean is an acceptable value.

183. (c) Hemoglobins are large globular proteins of molecular weight about 65,000. Each molecule of globin is composed of four polypeptide chain subunits and each peptide chain has an inserted iron-containing heme group.

184. (d) There are 141 amino acids present in the alpha chain of the hemoglobin molecule.

185. (d) When hemoglobin S is associated with C, D or thalassemia the clinical state may be as severe as hemoglobin S/S.

186. (b) Both beta thalassemia minor and iron deficiency anemia present as a hypochromic microcytic anemia. Differentiation between them is made by hemoglobin electrophoresis.

187. (c) Using starch gel electrophoresis at pH 8.6 hemoglobin E and hemoglobin A_2 have the same mobility. Hemoglobin A_2 rarely exceeds 8 per cent whereas hemoglobin E is usually between 25 and 30 per cent.

188. (d) Chloramphenicol, primaquine and fava beans are all known to induce hemolysis in G-6-PD deficient individuals. Favism is one of the gravest potential clinical consequences.

189. (b) Heinz bodies are particles of denatured hemoglobin and stromal protein, which are formed in the presence of oxygen. The mechanism by which Heinz bodies are formed and become attached to red cell stroma has been subject to considerable investigation and spec-

ulation. It has been
found that exposure of
red cells to certain
drugs results in the
formation of low levels
of hydrogen peroxide as
the drug interacts with
hemoglobin.

190. (a) Acanthocytes take their
name from the thorny
appearance of the red
cells, and are striking
in appearance.

191. (b) Homozygotes of pyruvate
     (d) kinase deficiency have
hemolytic anemia and
splenomegaly. Heterozy-
gotes are clinically and
hematologically normal.
The autohemolysis test
most commonly shows mod-
erate to marked auto-
hemolysis poorly cor-
rected by the addition
of glucose or adenosine.

192. (a) Glanzmann's thrombasthenia is characterized
by a prolonged bleeding
time, defective clot re-
traction, with the absence
of platelet aggregation
induced by A.D.P. collagen,
adrenaline and thrombin.

193. (d) The platelet count in
the human adult does not
appear to have any sex
differences and is re-
latively constant without
definite diurnal variation.

194. (d) Stomatocytes have been
described in a rare type
of hemolytic anemia. In
some smears they may ap-
pear as an artifact and
it is known that the
change can be produced
by a decreased pH.

195. (d) The Prussian blue reaction uses potassium
ferrocyanide to demon-
strate hemosiderin.

196. (b) Sodium meta-bisulphite
is a reducing agent and
hastens the sickling
process in sickle cell
anemia.

197. (a) The mean hemoglobin in
full term infants is
$16.5^{\pm}\ 3.0$ g/dl.

198. (c) Vitamin B_{12} deficiency
anemia red cells appear
as oval macrocytes.

199. (c) Microspherocytes are a
classic finding in
some of the hemolytic
anemias.

200. (b) A contain pipet "con-
     (c) tains" a specific vol-
ume and in order to
transfer the correct
volume it must be
rinsed in the diluting
solution after it has
drained.

201. (b) The MCV is 92 fl - use
the following formula:

$$\frac{Hct}{RBC} = MCV = \frac{0.26}{2.78 \times 10^{12}} = 92\ fl$$

202. (a) The MCH is 29.5 pg -
use the following
formula:

$$\frac{Hgb\ in\ grams/l}{RBC\ count} = \frac{82}{2.78 \times 10^{12}} = 29.5\ pg$$

203. (d) The MCHC is 31.9 g/dl -
use the formula:

$$\frac{Hgb}{Hct} = MCHC \ g/dl$$

$$\frac{8.2}{0.26} = 31.9 \ g/dl$$

204. (a) To calculate the plate-let count use the form-ula:

$$\frac{N \times DILUTION \times Depth}{area}$$

$$= \frac{200 \times 100 \times 10}{1}$$

= 200,000/cmm = 200×10^9/l

205. (b) Free hemoglobin binds with haptoglobin hence in hemolytic anemia the haptoglobin would be decreased.

206. (c) The blood smear must be fixed in methanol before staining with buffer diluted Giemsa stain.

207. (b) Glucose-6-phosphate dehydrogenase deficient red cells are sensitive to primaquine and results in the formation of Heinz bodies.

208. (c) The characteristic ab-normality that occurs in the 21 - 22 chromo-some group is the Phila-delphia chromosome and this is present in chro-nic myelogenous leukemia.

209. (b) Salicylates interfere with platelet aggrega-tion and prolong the bleeding time.

210. (a) Protamine sulphate neu-tralizes heparin but if given in excess it may have a "heparin like" effect.

211. (a) The bone marrow in
(b) vitamin B_{12} and folic
(c) acid deficiency shows
(d) erythroid hyperplasia with megaloblastic changes. The megalo-blasts have a nuclear-cytoplasmic asynchrony and there are giant metamyelocytes present.

212. (c) Howell-Jolly bodies are seen in blood films stained by Wright's stain, May-Grunwald Giemsa and Jenner-Giemsa stains, but the most specific stain would be the Feulgen reaction for desoxyribonucleic acid.

213. (b) Field's stain is an alternate to Giemsa stain for staining thick smears for malarial parasites.

214. (c) Tissue fluid contains thromboplastin so the sample is unsuitable for any coagulation studies.

215. (b) It is important that differentiation is made between rouleaux and agglutination. Where there is intense rouleaux formation as in myelomatosis, auto-agglutination may be stimulated.

216. (c) Aspirin interferes with platelet aggregation and prolongs the bleeding time.

217. (c)
     (d) Aluminum hydroxide is used to adsorb Factors II, VII, IX and X from *citrated* plasma. Barium sulphate is used to adsorb Factors II, VII, IX and X from *serum* or *oxalated* samples.

218. (d) Vitamin K deficiency, liver damage and reduced Factor VII concentration would all give a prolonged prothrombin time.

219. (a)
     (b) Acute leukemias and cirrhosis of the liver
     (c) give a reduced plate-
     (d) let count.
         Polycythemia vera and chronic myelogenous leukemia both give an increased platelet count.

220. (d) A method is said to be precise when the values obtained by it are consistently reproducible.

221. (d) Thrombasthenia refers to a functional defect in blood platelets.

222. (b) If the hematocrit is ⟩ 55 per cent the plasma volume of the sample will be reduced. In order that there is no dilution factor with the normal amount of anticoagulant the volume of the anticoagulant used should be reduced.

223. (d) Inspection of quality control data may reveal that the method being monitored is either within control bounds or without or lacks precision. The most important point is that all the quality control data be analyzed on a daily basis or whatever period the test demands and action is to be taken immediately if results are out of bounds.

224. (c) In hereditary spherocytosis, the disease is transmitted by either parent; the erythrocytes are thicker than normal and the red cells show an increase in osmotic fragility. The red cells would not be larger than normal.

225. (a) Afibrinogenemia, Factor VII deficiency, Factor X deficiency would prolong the prothrombin time and the activated partial thromboplastin time, neither test would be affected by thrombocytopenia.

226. (b) Thrombocytopenia is not present in a post-splenectomy blood smear; however, Howell-Jolly bodies, target cells and thrombocytosis are usual findings.

227. (b) If the bleeding time is prolonged, it should be followed up with a total platelet count. The bleeding time is

dependent on platelets both in number and in their function.

228. (b) A suitable diluent for manual platelet counts would be a 1 per cent ammonium oxalate solution. The erythrocytes will lyse and leave the platelets and white blood cells in solution.

229. (a) The normal range for the absolute lymphocyte count in an adult is 0.5 - 2.5 x 10^9/l or 500 - 2,500/μl.

230. (b) A relative neutrophilic granulocytosis is when the granulocyte percentage is elevated 80 per cent or an absolute count of 7.0 x 10^9/l.

231. (b) Leukopenia is when the total white cell count is depressed below 4.0 x 10^9/l.

232. (a) Rouleaux formation is
     (b) a characteristic finding
     (c) in multiple myeloma and the ESR; total protein and electrophoresis would also be abnormal.

233. (a) The absolute eosinophil count in the normal adult is 0.04 - 0.4 x 10^9/l.

234. (c) The unit of electrical resistance is the ohm.

235. (d) The smaller the bore of a syringe needle the larger is its identifying number;

e.g., a 21 gauge needle has a smaller bore than an 18 gauge needle.

236. (c) Mitosis consists of 4 phases, prophase, metaphase, anophase and telophase.

237. (a) An Angstrom unit is a unit for the measurement of the wavelength of light.

238. (b) Deliquescent chemicals absorb moisture from the air until they eventually dissolve, e.g., sodium hydroxide and phosphorus pentoxide.

239. (b) In the Embden-Meyerhoff pathway of glucose metabolism, glucose is catabolized anerobically to lactate.

240. (a) Most chromosomes have median or submedian constrictions (centromeres) but a few have terminal constrictions and are termed acrocentric.

241. (d) Hemophilia A, G-6-PD deficiency and Christmas disease are all sex-linked disorders.

242. (c) Erythropoietin, a plasma circulating factor, has the chemical properties of a glycoprotein and is produced mainly in the kidney.

243. (d) Erythrocyte, leukocyte and thrombocyte production is decreased

in pancytopenia.   and spleen.

244. (a) The center square milli-
          meter of an improved Neu-
          bauer hemacytometer is   SECTION B: HEADINGS
          subdivided into 400 squares
          and each square measures   (1)
          0.05 mm x 0.05 mm.   251. (b) Myeloblast

245. (b) An Auer body may be pres-   252. (d) Giant metamyelocyte
          ent in the cytoplasm of
          myeloblasts; they are   253. (a) Lymphoblast
          rod shaped and are per-
          oxidase positive.   254. (c) Myelocyte

246. (d) An atypical lymphocyte   (2)
          is usually large but   255. (e) Pappenheimer bodies
          can vary widely in size.
          It has an irregular   256. (a) Maurer's dots
          cytoplasmic margin with
          blunt pseudopods. The   257. (d) Neutrophils
          cytoplasm is very baso-
          philic and is quite often   258. (c) Schuffner's dots
          more intense at the edge
          of the cytoplasmic margin. 259. (b) Punctate basophilia
          The nucleus shows irregu-
          larly distributed chro-   260. (f) Heinz bodies
          matin.
                                      (3)
247. (a) Neutropenia is a charac-   261. (b) Von Willebrand's disease
          teristic finding in
          megaloblastic anemia.   262. (d) Factor XII

248. (a) Lymphocytosis is an   263. (e) Factor X
     (b) increase in the number
     (c) of lymphocytes above   264. (c) Christmas disease
          45 per cent or 4.0 x
          10^9/1 and occurs in   265. (a) Hemophilia A
          lymphatic leukemia,
          acute viral infections   (4)
          and infectious hepatitis.   266. (b) Hemoglobin F

249. (d) A femtoliter is 10^{-15} 267. (a) Hemoglobin A
          liter.
                                      268. (e) Hemoglobin D
250. (c) Extramedullary hema-
          topoiesis is the abnor-   269. (d) Hemoglobin A_2
          mal production of ery-
          throcytes, granulocytes   270. (c) Hemoglobin S
          and megakaryocytes out-
          side of the bone marrow,
          usually in the liver

SECTION C: TRUE OR FALSE

271. False   It is G-6-PD deficient
               erythrocytes that are
               sensitive to prima-
               quine and form Heinz
               bodies.

272. True

273. True

274. True

275. True

276. False   The Philadelphia
               chromosome is pres-
               ent in chronic mye-
               logenous leukemia.

277. True

278. False   Factor V is particu-
               larly labile when the
               blood is collected
               into sodium oxalate.

279. True

280. False   Tissue fluid contains
               thromboplastin and
               this would give
               erroneus coagulation
               results.

281. True

282. True

283. True

284. False   The Fuchs-Rosenthal
               is 0.2 mm deep.

285. True

286. False   The synonym for sickle
               cells is drepanocytes
               and they may be pres-
               ent in the peripheral
               blood of homozygous
               Hb-S disease.

287. True

288. True

289. False   Auer rods may be
               present in myelo-
               blasts.

290. True

291. True

292. True

293. True

294. False   Hypersegmented neu-
               trophils are charac-
               teristic of vitamin B_{12}
               deficiency.

295. True

296. True

297. True

298. False   Schuffner's dots are
               seen in *Plasmodium
               vivax*.

299. True

300. True

301. False   *Diphyllobothrium
               latum* infestation
               gives a bone marrow
               and peripheral blood
               picture that resembles
               pernicious anemia.

302. True

303. True

304. True

305. True

306. True

307. False   Acute lymphatic leu-
             kemia occurs mainly
             in children. Chronic
             lymphatic leukemia
             occurs mainly in the
             45 - 75 years of age.

308. False   Auer rods may be
             present in myelo-
             blasts in acute
             myelogenous leukemia.

309. True

310. True

311. False   It is particularly
             good for use in hot
             climates because the
             glycerin in the stain
             retards evaporation.

312. True

313. False   Myeloblasts and mono-
             blasts are both non-
             specific esterase
             positive and after
             treatment with sodium
             fluoride the non-
             specific esterase in
             monoblasts is inhibi-
             ted.

314. True

315. True

316. True

317. True

318. True

319. True

320. True

321. False   The S.I. unit for
             M.C.V. is femto-
             liter.

322. False   Electrical resistance
             is measured in ohms.

323. True

324. True

325. False   Erythropoietin is pro-
             duced mainly in the
             kidney.

326. True

327. False   Adult hemoglobin has
             2 alpha and 2 beta
             chains.

328. False   Oval macrocytes are
             associated with
             pernicious anemia
             Pyridoxine deficiency
             presents as a hypo-
             chromic-microcytic
             anemia.

329. True

330. True

331. True

332. False   Heinz bodies are best
             demonstrated with
             methyl violet stain.

333. False   Von Willebrand's plate-
             lets aggregate with
             epinephrine but not
             with ristocetin.

334. True

335. False   The di-potassium salt
             of E.D.T.A. has greater
             solubility.

336. False   *P. falciparum* has Maurer's dots, *P. vivax* may contain Schuffner's dots.

337. True

338. True

339. False   Resolving power is its ability to distinguish minute particles as being separate.

340. True

341. True

342. False   The thymus helps in the development of T-lymphocytes.

343. False   The Coulter 'S' uses an electronic impedance detection system.

344. False   Nanometer is 10^{-9} of a meter.

345. True

346. True

347. True

348. False   Pelger-Huet anomaly is seen in neutrophils.

349. True

350. True

351. True

352. True

353. False   Dohle bodies may be present in neutrophils. Auer rods may be present in myeloblasts.

354. False   The platelet count is greatly reduced.

355. True

356. True

357. True

358. True

359. True

360. True

361. False   The P.T. is prolonged in an extrinsic system deficiency.

362. True

363. True

364. True

365. True

366. True

367. True

368. True

369. True

370. True

SECTION D: MISSING WORDS

371. Fibrinogen, Factor II, V, VIII

372. Factor II, VII, IX, X

373. Vitamin B_{12} deficiency

374. Rouleaux formation

375. Standard deviation

376. 0.2 mm

377. Auer rods

378. Neutrophils

379. G-6-PD deficiency

380. Polychromatophilic cells

381. 0.1 mm

382. 0 - 20/cu mm

383. Agranulocytosis

384. Erythropoietin

385. Extramedullary hematopoiesis

386. Hemoglobinemia

387. Howell-Jolly bodies

388. G-6-PD deficient

389. Plasma cell

390. Picogram

391. Femtoliter

392. Pappenheimer bodies

393. 3.8 per cent trisodium citrate

394. Factor V

395. P.A.S. stain

396. Perl's Prussian blue reaction

397. G-6-PD deficient individuals

398. Protamine sulphate

399. Hereditary spherocytosis

400. Vitamin B_{12} deficiency

401. Folic acid deficiency

402. Megakaroycyte

403. Hemoglobin C disease

404. Hemoglobin D

405. 3:1

406. Neutrophils, eosinophils, basophils

407. Chronic myeloid leukemia

408. Plasma cell

409. E.D.T.A.

410. Children

411. Children, pertussis, infectious mononucleosis, infectious lymphocytosis

412. Infectious mononucleosis

413. Beef red cells

414. Platelets

415. Bleeding time

416. $150 - 400 \times 10^9/1$

417. Thrombasthenia

418. Hemoglobin A_2

419. Manual platelet counts

420. New methylene blue

SECTION E: SPECIAL QUESTIONS

421. (a) Chronic myeloid leukemia

      (b) Karyotyping - Philadelphia chromosome (Ph^1) is present.
           Bone marrow - shows a myeloid hyperplasia with a decreased
                          leukocyte alkaline phosphatase reaction.

Hemoglobin 9.7 g/dl		White cell differential	
RBC	$3.1 \times 10^{12}/1$	Neutrophils	33%
WBC	$170 \times 10^9/1$	Bands	7%
Platelets	$34 \times 10^9/1$	Metamyelocytes	9%
		Myelocytes	21%
		Promyelocytes	3%
		Blasts	1%
		Eosinophils	2%
		Basophils	10%
		Lymphocytes	4%
		Monocytes	10%

A provisional diagnosis of chronic myeloid leukemia can be made
from the data given because

(1) The total white cell count is greatly increased.
(2) The platelet count is markedly reduced.
(3) The white cell differential shows a marked left shift with
     promyelocytes present.
(4) There is a low blast count; therefore, it is not an acute
     form of the disease.
(5) There is an increase in the basophil count.

Confirmation of the diagnosis would be made by karyotyping and
the Philadelphia chromosome would be found.
A bone marrow examination would reveal a marked myeloid hyperplasia with a reduced leukocyte alkaline phosphatase reaction.

422. (a) Beta-thalassemia minor

      (b) Hemoglobin electrophoresis showing an increase in the A_2
           band.

Hemoglobin	10.0 g/dl
RBC	$5.85 \times 10^{12}/1$
WBC	$5.3 \times 10^{9}/1$
Mean cell volume	59 fl
Platelets	$170 \times 10^{9}/1$

White cell differential

Neutrophils	50%
Eosinophils	3%
Basophils	1%
Lymphocytes	44%
Monocytes	2%

The erythrocytes show a hypochromic-microcytic picture.

Using the data given,

(1) The mean cell volume is greatly reduced.
(2) The red cell count is increased.
(3) The hemoglobin is reduced.
(4) The blood smear shows hypochromasia and microcytosis.

There are two possible diagnoses, iron deficiency anemia and thalassemia minor.
Further studies of serum iron and serum ferritin and hemoglobin electrophoresis would indicate an increase in hemoglobin A_2 on cellulose acetate at pH 8.6.

423.   DISTRIBUTION OF COAGULATION FACTORS

	I	II	V	VII	VIII	IX	X	XI	XII
Fresh Normal Plasma	+	+	+	+	+	+	+	+	+
Stored Plasma	+	+	0	+	0	+	+	+	+
Adsorbed Plasma	+	0	+	0	+	0	0	+	+
Aged Serum	0	0	0	+	0	+	+	+	+

424.   COAGULATION MECHANISM

Intrinsic System

contact with foreign surface; platelets (PF3)

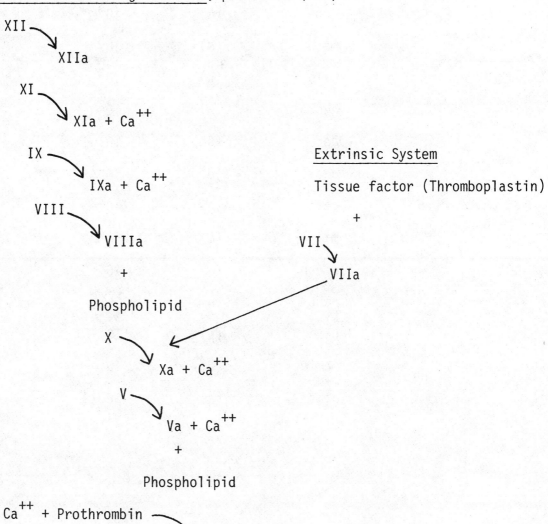

XII
  ↘
    XIIa

XI
  ↘
    XIa + Ca^{++}

IX
  ↘
    IXa + Ca^{++} Extrinsic System

VIII   Tissue factor (Thromboplastin)
   ↘
     VIIIa   +

       +   VII
                                         ↘
   Phospholipid   VIIa

X
 ↘
   Xa + Ca^{++}

V
 ↘
   Va + Ca^{++}

     +

   Phospholipid

Ca^{++} + Prothrombin
                      ↘
                        Thrombin

Fibrinogen ————→ Fibrin + XIII + Ca^{++}
                            ↓
                      Insoluble Fibrin

425.   THE METRIC SYSTEM PREFIXES

tera	(T)	10^{12}
giga	(G)	10^{9}
mega	(M)	10^{6}
kilo	(K)	10^{3}
hecto	(H)	10^{2}
deca	(da)	10^{1}
deci	(d)	10^{-1}
centi	(c)	10^{-2}
milli	(m)	10^{-3}
micro	(u)	10^{-6}
nano	(n)	10^{-9}
pico	(p)	10^{-12}
femto	(f)	10^{-15}
atto	(a)	10^{-18}

IMMUNOHEMATOLOGY

NEVILLE J. BRYANT
A.R.T.,F.A.C.B.S.
Technical Director
Serological Services Ltd.
TORONTO, ONTARIO, CANADA

QUESTIONS

SECTION A: MULTIPLE CHOICE

Choose the phrase, sentence or symbol which completes the statement or answers the question. More than one answer may be correct in each case.

1. The red cells in the circulation of a normal individual have an average life span of:
    (a) 21 days
    (b) 80 days
    (c) 100 - 120 days
    (d) 9 - 12 days

2. The majority of blood group genes are:
    (a) dominant
    (b) recessive
    (c) amorphic
    (d) none of the above

3. Of the total immunoglobulin, IgG constitutes:
    (a) 20 per cent
    (b) 45 per cent
    (c) 99 per cent

    (d) 85 per cent

4. B-cells:
    (a) are primarily involved in cell-mediated immunity
    (b) are primarily involved in humoral antibody synthesis
    (c) constitute 10 - 20 per cent of peripheral blood lymphocytes
    (d) (b) and (c) are correct

5. Antibodies which are produced in response to antigens of another of the same species are known as:
    (a) xenoantibodies
    (b) heterophile antibodies
    (c) alloantibodies
    (d) none of the above

6. The enzyme 'trypsin' splits the immunoglobulin molecule into:
    (a) 2 Fab fragments and 1 Fc fragment
    (b) 1 F(ab')$_2$ fragment and

several smaller fragments
   (c) 2 Fab(t) fragments and 1
       Fc(t) fragment
   (d) 2 Fab(t) fragments and 2
       Fc(t) fragments

7. Which of the following immunoglobulin classes represents antibodies which do not initiate the
   complement sequence?
   (a) IgG1
   (b) IgG2
   (c) IgG3
   (d) IgG4

8. ABH antigens are found on:
   (a) normoblasts
   (b) epidermal cells
   (c) spermatozoa
   (d) all of the above

9. Anti-A and anti-B:
   (a) are always present in neo-
       natal sera
   (b) are sometimes present in
       neonatal sera
   (c) are never present in neo-
       natal sera
   (d) reach maximum strength by
       age 3 months

10. There are two kinds of anti-Le^b
    sera, known as:
   (a) anti-Le^{bH} and anti-Le^{bL}
   (b) anti-Le^{b1} and anti-Le^{b2}
   (c) anti-Le^{bA} and anti-Le^{bB}
   (d) anti-Le^{bH} and anti-Le^{bA}

11. By age three months, over 80 per
    cent of children type as:
   (a) Le(a-b+)
   (b) Le(a+b-)
   (c) Le(a-b-)
   (d) Le(a+b+)

12. The component parts of the D
    antigen mosaic are known as:
   (a) A, B, C and D
   (b) C, D, E and F
   (c) 1, 2, 3 and 4
   (d) X, X, Y and Z

13. The majority of Rh anti-
    bodies are:
   (a) IgG
   (b) IgM
   (c) IgA
   (d) IgD

14. Hydatid cyst fluid:
   (a) strongly inhibits
       anti-P
   (b) will inhibit anti-Jk^a
   (c) contains P$_1$ and Le^a
       substance
   (d) will inhibit (in part)
       anti-P^k sera

15. Anti-S:
   (a) is commonly found as
       an immune antibody in
       multitransfused patients
   (b) is usually IgM
   (c) always binds complement
   (d) should be considered
       clinically significant

16. The M and N antigens:
   (a) are glycoproteins
   (b) appear to be dependent
       on sialic acid in
       appropriate linkages
       for their integrity
   (c) are well developed at
       birth
   (d) are poorly developed
       at birth

17. I antigens:
   (a) show a great range of
       strength in various
       individuals
   (b) are possessed by almost
       all healthy adults
   (c) are of constant strength
       in all individuals
   (d) are of constant strength
       in any one individual

18. The expression of HLA antigens
    is controlled by a region of
    chromosome number:
   (a) 1

    (b) 4
    (c) 9
    (d) 6

19. The first HLA antigen to be described was called Mac. Under current nomenclature, this antigen is known as:
    (a) HLA-A1
    (b) HLA-A2
    (c) HLA-A3
    (d) HLA-2

20. The antibodies most often implicated as the cause of hemolytic disease of the new-born are:
    (a) ABO and Kell
    (b) ABO and Rh
    (c) ABO and Lewis
    (d) ABO and Kidd

21. If a baby has had repeated intrauterine transfusions, erroneous results may be obtained in:
    (a) ABO grouping
    (b) Rh typing
    (c) the direct antiglobulin test
    (d) the indirect antiglobulin test

22. The take-up of antibody by the red cells is known as:
    (a) absorption
    (b) elution
    (c) adsorption
    (d) antigen absorption

23. The causative antibodies in 'cold' antibody autoimmune hemolytic anemia:
    (a) react best at room temperature or below
    (b) react best at 25°C - 37°C
    (c) may have a wide thermal range
    (d) react at 4°C only

24. In most cases of drug-induced hemolytic anemia, the immunoglobulin on the red cells is solely:
    (a) IgG1
    (b) IgG2
    (c) IgM
    (d) IgG4

25. The amount of ACD-A required to prevent the clotting of 100 ml of blood is:
    (a) 63.5 ml
    (b) 67.5 ml
    (c) 15 ml
    (d) 35 ml

26. The specific gravity of the copper sulphate solution used for the determination of hemoglobin levels in male donors is:
    (a) 1.053
    (b) 1.055
    (c) 1.057
    (d) 1.059

27. The hemoglobin requirements for female blood donors is:
    (a) 10.5 mg/dl
    (b) 12.5 mg/dl
    (c) 13.5 mg/dl
    (d) 11.5 mg/dl

28. Blood donations collected into heparin can be stored for:
    (a) 21 days
    (b) 28 days
    (c) 35 days
    (d) 48 hours

29. If the hermaetic seal has been broken during the preparation of red blood cells (red cell concentrates), the red cells must be transfused within:
    (a) 48 hours
    (b) 6 hours
    (c) 24 hours
    (d) 72 hours

30. Washed red blood cells:
    (a) may be used in cases of
        paroxysmal nocturnal
        hemoglobinuria
    (b) may be stored for 21
        days at 2 - 6°C
    (c) are prepared by manual
        washing or with the use
        of special cell-washing
        instruments
    (d) should not be stored,
        but rather should be
        prepared especially for
        a proposed transfusion

31. Factor IX concentrates may be
    useful in cases of:
    (a) liver disease
    (b) congenital Factor VII
        deficiency
    (c) congenital Factor X
        deficiency
    (d) congenital Factor IX
        deficiency

32. When low ionic strength solu-
    tion is used as a suspending
    medium in the antiglobulin
    test, the usual recommended
    incubation time is:
    (a) 30 minutes
    (b) 1 hour
    (c) 45 minutes
    (d) 10 minutes

33. Which of the following antigens
    is weakened or inactivated by
    proteolytic enzymes?
    (a) Jk^a
    (b) Ch^a
    (c) C^w
    (d) i

34. The specificity of the lectin
    derived from the plant *Ulex
    europaeus* is:
    (a) anti-A_1
    (b) anti-N
    (c) anti-T
    (d) anti-H

35. The spontaneous agglutination
    of all red cells (irrespective
    of blood group) by a given
    serum is known as:
    (a) polyagglutination
    (b) panagglutination
    (c) prozone phenomenon
    (d) none of the above

36. The latent receptor, T:
    (a) is contained in all
        human red cells
    (b) is contained in 50
        per cent of all human
        red cells
    (c) can be activated by
        various strains of
        bacteria
    (d) can be activated by
        the enzymes derived
        from certain strains
        of bacteria

37. Rouleaux formation is encountered:
    (a) if red cells are allowed
        to sediment in their own
        plasma, especially in
        individuals with a high
        sedimentation rate
    (b) in certain disease states
        involving high levels of
        immunoglobulin
    (c) in patients with serum
        protein abnormalities
    (d) if a patient is on
        fibrinogen therapy

38. Febrile transfusion reactions
    may be due to:
    (a) leukocyte antibodies
    (b) platelet antibodies
    (c) pyrogens
    (d) none of the above

39. The antigens and antibodies
    known or suspected of being
    associated with anaphylactoid
    transfusion reactions include:
    (a) IgG-anti-IgG
    (b) IgM-anti-IgM
    (c) IgA-anti-IgA

(d) IgE-anti-IgE

40. The probability of stimulating
    one or more antibodies to red
    cell antigens after one blood
    transfusion has been estimated
    to be about:
    (a) 10 per cent
    (b) 1 per cent
    (c) 5 per cent
    (d) 25 per cent

41. The quantity of sodium chloride
    required to prepare half ($\frac{1}{2}$) a
    liter of physiological saline
    is:
    (a) 67.5 ml
    (b) 0.9 grams
    (c) 4.5 milligrams
    (d) 4.5 grams

42. Which of the following tests
    is not generally performed on
    donor blood?
    (a) The direct antiglobulin
         test
    (b) Tests for HB_sAg
    (c) The antibody screening
         test
    (d) Test for antibodies to
         Treponema pallidum

43. The Betke-Kleihauer test:
    (a) is used primarily to
         detect maternal red
         cells in the fetal
         circulation
    (b) is an alkaline elution
         test
    (c) is used primarily to
         detect fetal red cells
         in the maternal circu-
         lation
    (d) is an acid elution test

44. Mother: Rh: 1,2,-3,-4,5
    Child 1: Rh: 1,2,3,4,5
    Child 2: Rh: 1,2,-3,4,5
    Assuming that neither child
    is extramarital, which of the
    following is the father's
    genotype?
    (a) $R^o r$
    (b) $R^1 R^2$
    (c) $R^2 r$
    (d) $R^1 r$

45. In man, a full chromosome
    complement numbers:
    (a) 46 pairs of chromosomes
    (b) 23 pairs of chromosomes
    (c) 46 single chromosomes
    (d) 46 autosomal chromosomes

46. A 'zygote' is formed as a
    result of:
    (a) meiosis
    (b) fertilization
    (c) mitosis
    (d) none of the above

47. The antigens K and k are:
    (a) alleles
    (b) antithetical
    (c) amorphs
    (d) recessive

48. According to the numerical
    nomenclature in the Kell
    system:
    (a) K is K2
    (b) k is K3
    (c) Kp^a is K4
    (d) Js^a is K6

49. The majority of bloods from
    black donors are of pheno-
    type:
    (a) Fy(a-b+)
    (b) Fy(a-b-)
    (c) Fy(a+b-)
    (d) Fy(a+b+)

50. The term 'genotype' refers
    to:
    (a) the products of a gene
    (b) the total sum of genes
         present on a chromo-
         some (with respect to
         one or more than one

characteristic) that pro-
duce detectable products

(c) the total sum of genes
present on a chromosome
(with respect to one or
more than one character-
istic) regardless of
whether or not they pro-
duce detectable products

(d) the antigens on the red
cells

51. The cell alteration that is
concerned with cell division
by which the body grows and
replaces discarded cells is
known as:
(a) reproduction
(b) fertilization
(c) mitosis
(d) meiosis

52. The placental transfer of
antibodies from mother to
fetus is an example of:
(a) naturally acquired passive immunity
(b) naturally acquired active
immunity
(c) artificially acquired
passive immunity
(d) artificially acquired
active immunity

53. IgM consists of:
(a) 10 basic structural units
(b) 1 basic structural unit
(c) 5 basic structural units
(d) 2 basic structural units

54. Secretory IgA:
(a) is made up of two basic
structural units with a
J-chain
(b) is known to fix complement
(c) is transported across
the human placenta
(d) is detectable in cord
serum

55. The alternative pathway of
complement activation could
be initiated by:
(a) red cell antibodies
(b) IgA antibodies
(c) IgG antibodies
(d) (b) and (c) are correct

56. With anti-H, the order of
reactivity of red cells of
various ABO groups (from the
strongest to the weakest
reaction) usually follows
the pattern:
(a) A_1 - A_2 - B - O - A_1B - A_2B
(b) O - A_2 - A_2B - B - A_1 - A_1B
(c) A_1B - A_1 - B - A_2B - A_2 - O
(d) A_2 - B - A_1B - A_2B - A_1 - O

57. Secretion of ABH substances is
controlled by the gene:
(a) A, B and H
(b) se
(c) Se
(d) X

58. Anti-A_1:
(a) is present in all group
O and group B individuals
(b) is often IgG in group B
individuals
(c) always occurs as a separate antibody in A_2B
individuals
(d) is usually clinically
significant

59. Anomalous results in ABO testing may be caused by:
(a) disease
(b) irregular antibodies
(c) unwashed red cells
(d) all of the above

60. The inheritance of Lewis
substances is controlled
by the genes:
(a) Le^a and Le^b
(b) Le and le
(c) Jk^a and Jk
(d) Se and se

61. Most Lewis antibodies are:
    (a) IgG
    (b) IgM
    (c) IgA
    (d) IgD

62. An individual whose serum possesses potent Lewis antibodies should be transfused with blood of phenotype:
    (a) Le(a-b+)
    (b) Le(a-b-)
    (c) Le(a+b-)
    (d) Le(a+b+)

63. The *Rh* complex has been assigned to chromosome number:
    (a) 6
    (b) 1
    (c) 2
    (d) 14

64. The antigen K1 is found in:
    (a) 7 - 9 per cent of random whites
    (b) 8 - 10 per cent of random blacks
    (c) 20 - 30 per cent of random whites
    (d) 90 per cent of random whites

65. The Fy^a and Fy^b antigens:
    (a) are thought to be associated with susceptibility to malaria
    (b) are highly antigenic
    (c) are unaffected by enzyme treatment of the red cells
    (d) none of the above

66. The antibodies of the Kidd system are:
    (a) clinically significant
    (b) clinically insignificant
    (c) usually complement binding
    (d) usually found in conjunction with other red cell antibodies

67. There is evidence of linkage between the *Lutheran* locus and the:
    (a) *Rh* locus
    (b) *Lewis* locus
    (c) *Secretor* locus
    (d) *Hh* locus

68. Anti-Lu^a usually reacts best at:
    (a) 37°C
    (b) 20°C
    (c) 12°C
    (d) 0°C

69. The *M* and *N* genes give rise to:
    (a) three genotypes and three phenotypes
    (b) four genotypes and three phenotypes
    (c) the phenotypes *MM, MN* and *NN*
    (d) the phenotypes M, MN and N

70. Anti-P$_1$:
    (a) is found in almost 90 per cent of pregnant women
    (b) is never found as a non-red-cell-immune antibody
    (c) may bind complement when reactive at 37°C
    (d) is usually a warm-reacting IgG antibody

71. With respect to the Ii blood group system, most infants appear to be of phenotype:
    (a) II
    (b) i
    (c) I
    (d) I-i-

72. Which of the following is not an HTLA antibody?
    (a) anti-Kn^a
    (b) anti-McC^a
    (c) anti-Wr^a
    (d) anti-Cs^a

73. Individuals who are HLA-B17-positive have red cells possessing:
    (a) the Bg^a antigen
    (b) the Bg^b antigen
    (c) the Bg^c antigen
    (d) none of the above

74. The complement components involved in 'warm' antibody auto-immune hemolytic anemia are:
    (a) C3d and C4d
    (b) C3c and C4a
    (c) C5 and C6
    (d) C1 and C2

75. When a fetus is ABO incompatible with the mother, immunization due to Rh through pregnancy is:
    (a) more common
    (b) less common
    (c) equally common
    (d) more rapid

76. The procedure whereby a unit of blood is withdrawn from a donor to obtain plasma, followed by the reinfusion of the donor's red cells is known as:
    (a) cell separation
    (b) leukapheresis
    (c) thrombapheresis
    (d) plasmapheresis

77. Selective transfusion of specific blood components is preferable to the routine use of whole blood because:
    (a) a concentrated form of the required fraction can be administered
    (b) the risk of circulatory overload is reduced
    (c) many patients can be treated from a single donation
    (d) all of the above

78. The enzyme papain is prepared from:
    (a) *Chorica papaya*
    (b) *Ficus corica*
    (c) *Ananas sativus*
    (d) Pig's stomach

79. Rouleaux formation is inhibited by:
    (a) saline
    (b) glycine
    (c) anticoagulants
    (d) sodium salicylate

80. The type of red cell destruction in which the red cells rupture within the blood stream with consequent liberation of hemoglobin into the plasma is known as:
    (a) internal destruction
    (b) intravascular destruction
    (c) external destruction
    (d) extravascular destruction

81. If you have a 30 per cent solution and you require a 5 per cent solution of the same substance, how much of a 5 per cent solution could you prepare with 0.5 ml of the 30 per cent solution?
    (a) 3 ml
    (b) 3.5 ml
    (c) 2.5 ml
    (d) 30 ml

82. False positive antiglobulin reactions may be caused by:
    (a) inadequate washing of red cells
    (b) bacterial contamination of the red cells
    (c) underincubation of the

cell-serum mixture
(d)   the use of EDTA blood
      samples

83.   An $Rh_0(D)$-negative woman has
      delivered an $Rh_0(D)$-positive
      child, and the fetal-maternal
      bleed is estimated to be 10.0
      ml. How many 300 μl vials of
      Rh immune globulin should this
      woman receive?
      (a)   1
      (b)   2
      (c)   3
      (d)   4

84.   To minimize the risk of bacter-
      iogenic reactions:
      (a)   blood should remain at
            refrigerator temperature
            at all times during stor-
            age
      (b)   the blood container should
            not be opened or punctured
            to obtain a specimen
      (c)   components prepared by
            'open' procedures must be
            used within 72 hours
      (d)   the recommended storage
            time must not be exceeded
      (e)   blood should be examined
            visually before issue
            and after storage for an
            unusual color or the pres-
            ence of hemolysis

85.   Which of the following diseases
      can be transmitted by trans-
      fusion?
      (a)   Chagas' disease
      (b)   Infectious mononucleosis
      (c)   Leishmaniasis
      (d)   Hypotension

86.   An extract from the seeds of
      Salvia sclaera, when diluted:
      (a)   reacts strongly with Tn
            red cells
      (b)   reacts strongly with T-
            activated red cells
      (c)   reacts strongly with Tk-

activated red cells
(d)   does not react with
      T-activated red cells

87.   Panagglutination is frequently
      the result of:
      (a)   bacterial action
      (b)   the exposure of the T
            receptor on the red
            cells
      (c)   Tk-activation
      (d)   Tn-activation

88.   When bovine albumin solutions
      are contaminated:
      (a)   the solution becomes
            cloudy
      (b)   the solution becomes
            colorless
      (c)   no cloudiness occurs
      (d)   the solution becomes
            darker in color

89.   A satisfactory bacterio-
      static agent for stored
      serum is sodium azine with
      a final concentration of:
      (a)   0.1 per cent
      (b)   0.01 per cent
      (c)   0.001 per cent
      (d)   1 per cent

90.   Leukocyte concentrates:
      (a)   can be stored for
            72 hours at $4°C$
      (b)   are prepared from
            single units of blood
            by manual methods
      (c)   should not be stored
            but should be infused
            as soon as possible
            after collection
      (d)   are only prepared by
            leukapheresis techniques

91.   Frozen red blood cells which
      are prepared in high concen-
      tration glycerol must be
      stored at:
      (a) $-150°C$ or lower
      (b) $-65°C$ or lower and

preferably at -80°C
(c) -20°C or lower
(d) 4°C

92. A full donation of blood (450 ± 45 ml plus up to 30 ml for processing tubes) may be taken from otherwise eligible donors weighing:
(a) 110 kg or more
(b) 20 kg or more
(c) 60 kg or more
(d) 50 kg or more

93. Autologous blood may be used to:
(a) provide blood products to patients who react adversely to their own blood
(b) provide blood to patients of extremely rare blood type
(c) provide blood to patients with unexpected antibodies for whom compatible blood cannot be found
(d) all of the above

94. The risk of feto-maternal hemorrhage is increased by:
(a) stillbirth
(b) spontaneous miscarriage
(c) amniocentesis
(d) manual removal of the placenta

95. In cases of hemolytic disease of the newborn, exchange transfusion of the baby is performed to:
(a) lower the serum bilirubin
(b) remove the baby's red cells which have been sensitized with antibody
(c) provide substitute compatible red cells with adequate oxygen-carrying capacity

(d) reduce the amount of irregular antibody in the baby

96. Antibodies which are directed against an individual's own tissues are known as:
(a) alloantibodies
(b) autoantibodies
(c) isoantibodies
(d) xenoantibodies

97. The Donath-Landsteiner antibody commonly has the specificity:
(a) anti-D
(b) anti-Pr
(c) anti-P_1
(d) anti-P

98. The frequency of febrile reactions to blood transfusion in patients with leukocyte antibodies is:
(a) greater than 50 per cent
(b) greater than 90 per cent
(c) less than 50 per cent
(d) less than 10 per cent

99. HLA antigen typing has proven useful:
(a) in organ transplantation
(b) as an aid in the differential diagnosis of certain disease states
(c) in parentage disputes
(d) all of the above

100. The genes of the Xg blood group system are carried on:
(a) the autosomes
(b) chromosome number 6
(c) chromosome number 1
(d) the X chromosome

101. To be catagorized as a 'low-frequency' antigen, the following criteria must be satisfied:
(a) the antigen must have an incidence of not more than 1 in 100 in the

population
(b) the antigen must be a dominant character
(c) the antigen must be defined by a specific antibody
(d) the antigen must be extant

102. That part of the I antigen which is developed after the first eighteen months of life is known as:
(a) I^F
(b) I-cord
(c) I^T
(d) I^D

103. Anti-I:
(a) is contained by most normal sera
(b) is contained by some normal sera
(c) is not contained by normal sera
(d) is usually stimulated by transfusion

104. The P_1 antigen:
(a) is inherited as a dominant mendelian character
(b) is inherited as a recessive mendelian character
(c) is an amorphic antigen
(d) is the product of an amorphic gene

105. In paroxysmal cold hemoglobulinuria, the patient's serum contains an antibody which classically has the specificity:
(a) anti-P_1
(b) anti-P
(c) anti-PP_1P^k
(d) anti-p^k

106. Anti-M:
(a) occurs more commonly in adults than in infants

(b) is usually IgG
(c) reacts well with enzyme-treated red cells
(d) is found in an extract of the seeds of *Ulex europaeus*

107. The MNSs blood group system was discovered:
(a) through the presence of anti-M antibodies in a recipient of transfusion
(b) through the presence of anti-M, which causes hemolytic disease of the newborn
(c) through the injection of human red cells into rabbits
(d) at the same time as the P antigen was discovered

108. Anti-Lu^a:
(a) commonly causes hemolytic transfusion reactions
(b) has not been clearly incriminated as the cause of hemolytic disease of the newborn
(c) has caused delayed hemolytic transfusion reactions
(d) has commonly been shown to be the cause of hemolytic disease of the newborn

109. Anti-Lu3:
(a) is 'separable' anti-Lu^a plus anti-Lu^b
(b) appears to be made by individuals of the recessive type of Lu(a-b-)
(c) appears to be made by individuals of the

dominant type of
Lu(a-b-)
(d) (a) and (c) are correct

110. The majority of black and
white individuals are of
Lutheran phenotype:
(a) Lu(a-b+)
(b) Lu(a-b-)
(c) Lu(a+b-)
(d) Lu(a+b+)

111. Kidd antibodies:
(a) react best in the in-
direct antiglobulin
test
(b) are generally enhanced
by first enzyme-treat-
ing the red cells with
ficin or papain
(c) commonly show dosage
effect
(d) deteriorate rapidly on
storage

112. The antigen Jk^a is found in:
(a) 20 per cent of whites
(b) 99 per cent of whites
(c) 77 per cent of whites
(d) 32 per cent of whites

113. The *Duffy* locus has been
assigned to chromosome
number:
(a) 12
(b) 6
(c) 4
(d) 1

114. Under the numerical nomenclature for the Duffy system,
the antigen Fy^b is:
(a) Fy2
(b) Fy3
(c) Fy1
(d) Fy4

115. The antibody which reacts
with all red cells carrying
Kell antigens is known as:
(a) anti-K^o

(b) anti-Ku
(c) anti-Kk$Js^a$$Js^b$
(d) anti-Kn^a

116. Anti-K and anti-k are
usually:
(a) IgM
(b) IgA
(c) IgG
(d) IgE

117. Rh antigens have been
detected:
(a) in saliva
(b) in amniotic fluid
(c) on platelets
(d) none of the above

118. The Rh antigens:
(a) are well developed
at birth
(b) are poorly developed
at birth
(c) may not reach adult
strength until age
seven
(d) are not detectable
with anti-Rh at birth

119. The most common Rh antibody
formed (from the following
choices) is:
(a) anti-c
(b) anti-E
(c) anti-G
(d) anti-C

120. Treatment of red cells with
enzyme papain:
(a) produces clustering
of the Rh antigen
(b) has no effect on the
Rh antigen
(c) destroys the Rh anti-
gen
(d) enhances the Rh anti-
gen

121. Lewis antibodies:
(a) are not found in
pregnant women

(b) cause hemolytic disease
     of the newborn
(c) do not cause hemolytic
     disease of the newborn
(d) are predominantly IgG

122. An individual whose saliva
      contains H substance but no
      Lewis substance would be
      classified as saliva type:
      (a) Les Sec
      (b) Les nS
      (c) nL Sec
      (d) nL nS

123. The strength of anti-A and
      anti-B antibodies:
      (a) is the same in all
           individuals
      (b) varies considerably
           in different indivi-
           duals
      (c) is dependent on the
           immunoglobulin class
           of the antibodies
      (d) only shows a differ-
           ence when comparing
           adult and cord samples

124. The difference between A_1
      and A_2 is believed to be:
      (a) qualitative only
      (b) quantitative only
      (c) both quantitative and
           qualitative
      (d) none of the above

125. Individuals who possess the
      A antigen on their red cells:
      (a) have anti-A in their
           serum
      (b) have anti-B in their
           serum
      (c) have anti-A and anti-B
           in their serum
      (d) have neither anti-A
           nor anti-B in their
           serum

126. Which of the following factors
      influence antigen-antibody

reactions *in vitro*?
(a) Antibody size
(b) Ionic strength of
     the surrounding medium
(c) The number of antibody
     molecules present
(d) All of the above

127. Complement can be destroyed
      in vitro by which of the
      following substances or
      conditions?
      (a) Heating the serum
           to 56°C for 30 minutes
      (b) Anticoagulants
      (c) Storage at 37°C for
           72 hours
      (d) All of the above

128. C1 (first component of
      complement) is a macromo-
      lecular complex of three
      subcomponents, known as:
      (a) C1p, C1q, C1r
      (b) C1s, C1t, C1q
      (c) C1q, C1r, C1s
      (d) C1a, C1b, C1c

129. The nucleus of a somatic
      cell is *primarily* concerned
      with:
      (a) phagocytosis
      (b) oxidative processes
      (c) body growth and cell
           division
      (d) none of the above

130. A cell which is not actively
      dividing is said to be in:
      (a) interphase
      (b) prophase
      (c) anaphase
      (d) telophase

131. The position occupied by a
      gene on a chromosome is
      known as:
      (a) the triplet
      (b) the codon
      (c) the locus
      (d) none of the above

132. The pentose sugar in RNA is:
    (a) fucose
    (b) ribose
    (c) galactose
    (d) deoxyribose

133. The postmitotic period during which there is no DNA synthesis is known as:
    (a) gap 1 (G_1)
    (b) gap 2 (G_2)
    (c) S
    (d) gap 3 (G_3)

134. Which mendelian law states that two members of a single pair of genes are never found in the same gamete?
    (a) Unit inheritance
    (b) Dependent assortment
    (c) Independent assortment
    (d) Segregation

135. When the centromere of a chromosome is very close to but not quite at one end, the chromosome is classified as:
    (a) metacentric
    (b) acrocentric
    (c) submetacentric
    (d) telocentric

136. What percentage of the total volume of blood does plasma constitute?
    (a) 10 - 20 per cent
    (b) 30 - 40 per cent
    (c) 89 - 90 per cent
    (d) 55 - 60 per cent

137. Which of the following sugars is not part of the basic precursor substance of all antigens studied so far?
    (a) D-galactose
    (b) N-acetyl galactosamine
    (c) N-acetyl glucosamine
    (d) L-fucose

138. The addition of which of the following sugars to the terminal sugar of the basic precursor substance determines H antigen specificity?
    (a) L-fucose
    (b) N-acetyl galactosamine
    (c) D-galactose
    (d) N-acetyl glucosamine

139. The lowest molecular weight limit for a substance to be a good antigen is considered to be:
    (a) 5000 - 7000 MW
    (b) 40,000 - 50,000 MW
    (c) 100,000 - 120,000 MW
    (d) 300 - 500 MW

140. The portion of the immunoglobulin molecule thought to determine antibody specificity is located in the:
    (a) constant portion of the molecule
    (b) variable portion of the molecule
    (c) hinge region of the molecule
    (d) none of the above

141. The antibody formed in the secondary response is usually:
    (a) IgM
    (b) IgG
    (c) IgA
    (d) IgD

142. The four ABO alleles, A_1, A_2, B and O give rise to:
    (a) three genotypes and three phenotypes
    (b) four genotypes and ten genotypes
    (c) ten genotypes and four phenotypes
    (d) ten genotypes and six phenotypes

143. The serum of which of the following usually contains anti-A_1?
    (a) A_2
    (b) A_{int}
    (c) A_m
    (d) A_3

144. Individuals with acquired B antigen:
    (a) have normal anti-B in their serum
    (b) secrete A, B and H substances in their saliva
    (c) have anti-B-like antibodies in their serum
    (d) are always non-secretors

145. The A and B antigens:
    (a) are fully developed at birth
    (b) increase in strength during fetal life
    (c) are detectable long before birth
    (d) all of the above

146. Pure anti-H:
    (a) is found as a non-red-cell-immune antibody in all individuals
    (b) is found in an extract of the seeds of *Dolichos biflorus*
    (c) is found in Bombay (O_h) individuals
    (d) is found in a number of seed extracts, all of which are commonly used in the laboratory

147. Which of the following are usually used in forward (direct) ABO grouping?
    (a) Anti-A and anti-B only
    (b) Anti-A, anti-B and anti-A,B

(c) A_1 cells and B cells only
(d) A_1 cells, B cells and O cells

148. The genes *le*, *h* and *se* are:
    (a) amorphic
    (b) dominant
    (c) recessive
    (d) none of the above

149. Anti-Le^a can be produced by:
    (a) secretors who are Le(a-b+)
    (b) non-secretors who are le(a-b+)
    (c) secretors who are Le(a-b-)
    (d) non-secretors who are *Lele*

150. Anti-Le^a has been produced in:
    (a) chickens
    (b) rabbits
    (c) goats
    (d) all of the above

151. Le(a-) parents can produce:
    (a) Le(a-) offspring only
    (b) Le(a+) offspring only
    (c) Le(a-) or Le(a+) offspring
    (d) Le(b+) offspring only

152. Anti-Le^x:
    (a) reacts with the same proportion of adult and cord red cells
    (b) fails to react with O, A_1 and A_2 red cells
    (c) is considered to be a specific agglutinin with a corresponding receptor, X
    (d) is not inhibited by saliva from Le(a-b-) non-secretors

153. The guinea-pig anti-rhesus antibody is known as:
    (a) anti-Rh
    (b) anti-rh
    (c) anti-Rh$_1$
    (d) anti-LW

154. According to the Wiener nomenclature and/or genetic theory of Rh inheritance:
    (a) there are three closely linked loci, each with a primary set of allelic genes
    (b) the alleles are named R^1, R^2, r, R^O, r', r'', R^z and r^x
    (c) there are an infinite number of alleles at a single complex locus, each determining its own agglutinogen, which comprise multiple factors
    (d) the antigens are named D, C, E, c and e

155. The structure of the Rh antigen is maintained by surrounding lipid. This lipid:
    (a) carries the antigenic determinants
    (b) determines the antigenicity of the molecule
    (c) may be essential for the conformation of the antigen
    (d) none of the above

156. The D^u antigen:
    (a) is a weak form of the D antigen, giving some but not all of the reactions of normal D
    (b) is always genetically determined
    (c) is not detectable in the indirect antiglobulin test
    (d) is clinically insig-nificant

157. D^u red cells:
    (a) react with 'genuine' saline anti-D only
    (b) are classified as Rh$_O$(D)- positive in recipients of transfusion
    (c) react with anti-D^u
    (d) none of the above

158. The Rh$_{null}$ condition:
    (a) refers to the lack of C and e antigens
    (b) refers to individuals with normal red cells
    (c) may be due to an amorphic gene at the Rh complex locus
    (d) is formed in response to transfusion or pregnancy

159. The red cells of individuals who are Rh$_{null}$:
    (a) appear as stomatocytes
    (b) lack some membrane component
    (c) survive normally
    (d) (a) and (b) are correct

160. Rh antibodies:
    (a) are capable of causing severe hemolytic disease of the newborn
    (b) are capable of causing severe hemolytic transfusion reactions
    (c) are clinically significant
    (d) all of the above

161. False negative reactions in Rh typing may be caused by:
    (a) a reagent antibody which recognizes only a compound antigen
    (b) the presence of a contaminating antibody in the test

reagent
(c) panagglutination
(d) polyagglutination

162. The K^o gene:
(a) can be considered to
be an allele at the
Kell locus
(b) produces no Kell antigens
(c) could be a rare allele
at a Kell operator
site which depresses
the activity of its
neighboring K, Kp and
Js sites
(d) all of the above

163. In a person who is K+,
Kp(a+):
(a) the k antigen is
weaker than normal
when produced by the
same gene complex
which produces Kp^a
(b) the k antigen is
stronger than normal
when produced by the
same gene complex
which produces Kp^a
(c) the K antigen is weaker
than normal when pro-
duced by the same gene
complex which produces
Kp^a
(d) all Kell antigens are
weaker than normal

164. Which of the following antibodies is compatible with
McLeod red cells?
(a) anti-Claas
(b) anti-K^o
(c) anti-K10
(d) anti-Ku

165. The Fy^a antigen occurs in:
(a) 10 per cent of whites
(b) 66 per cent of whites
(c) 98 per cent of whites
(d) 30 per cent of whites

166. The gene Fy^x:
(a) is the white (Caucasian)
equivalent of the Fy
gene
(b) is an independent,
modifying gene which
affects the expression
of the Fy^a gene
(c) is independent of the
Fy gene
(d) none of the above

167. The Fy^a and Fy^b antigenic
determinants:
(a) are thermostable
(b) exist naturally in
a soluble form
(c) are inactivated by
heating red cells
to 56°C for 10 minutes
(d) are not affected by
formaldehyde treatment

168. Anti-Fy^a and anti-Fy^b are
usually:
(a) IgG
(b) IgM
(c) IgA
(d) IgD

169. The Fy3 antigen:
(a) is the product of
an allele, Fy^x at
the $Duffy$ locus
(b) is unaffected by
enzyme treatment
of the red cells
(c) reacts with anti-Fy^b
(d) all of the above

170. Anti-Fy^a and anti-Fy^b are:
(a) clinically signifi-
cant antibodies
(b) clinically insigni-
ficant antibodies
(c) unable to cause hemolytic disease of the
newborn
(d) never involved in delayed hemolytic trans-
fusion reaction

171. The phenotype:
    (a) Jk(a+b+) is most common among whites
    (b) Jk(a-b+) is most common among whites
    (c) Jk(a+b-) is most common among blacks
    (d) Jk(a+b-) is most common among whites

172. Anti-Jk^a and anti-Jk^b:
    (a) are usually IgM
    (b) are usually IgG
    (c) may be IgM
    (d) are usually IgA

173. The Jk^a and Jk^b antigens:
    (a) are poorly developed at birth
    (b) are well developed at birth
    (c) are useful anthropological markers
    (d) occur infrequently in Polynesians

174. Anti-Jk3:
    (a) behaves as 'inseparable' anti-Jk^a plus anti-Jk^b
    (b) is known to be cross-reacting anti-Jk^a plus anti-Jk^b
    (c) is usually non-red-cell-immune
    (d) is commonly found in individuals of phenotype Jk(a+b+)

175. The Lu(a-b-) phenotype is sometimes inherited:
    (a) as a 'recessive' character
    (b) due to homozygosity for the rare allele, *Lu*
    (c) as a 'dominant' character
    (d) all of the above

176. The allele which converts the Lu precursor substance into a form such that it is unable to affect the production of Lu antigens is called:
    (a) *Lu*
    (b) *In(Lu)*
    (c) *Lu(De1)*
    (d) Lu(a-b-)

177. Anti-Lu^b:
    (a) is found not uncommonly in Lu(a-b-) individuals following transfusion or pregnancy
    (b) is usually IgM
    (c) commonly causes *in vitro* lysis
    (d) is usually non-red-cell-immune

178. Which of the following is used as a positive control in typing for the Lu^b antigen?
    (a) Lu(a-b+) red cells
    (b) Lu(a+b+) red cells
    (c) Lu(a+b-) red cells
    (d) Red cells resulting from the genotype *LuLu*

179. The Lu^b antigen of Lu(a-b+) cord red cells is:
    (a) weaker than that of adults
    (b) stronger than that of Lu(a+b+) infants
    (c) stronger than that of adults
    (d) fully developed at birth

180. Blood samples which give negative reactions with anti-U also give negative reactions with:
    (a) anti-M and anti-N
    (b) anti-S and anti-s
    (c) anti-S only
    (d) anti-M only

181. The so-called Miltenberger
     subsystem involves:
     (a) four classes of reac-
         tion pattern
     (b) five classes of reac-
         tion pattern
     (c) antigens which are all
         reactive with anti-Mi^a
     (d) antigens which are all
         reactive with anti-S

182. Anti-N:
     (a) will agglutinate M-
         positive red cells at
         temperatures of 23°C
         or lower
     (b) is usually non-red-cell-
         immune
     (c) has never caused hemo-
         lytic disease of the
         newborn
     (d) is found almost exclu-
         sively in S-s- indivi-
         duals

183. Anti-s:
     (a) is commonly found as
         an immune antibody in
         multitransfused patients
     (b) is usually IgG
     (c) always binds complement
     (d) is clinically insigni-
         ficant

184. Anti-M and anti-N reagent
     antisera:
     (a) may be prepared from
         human serum
     (b) may be prepared from
         goat serum
     (c) usually react best in
         the indirect anti-
         globulin test
     (d) usually react best with
         enzyme-treated red
         cells

185. In light of the discovery
     that P-negative individuals
     share a powerful antigen
     with P-positive individuals

and do not lack an antigen
of the P blood group system,
as was originally thought,
the P-negative phenotype
became known as:
     (a) P_1
     (b) Tj(a-)
     (c) P_2
     (d) P_3

186. The P_1 antigen:
     (a) is inhibited by the
         gene *In(Lu)*
     (b) occurs in a wide
         variety of strengths
     (c) is more common than
         the P_2 antigen
     (d) all of the above

187. The immunodominant sugar
     of the P_1 antigen is:
     (a) L-fucose
     (b) *N*-acetyl galactosamine
     (c) *N*-acetyl glucosamine
     (d) D-galactose

188. Anti-P_1:
     (a) can cause severe
         adverse transfusion
         reactions
     (b) commonly causes the
         destruction of P_1
         red cells *in vivo*
     (c) can always be regarded
         as clinically signi-
         ficant
     (d) has been implicated as
         the cause of hemolytic
         disease of the newborn

189. The differences between the
     I antigen of cord and adult
     red cells:
     (a) are qualitative only
     (b) are quantitative only
     (c) are both qualitative
         and quantitative
     (d) have not been class-
         ified

190. Red cells which have a small

amount of I antigen are classified as:
- (a) I_1
- (b) i_1
- (c) i_2
- (d) I_2

191. I substance has been found in:
- (a) saliva
- (b) human milk
- (c) amniotic fluid
- (d) urine

192. Anti-I:
- (a) is found as a weak cold agglutinin in the serum of most normal individuals
- (b) is usually clinically insignificant
- (c) is usually IgM
- (d) commonly binds complement

193. Anti-i:
- (a) is commonly encountered as an alloantibody
- (b) has been found in individuals suffering from infectious mononucleosis as a transient antibody
- (c) is a warm-reacting, IgG antibody
- (d) is usually a cold-reacting, IgM antibody

194. Anti-I:
- (a) has been implicated as the cause of hemolytic disease of the newborn
- (b) is clinically significant when reactive at 4 - 20°C *in vitro*
- (c) is clinically significant when reactive at 30 - 37°C *in vitro*
- (d) produces varying degrees of red cell destruction *in vivo*

which is well correlated with the *in vitro* thermal range

195. The I antigen:
- (a) occurs as a glycoprotein in secretions
- (b) could be a branched carbohydrate chain attached at an early stage in the biosynthetic pathway of the ABO antigens
- (c) develops during the first eighteen months of life
- (d) all of the above

196. The Bg antigens are, in reality, HLA antigens which demonstrate weakly on the red cells. The Bg^a antigen is known to correspond to:
- (a) HLA-A2
- (b) HLA-B7
- (c) HLA-Bw17
- (d) HLA-A28

197. Anti-Ch^a (Chido):
- (a) is neutralized by the plasma and serum of Ch(a+) individuals
- (b) is neutralized by the saliva of Ch(a+) individuals
- (c) is absorbed by the leukocytes of Ch(a+) individuals
- (d) reduces the survival of Ch(a+) red cells *in vivo*

198. The antigen Rg^a (Rogers):
- (a) occurs in about 10 per cent of whites
- (b) is an antigen on C4 molecules
- (c) occurs in more than

95 per cent of whites
(d) none of the above

199. Which of the following statements is correct?
(a) The gene locus origi-
nally known as *LA* is
now known as *HLA-B*
(b) The gene locus origi-
nally known as *Four* is
now known as *HLA-A*
(c) The gene locus origi-
nally known as *MLC* is
now known as *HLA-D*
(d) The gene locus origi-
nally known as *AK* is
now known as *HLA-B*

200. There is a dramatic association between HLA-B27 and the
disease:
(a) Syphillis
(b) Ankylosing spondylitis
(c) Influenza
(d) None of the above

201. HLA antibodies are characteristically:
(a) IgG
(b) IgM
(c) IgA
(d) IgD

202. Cytotoxic HLA antibodies:
(a) do not occur in preg-
nant women
(b) occur in about 80 per
cent of women after
the first pregnancy
(c) occur in about 95 per
cent of women after
three pregnancies
(d) occur in about 55 per
cent of women after
three pregnancies

203. Causative antibodies in
'warm' antibody autoimmune
hemolytic anemia:
(a) usually react well at
37°C

(b) usually react more
strongly at 20°C
than at 37°C
(c) react as well or
better at 37°C than
at lower tempera-
tures
(d) are usually IgG

204. Which of the following
antibodies are associated
with autoimmune hemolytic
anemia of the warm anti-
body type?
(a) Anti-K
(b) Anti-U
(c) Anti-Rh$_0$(D)
(d) anti-Jk^a

205. When fresh serum is used,
the complement components
detected *in vitro* in cold
antibody type autoimmune
hemolytic anemia include:
(a) C4c, C4d, C3c and
C3d
(b) C3d and C4d only
(c) C3c and C4c only
(d) C3c and C4d only

206. Most antibodies in cold
type autoimmune hemolytic
anemia have the specificity:
(a) anti-Pr
(b) anti-I
(c) anti-i
(d) anti-Rh

207. The tests used to detect
paroxysmal nocturnal hemoglobinuria are:
(a) the indirect anti-
globulin test
(b) the Ham test
(c) the sucrose hemolysis
test
(d) the direct antiglobulin
test

208. The drug penicillin can cause
a positive direct antiglobulin

test and hemolytic anemia
by the:
- (a) immune complex
  mechanism
- (b) drug adsorption
  mechanism
- (c) non-immunologic
  protein adsorption
  mechanism
- (d) aldomet mechanism

209. The destruction of red cells
transfused to a patient
with autoimmune hemolytic
anemia may be:
- (a) greater than the
  destruction of the
  patient's own cells
  at first, but will
  eventually equalize
- (b) less than the
  destruction of the
  patient's own cells,
  and will not equalize
- (c) equal to the destruction of the patient's
  own cells, but will
  decrease with time
- (d) none of the above

210. Immune anti-A and anti-B
in group B and group A
subjects, respectively, is
usually:
- (a) IgG
- (b) IgA
- (c) IgM
- (d) IgG4

211. Routine laboratory tests
performed on a mother's
first prenatal specimen
should include:
- (a) ABO grouping
- (b) Rh typing
- (c) antibody screening
- (d) (a) and (b) are correct

212. Anti-Le^a and anti-Le^b:
- (a) commonly cause hemolytic disease of the

newborn
- (b) do not cause hemo-
  lytic disease of the
  newborn
- (c) occur relatively
  commonly during preg-
  nancy
- (d) do not occur during
  pregnancy

213. If a mother is $Rh_o(D)$-negative
with no irregular antibodies
and tests on the father reveal him also to be $Rh_o(D)$-
negative:
- (a) hemolytic disease of
  the newborn can be
  discounted
- (b) hemolytic disease of
  the newborn due to
  Rh can be discounted
- (c) hemolytic disease of
  the newborn due to
  $Rh_o(D)$ can be dis-
  counted
- (d) hemolytic disease of
  the newborn due to
  'other' antigens is
  more likely

214. Amniocentesis is indicated:
- (a) if a mother has an
  antiglobulin titer
  of 32 or higher for
  a significant anti-
  body
- (b) if a mother has an
  antiglobulin titer
  of 4 or higher for
  a significant anti-
  body
- (c) if a mother has a
  history of producing
  children suffering
  from hemolytic disease
  of the newborn
- (d) (b) and (c) are correct

215. Blood used for intrauterine
transfusion:
- (a) is normally group O

Rh$_0$(D)-negative
(b)   is normally group O
Rh$_0$(D)-positive
(c)   is given as whole
blood
(d)   is given as packed
red cells

216.   Rh immune globulin is given
to Rh$_0$(D)-negative women:
(a)   who have had first
trimester amniocentesis
(b)   whose serum contains
anti-Rh$_0$(D)
(c)   who have had an ectopic
pregnancy
(d)   who have had abortions

217.   Except in special circumstances and with the written
consent of a physician, the
interval between blood donations must be a minimum of:
(a)   eight months
(b)   eight weeks
(c)   ten weeks
(d)   four weeks

218.   Citrate toxicity in patients
undergoing discontinuous
leukapheresis or plateletpheresis can be avoided:
(a)   by using half-strength
ACD-A or sodium citrate
(b)   by using ACD-B solution
(c)   by using concentrated
ACD-A solution
(d)   by using CPD instead
of ACD

219.   The procedure whereby platelets are separated centri-
fugally from whole blood
with the continuous or intermittent return of platelet-
poor whole blood to the donor
is known as:
(a)   leukapheresis
(b)   plateletpheresis
(c)   plasmapheresis
(d)   thrombapheresis

220.   In the testing of blood
donations, it is important
to perform the following
tests on the donor's serum:
(a)   antibody screening
(b)   syphilis testing
(c)   ABO and Rh typing
(d)   hepatitis testing

221.   To be issued as whole
blood, a unit must contain:
(a)   between 405 and 495
ml of blood
(b)   between 450 and 460
ml of blood
(c)   between 400 and 450
ml of blood
(d)   exactly 480 ml of
blood

222.   In the preparation of
platelet concentrates:
(a)   the donation time
should not exceed
eight minutes
(b)   the units to be used
must be kept at room
temperature at all
times before and
during platelet sepa-
ration
(c)   the preparation must
begin no more than
four hours after
donation
(d)   donations from individuals who are
taking aspirin-contain-
ing compounds are
acceptable

223.   Leukocyte-poor red blood
cells:
(a)   can be stored for 21
days at 2 - 6°C if a
'closed' system is
used in preparation
(b)   should not be stored
but should be infused
as soon as possible
after collection

(c) can be prepared by
     filtration
(d) (b) and (c) are correct

224. Stored plasma:
(a) may be prepared from
     the supernatant plasma
     after cryoprecipitate
     production
(b) may be stored at 2 -
     6°C for 26 days from
     phlebotomy
(c) may be stored at -18°C
     for five years
(d) may be stored at 2 -
     6°C for five years

225. Human serum albumin:
(a) should be stored
     frozen
(b) is prepared from
     normal human plasma
     by cold ethanol
     plasma fractionation
(c) can be stored at room
     temperature for three
     years
(d) is not indicated in
     cases of chronic
     nephrosis

226. Cryoprecipitated antihemo-
      philic factor is indicated
      in cases of:
(a) von Willebrand's disease
(b) disseminated intra-
     vascular coagulation
(c) transfusional dilution
     in massive transfusion
(d) all of the above

227. Isotonic saline is prepared
      by:
(a) dissolving 9.5 g of
     sodium chloride in one
     liter of distilled
     water
(b) dissolving 8.5 g of
     sodium chloride in one
     liter of distilled
     water

(c) dissolving 8.5 g of
     potassium chloride
     in one liter of dis-
     tilled water
(d) dissolving 8.5 g of
     sodium chloride in
     two liters of dis-
     tilled water

228. Preparations of bovine
      albumin vary greatly in
      their potentiating effect,
      apparently depending on
      the:
(a) storage of the solution
(b) polymer content
(c) species origin of the
     solution
(d) none of the above

229. Which of the following
      antibodies are enhanced
      in their reactions when
      enzyme-treated red cells
      are used?
(a) Anti-M
(b) Anti-I
(c) anti-P_1
(d) (b) and (c) are
     correct

230. The characteristics of
      the reactions of T-activated
      red cells are:
(a) the cells are agglu-
     tinated by most sera
     from newborn infants
(b) the reactions are
     strongest at 37°C
(c) the reactions are
     strongest with fresh
     serum
(d) the cells react better
     with serum containing
     anti-A than with those
     that do not

231. Polyagglutination due to
      Tn-activation:
(a) is persistent rather
     than transient (as

with T and Tk-activation)

(b) is transient rather than persistent

(c) is associated with gross infection

(d) may be found in people described as always healthy

232. Wharton's jelly:
(a) is usually present in cord samples which have been collected by cutting the umbilical cord and allowing the blood to drain into the tube

(b) is usually present in samples which have been collected from the umbilical vein

(c) may cause red cells to agglutinate spontaneously

(d) is present in all adult samples

233. Prozone phenomenon:
(a) is sometimes observed in titration of antibodies in which the antibody apparently reacts more strongly with serum when it is undiluted than when it is diluted

(b) has been attributed to lack of proportions between antigen and antibody

(c) may be due to the use of fresh serum containing complement

(d) is sometimes seen in the antiglobulin test as a result of partial neutralization of the antiglobulin reagent

234. The non-specific reactions (agglutination) of red cells caused by colloidal silica:
(a) may be seen when solutions are stored in glass bottles

(b) may be seen when tests are performed on glass slides

(c) may be seen when solutions are stirred with a glass rod

(d) all of the above

235. Adverse reactions to transfusion have been recorded in:
(a) 6.6 per cent of recipients

(b) 1 per cent of recipients

(c) 55 per cent of recipients

(d) 20 per cent of recipients

236. The reaction of anti-A or anti-B with their corresponding antigens *in vivo* would be an example of:
(a) internal destruction

(b) intravascular destruction

(c) external destruction

(d) extravascular destruction

237. The most common signs of extravascular red cell destruction are:
(a) fever and jaundice

(b) fever and hemoglobinemia

(c) chills and jaundice

(d) chills and fever

238. Hemolytic transfusion reactions can be caused by:
(a) the transfusion of incompatible red

cells to a patient
whose plasma contains
an antibody directed
against an antigen on
the transfused red cells
(b) the injection of water
into the circulation
(c) the injection of blood
into the circulation
under pressure
(d) the transfusion of blood
containing antibody

239. In a delayed transfusion reaction, the causative antibody is generally too weak
to be detected in routine
crossmatching, but becomes
detectable:
(a) 60 - 90 days after
transfusion
(b) 3 - 6 hours after
transfusion
(c) 3 - 7 days after
transfusion
(d) 120 days after
transfusion

240. Bacteriogenic transfusion
reactions may be caused by:
(a) pyrogens
(b) contamination at the
time of blood collec-
tion
(c) flaws in the blood
container
(d) all of the above

241. The reaction to circulatory
overload is characterized by:
(a) coughing
(b) cyanosis
(c) difficulty in breathing
(d) all of the above leading to congestive heart
failure

242. The amount of CPD anticoagulant in a unit of blood is:
(a) 67.5 ml
(b) 63.0 ml

(c) 70.0 ml
(d) 65.0 ml

243. In the auto-absorption
procedure for the removal
of cold auto-agglutinins
from serum, pretreatment
of the patient's red cells
with one of the following
reagents is often helpful:
(a) 2-mercaptoethanol
(b) phosphate buffered
saline at pH 9.0
(c) ficin
(d) albumin

244. With respect to broad-
spectrum antiglobulin
reagent:
(a) the antibodies in
this reagent that
attach to the Fc
portion of human
antibodies are IgM
(b) this reagent is
sensitive enough to
detect as few as 10 -
20 antibody molecules
per red cell
(c) all batches of the
reagent are identi-
cally manufactured to
ensure rigid quality
control
(d) red cells from a
patient with cold
hemagglutinin disease
may be agglutinated
by the anti-complement
fraction of this reagent

245. A blood sample was received
for crossmatching. The
blood group was found to be
A $Rh_0(D)$-positive and the
antibody screen and direct
antiglobulin tests were
found to be negative. Six
units of group A $Rh_0(D)$-
positive blood were cross-
matched and one unit was

found to be weakly incompatible in the antiglobulin test.
The same result was obtained
when the test was repeated on
this unit. In this situation,
which of the following should
be done *first*?
  (a) Repeat the ABO grouping
       on the incompatible
       unit using a more sen-
       sitive technique
  (b) Set up an antibody in-
       vestigation panel made
       up of red cells which
       possess low-frequency
       antigens and test these
       against the patient's
       serum
  (c) Perform a direct anti-
       globulin test on the
       donor blood
  (d) obtain a new specimen
       of blood from the
       patient and repeat the
       crossmatch with a new
       serum sample

246. A 26 year old AB Rh_0(D)-
      negative female requires
      a transfusion. There are
      no AB Rh_0(D)-negative donor
      units available. Which of
      the following should be
      chosen for transfusion?
        (a) A Rh_0(D)-negative
             blood
        (b) O Rh_0(D)-negative red
             cells
        (c) B Rh_0(D)-negative
             blood
        (d) A Rh_0(D)-negative red
             cells
        (e) A Rh_0(D)-positive red
             cells

247. A patient has a mixture of
      antibodies, and preliminary
      testing suggests that one of
      them is IgM anti-Le^a. Which
      of the following tests would
      help to identify any other

antibodies which might be
present?
  (a) Treatment of the
       serum with 2-mercap-
       toethanol
  (b) Performing the tests
       at 56°C
  (c) Addition of saliva
       from a Le(a+b-)
       individual
  (d) Enzyme treating the
       panel red cells
  (e) Heat the serum to 56°C
       for 30 minutes

248. When testing blood samples
      from individuals with weak
      subgroups of A, the following
      may be observed: .
        (a) the red cells may
             react with anti-A,B
        (b) the red cells may
             type as group O
        (c) the serum may contain
             anti-A_1
        (d) an increase in the
             incidence of immune
             antibodies

249. With respect to the sugar-
      water test:
        (a) it is a screening
             test for paroxysmal
             nocturnal hemoglobinuria
        (b) it is a screening
             test for paroxysmal
             cold hemoglobinuria
        (c) if the test is per-
             formed on the blood
             of a patient who has
             been recently trans-
             fused, the results
             may be unreliable
        (d) the principle of this
             test is often used to
             prepare complement-
             coated red cells

250. In a centrifuge the relative
      centrifugal force does not
      depend on:

(a) the number of revolu-
     tions per minute
(b) the radius of the cen-
     trifuge head
(c) the viscosity of the
     contents of the tube
(d) the diameter of the
     sample container

SECTION B: HEADINGS

*For each numbered word or phrase,
select the heading that is most
closely related to it.*

(1) (a) Isotonic saline
     (b) Bovine albumin
     (c) Low ionic strength
          solution
     (d) Proteolytic enzyme
     (e) Complement
     (f) Lectin

251. Prepared from beef blood.
      ANSWER: _____

252. Plant agglutinin.
      ANSWER: _____

253. The antigen Fy^a is weakened
      or inactivated by this.
      ANSWER: _____

254. The solution is of the same
      osmotic pressure as the
      contents of the human red
      cell.
      ANSWER: _____

255. The refractive indices of
      bacteria and this solution
      are very similar.
      ANSWER: _____

256. The solution acts to increase
      the rate of uptake of certain
      antibodies.
      ANSWER: _____

257. This solution is sometimes
      added to the test system
      in order to demonstrate a
      hemolytic antibody.
      ANSWER: _____

258. *Dolichos biflorus* is an
      example.
      ANSWER: _____

259. Prepared with sodium chlor-
      ide and distilled water.
      ANSWER: _____

260. A 22 per cent solution is
      better than normal serum
      at enhancing agglutination
      of IgG anti-Rh.
      ANSWER: _____

261. Trypsin is an example.
      ANSWER: _____

262. This solution may be ob-
      tained from human or ani-
      mal serum.
      ANSWER: _____

263. The use of this solution
      tends to give false posi-
      tive results with greater
      frequency than with other
      solutions.
      ANSWER: _____

264. One is an extract from the
      pineapple.
      ANSWER: _____

265. Concentrations of 30 per
      cent have a tendency to
      cause rouleaux formation.
      ANSWER: _____

(2) (a) Anti-I
     (b) Anti-i
     (c) Anti-I^T

266. Possessed by most normal
      sera.
      ANSWER: _____

267. Fetal red cells react more strongly than cord red cells.
ANSWER: _____

268. Has not been described as an alloantibody.
ANSWER: _____

269. The red cells of phenotype I-i- react weakly with this antibody.
ANSWER: _____

270. Has once been implicated as the cause of hemolytic disease of the newborn.
ANSWER: _____

SECTION C: TRUE OR FALSE

Mark the following statements either TRUE (T) or FALSE (F).

271. A gene is a sequence of codons which contain the code for a single amino acid.

272. The action of ribosomes in protein synthesis is specific - certain ribosomes being committed to produce only certain kinds of protein.

273. A somatic cell is said to be 'diploid' in nature.

274. A 'mutation' is a qualitative or quantitative change in a gene which may result in the formation of a 'new' gene.

275. The injection of an antibody which survives and protects temporarily in the host is known as 'active' immunity.

276. IgM is the only immunoglobulin that is transferred across the placenta.

277. Treatment of IgA with 2-mercaptoethanol does not affect the serological activity of these antibodies.

278. The antibody formed initially in the primary immune response is always IgM.

279. Individuals of the Bombay phenotype test as group O even when normal A and/or B genes have been inherited.

280. The term 'secretor' refers only to individuals who are homozygous for the Se gene.

281. Anti-A_1 reactivity below 25°C is considered to be clinically significant.

282. When performing tests with respect to the ABO blood group system, controls may be considered unnecessary.

283. Red cells acquire their Lewis phenotype by adsorption of Lewis substances from the plasma.

284. Individuals who are of genotype $lele$ are either of phenotype Le(a-b+) or Le(a+b-).

285. The $Sese$ locus controls the secretion of Lewis substances.

286. Transfused Le(a+) and Le(b+) red cells lose their Lewis antigens within a few days after transfusion and become Le(a-b-).

287. R_1 is made up of at least three factors, called rh', Rh_0 and rh".

288. There is a specific anti-D^u serum.

289. The *LW* and *Rh* genes are inherited together.

290. Rh antibodies commonly bind complement.

291. The Sutter groups are related to the Kell blood group system.

292. Certain Kell antigens are found exclusively in whites or exclusively in blacks.

293. Non-red-cell-immune antibodies in the Kell system are extremely common.

294. Anti-K cannot cause hemolytic disease of the newborn.

295. The gene which is responsible for the Fy(a-b-) phenotype is called *Fy*.

296. The *Fy^b* gene is recessive.

297. Numerous examples of non-red-cell-immune anti-Fy^a have been reported.

298. Duffy antisera react best in the two-stage papain test.

299. *Jk^a* and *Jk^b* are inherited as mendelian co-dominants.

300. Anti-Jk^a and anti-Jk^b deteriorate rapidly on storage *in vitro*.

301. In some instances, the addition of complement may prove helpful in detecting very weak Kidd antibodies.

302. Anti-Jk^a and anti-Jk^b deter-

iorate rapidly *in vivo*.

303. The Lu(a-b-) phenotype may be inherited as a recessive or a dominant character.

304. With the use of anti-Lu^a and anti-Lu^b, four phenotypes can be distinguished.

305. In the heterozygote, the Lu^a antigen is only weakly expressed at birth.

306. Tests for the presence of the Lu^a antigen are usually performed at 37°C, unless an incubator is not available.

307. Sialic acid is an essential part of the M and N receptors.

308. Strong dosage effect can occur with anti-M.

309. Examples of anti-M have been reported that are dependent on an acid pH for their reactivity.

310. The reaction strength between anti-N and M-positive red cells is influenced by the Ss group of the red cells.

311. The inhibitor locus *In(Lu)* is linked to the *P* locus.

312. Anti-P$_1$ is frequently found in pregnant women who are of phenotype P$_2$. This fact is connected with alloimmunization in pregnancy.

313. Anti-P reacts equally strongly with P$_1$ and P$_2$ red cells.

314. Anti-P$_1$ has been implicated in hemolytic disease of the newborn.

315. The I antigen of normal individuals has been found to be of varying strength.

316. I inhibiting substances have not been found in urine.

317. Hydatid cyst fluid has been found to inhibit some anti-I sera.

318. The detection and identification of anti-I and anti-i require the testing of both cord and adult red cells.

319. The antigen 'Cad' has been shown to be a very strong form of Sd^a.

320. Cad red cells are agglutinated by *Dolichos biflorus* seed extracts, regardless of the ABO blood group of the cells.

321. Antigens of high frequency in the population are also known as 'private' antigens.

322. HLA antibodies can form troublesome contaminants in red cell typing sera.

323. Cross reactions commonly occur in practical testing with HLA antisera.

324. Absorption is the take-up of antibody by the red cells.

325. In cold antibody type autoimmune hemolytic anemia, cold agglutinins have been described which are solely IgG.

326. In certain cases of autoimmune hemolytic anemia, the direct antiglobulin test may be negative.

327. Transfusion should be avoided wherever possible to patients with autoimmune hemolytic anemia.

328. Hemolytic disease of the newborn is caused by blood group incompatibility between the mother and the fetus.

329. Antibodies other than those of the ABO and Rh blood group systems do not cause hemolytic disease of the newborn.

330. The ABO form of hemolytic disease of the newborn does not occur in the first pregnancy.

331. In ABO hemolytic disease of the newborn, group O red cells of the same Rh type as the baby should be used for transfusion.

332. Autologous blood can be collected by the salvage of blood lost during surgery.

333. Blood or blood products which are intended for autologous use yet which are not used are usually reassigned for homologous use.

334. Blood products intended for autologous use need not be subject to any of the routine tests per-

formed on blood intended for homologous use.

335. The anticoagulant CPD gives better viability of red cells than ACD after the regular period of storage.

336. The optimum storage conditions for platelet storage appear to be a temperature of 22°C, with continuous gentle agitation.

337. Platelet transfusions are primarily useful for patients with idiopathic thrombocytopenic purpura.

338. If fresh frozen plasma is to be prepared from a unit of blood, the duration of the donation must not exceed eight minutes.

339. Fibrinogen is rarely used because it has a post-transfusion hepatitis risk of at least 25 per cent.

340. Bovine albumin should be stored at 4°C and should not be frozen.

341. One-stage enzyme techniques tend to be more sensitive than two-stage enzyme techniques.

342. The enzyme 'trypsin' agglutinates most red cells after brief periods of incubation with normal sera - although after about one hour at 37°C, 99 per cent of these will have become negative.

343. When animal serum is used as a source of complement, it is not necessary to absorb out heteroagglutinins.

344. In cases of panagglutination, all red cells are agglutinated by a given serum except those of the individual from whom the serum was derived.

345. Polyagglutination refers to the agglutination of a serum sample by many samples of red cells.

346. Three to five saline washes usually eliminates the reaction caused by Wharton's jelly.

347. A prozone phenomenon could be due to the presence of both IgM (agglutinating) and IgG (blocking) antibodies in the same serum.

348. The most common type of adverse transfusion reaction is characterized by shivering without recorded fever.

349. Probably the most common cause of severe anaphylactic reaction following transfusion is the interaction between transfused IgA and class-specific anti-IgA in the recipient's plasma.

350. The most common cause of hemolytic transfusion reaction involving intravascular red cell destruction is the administration of the wrong blood to a recipient due to inadequate identification, clerical error, etc.

351. Syphilis can be transmitted by blood transfusion even after prolonged storage of the blood.

352. The most common genotype of individuals with the phenotype DCcEe is R^2r.

353. The potassium content of red cells decreases during storage.

354. By raising the dielectric constant of a medium, red cells are able to approach one another more closely.

355. The phenotype Le(a+b-) indicates that the individual is homozygous for the *Lewis* gene.

356. Individuals who possess the Le^a antigen are secretors of ABH substances.

357. If an individual has a positive V.D.R.L. test, his/her blood may be used for transfusion.

358. An individual of genotype R^1r will have red cells which are reactive with anti-ce.

359. T-cells are involved in cell-mediated immunity.

360. The 'Bombay' phenotype refers to individuals who have a powerful H gene.

361. 20 per cent of individuals who are of genotype *lele* are secretors of ABH substances.

362. Rh antigens have not been detected on platelets.

363. The antigen Js^a is part of the Kell blood group system.

364. The Fy^a and Fy^b receptors are thought to be associated with susceptibility to malaria.

365. The Lu^a antigen is only weakly expressed on the red cells at birth.

366. Anti-I is classified as a heterophile antibody.

367. In 'warm' antibody type autoimmune hemolytic anemia, IgG can usually be detected on the red cells of the patient.

368. The anemia seen in hemolytic disease of the newborn is usually accompanied by an increase in reticulocytes and nucleated red cells.

369. The pH of blood stored in ACD is higher than that of blood stored in CPD.

370. Complement is inhibited at a temperature of 56°C.

SECTION D: QUESTIONS AND ANSWERS

Answer the following questions.

371. Name the four organic bases that exist in DNA.
ANSWER: _____

372. Give the term used to describe a full set of chromosomes (and therefore genes) inherited as a unit from one parent.
ANSWER: _____

373. Name the three formed elements of blood.
ANSWER: _____

374. What is the average life span of human platelets?
ANSWER: _____

375. Give the molecular weight of IgM.
ANSWER: _____

376. Give the term used to describe red cell destruction that takes place outside of the blood vessels within the reticuloendothelial system (liver, spleen).
ANSWER: _____

377. What percentage of individuals secrete substances in their saliva which have the same specificity as the antigens (ABO) on their red cells?
ANSWER: _____

378. Give the Lewis phenotype of individuals who inherit the *le* gene.
ANSWER: _____

379. What is the most common Rh antibody formed?
ANSWER: _____

380. What percentage of individuals who are Rh-negative will form anti-Rh_0(D) following transfusion with Rh-positive blood?
ANSWER: _____

381. What is the immunoglobulin class of most Rh antibodies?
ANSWER: _____

382. What is the symbol used to denote the Kell phenotype which lacks all Kell antigens?
ANSWER: _____

383. Give the numerical nomenclature equivalent for the antigen Fy^b.
ANSWER: _____

384. Give the antigen that is antithetical to Jk^a.
ANSWER: _____

385. Describe the typical type of reaction seen with anti-Lu^a when tested against Lu^a-positive red cells.
ANSWER: _____

386. Patients on renal dialysis may develop anti-N which is reactive at 4°C and 20°C but never at 37°C. Name the antigen that is responsible for the development of this antibody.
ANSWER: _____

387. What is the usual immunoglobulin class of anti-M antibodies which react more strongly in albumin or serum than in saline?
ANSWER: _____

388. To which blood group system does the Di^a antigen belong?
ANSWER: _____

389. What is the term used to describe antibodies which are directed against an individual's own tissues?
ANSWER: _____

390. Name the most common type of autoimmune hemolytic anemia.
ANSWER: _____

391. Under normal circumstances, what is the required interval between blood donations?
ANSWER: _____

392. What is the minimum hemoglobin requirement for male blood donors?

ANSWER: _____

393. Name the blood component that would be best recommended in cases of coagulation factor deficiencies (other than Factors V and VIII).
ANSWER: _____

394. Name the blood component that would be best recommended in cases of congenital Factor VII deficiency.
ANSWER: _____

395. What is the effect of proteolytic enzymes on the antigen Rg^a?
ANSWER: _____

396. Give the term used to describe that form of pseudoagglutination in which the red cells give the appearance of 'stacks of coins.'
ANSWER: _____

397. Give the term used to describe the phenomenon in which an antibody reacts more strongly with serum when it is diluted than when it is undiluted.
ANSWER: _____

398. What is the most common cause of febrile transfusion reactions?
ANSWER: _____

399. Name the procedure in which antibodies are removed from the red cells.
ANSWER: _____

400. What period of time must elapse after the termination of a pregnancy before the individual can be accepted as a blood donor?
ANSWER: _____

401. What is the specific gravity of the copper sulphate solution used to determine adequate hemoglobin levels in a male donor?
ANSWER: _____

402. Give the specificity of *Ulex europaeus* lectin.
ANSWER: _____

403. Give the term used to describe alternative forms of a gene at a particular locus.
ANSWER: _____

404. Give the term used to describe a female member of a family through whom the family comes to be genetically studied.
ANSWER: _____

405. Name the process of cell division through which the body grows and replaces discarded cells.
ANSWER: _____

406. At what age does IgM concentration reach adult levels?
ANSWER: _____

407. What is the term used to describe a dual population of red cells in a single individual?
ANSWER: _____

408. Name the complement components which do not participate in the alternative pathway of complement activation.
ANSWER: _____

409. In certain antibody mixtures

containing two antibodies, both antibodies are sometimes bound to red cells which lack one of the corresponding antigens. Give the term that describes this phenomenon.
ANSWER: _____

410. What type of immunity are T-cells (T-lymphocytes) primarily involved in?
ANSWER: _____

411. Give the term used to describe individuals who secrete ABH substances in saliva.
ANSWER: _____

412. What blood group substance is secreted by *all* secretors?
ANSWER: _____

413. Give the term used to describe a gene which produces no detectable product.
ANSWER: _____

414. To which chromosome has the *Rh* complex been assigned?
ANSWER: _____

415. What is the most common Kidd phenotype in black individuals?
ANSWER: _____

416. Name the antibody which reacts with red cells possessing the antigen which is antithetical to Lu9.
ANSWER: _____

417. Which antibody specificity has been reported to be in an extract of the seeds of *Iberis amara?*
ANSWER: _____

418. Give the term used to describe genes which produce a product only when they occur in the homozygous state.
ANSWER: _____

419. What is the immunodominant sugar of the P_1 antigen?
ANSWER: _____

420. Give the term used to describe the take-up of antibody by the red cells.
ANSWER: _____

SECTION E: SPECIAL QUESTIONS

421. Give the most probable genotypes in the following cases in the Wiener, Fisher-Race and Rosenfield nomenclatures:

	REACTIONS WITH ANTI-					WIENER	FISHER-RACE	ROSENFIELD
	C	D	E	c	e			
A)	+	+	+	+	+	_____	_____	_____
B)	+	+	-	-	+	_____	_____	_____
C)	-	+	+	+	-	_____	_____	_____
D)	-	-	-	+	+	_____	_____	_____
E)	-	-	+	+	+	_____	_____	_____
F)	+	-	+	+	+	_____	_____	_____
G)	+	-	-	+	+	_____	_____	_____
H)	-	+	-	+	+	_____	_____	_____
I)	-	+	+	+	+	_____	_____	_____
J)	+	+	+	-	-	_____	_____	_____

422. Select from the following list the antibodies which are capable of crossing the placenta (in the vast majority of cases):
    A) anti-c
    B) anti-P_1
    C) anti-A_1
    D) anti-M
    E) anti-s
    F) anti-k
    G) anti-Le^a
    H) anti-Fy^a
    I) anti-I
    J) anti-Le^b

423. State which blood group system the following antigens are part of:
    A) f
    B) k
    C) Jk^b
    D) Levay
    E) Rautenberg
    F) Hu
    G) Tj^a
    H) Yt^a
    I) Ri^a
    J) U

424. Examine the antibody identification panel on page 248 and identify

the following antibody(ies):

CELL NUMBER	SALINE (RT)	ENZYME	ANTIGLOBULIN
1	0	0	0
2	0	0	+
3	0	0	+
4	+	0	+
5	0	0	+
6	0	0	0
7	0	0	+
8	0	0	+
9	0	0	0
10	0	0	+
CORD	-	-	-

425. Using the same antibody identification panel on page 248, identify
the following antibody(ies):

CELL NUMBER	SALINE	ENZYME	ANTIGLOBULIN
1	0	0	2+
2	1+	0	4+
3	3+	0	4+
4	3+	2+	4+
5	1+	2+	0
6	0	0	0
7	3+	0	0
8	0	0	0
9	1+	0	0
10	0	2+	4+
CORD	0	2+	4+

BLOOD GROUP SYSTEM	Rh/Hr					MNSs				P	LEWIS		KELL		DUFFY		KIDD	
CELL NUMBER	D	C	E	c	e	M	N	S	s	P₁	a	b	K	k	a	b	a	b
1	0	+	0	0	+	+	+	0	0	+	0	0	0	+	0	0	+	+
2	+	+	0	0	+	+	+	0	+	+	0	+	0	+	+	+	0	+
3	+	+	0	0	+	0	+	+	0	+	+	0	+	+	+	+	0	+
4	+	0	+	+	0	+	0	0	+	0	+	0	0	+	+	0	+	+
5	0	0	+	+	0	+	+	0	+	+	0	+	0	+	+	+	0	+
6	0	0	0	+	+	0	+	0	+	+	0	0	0	+	0	0	+	0
7	0	0	0	+	+	+	+	0	+	+	+	0	+	0	+	0	+	+
8	0	0	0	+	+	+	+	+	+	+	0	0	0	+	0	0	+	+
9	0	0	0	+	+	+	+	+	0	+	0	+	+	+	+	+	0	+
10	+	+	+	+	+	0	+	+	+	+	0	0	0	+	+	0	0	+
CORD	-	-	-	-	-	-	-	-	-	-	0	0	-	-	-	-	-	-

ANTIBODY IDENTIFICATION PANEL

+ = Positive reaction
0 = Negative reaction
- = Not tested

ANSWERS

SECTION A: MULTIPLE CHOICE

1. (c) The red cells in the circulation have an average
life span of 100 - 120
days.

2. (a) The majority of blood
group genes are dominant.
Recessive genes are those
which express *only* when
they occur in the homo-
zygous state. (NOTE:
Strictly speaking, it
is the *trait* (the
phenotypic expression of
a gene) rather than the
gene itself which is
dominant or recessive,
but the terms 'dominant,
and, recessive genes'
are in common use).
There are several examples
of amorphic genes (e.g.,
O, *le*, *se*, *h*, etc. but
these do not constitute
the majority.

3. (d) IgG constitutes 85 per

cent of the total
immunoglobulin.

4. (d) B-cells are primarily
involved in humoral
antibody synthesis,
and constitute 10 -
20 per cent of periph-
eral blood lymphocytes.
T-cells are primarily
involved in cell-mediated
immunity.

5. (c) Antibodies which are produced in response to
antigens of another of
the same species are
known as alloantibodies.
If antibodies are pro-
duced in response to
antigens of another
(different) species,
these are known as
'xenoantibodies' or
'heterophile' antibodies.

6. (c) The enzyme 'trypsin'
splits the immunoglobulin
molecule into two Fab(t)

249

fragments and one Fc(t) fragment.

7. (d) IgG4 is the only immuno- globulin of the IgG class that does not initiate the complement sequence.

8. (d) ABH antigens are found on normoblasts, epidermal cells, spermatozoa, plate- lets, white cells, epithe- lial cells and cancer cells. The antigens are also found in serum and in most secretions and tissues of the human body. They are also found in animals, plants and bac- teria.

9. (b) Anti-A and anti-B are sometimes present in neo- natal sera, though in- frequently. These anti- bodies usually reach a maximum strength at 5 - 10 years of age.

10. (a) The two kinds of anti-Le^b sera are known as anti- Le^{bH} and anti-Le^{bL}. Anti- Le^{bH} is neutralized by the saliva of all ABH secre- tors and reacts only with A$_2$ and O red cells, where- as anti-Le^{bL} is not neu- tralized by the saliva of ABH secretors, but is neu- tralized by the saliva of Le(a-b+) individuals and reacts with the red cells of all blood groups.

11. (b) By age three months, over 80 per cent of children type as Le(a+b-). At birth, children type as Le(a-b-), and the adult frequency of Lewis antigens does not occur until about

age seven.

12. (a) The component parts of the D antigen mosaic are known as A, B, C and D.

13. (a) The majority of Rh antibodies are IgG. A *few* may contain IgM antibody (almost always accompanied by IgG antibody) and rare anti-D sera contain a minor IgA component.

14. (d) Hydatid cyst fluid will inhibit (in part) anti-P^k sera. Anti-P is only very weakly inhibited. Hydatid cyst fluid will not inhibit anti-Jk^a or anti-Le^a sera.

15. (a) Anti-S is commonly found as an immune antibody in multitrans- fused patients. The antibody is usually IgG. Only some examples of the antibody have the ability to bind complement, and, since the antibody has caused both hemolytic disease of the newborn and hemolytic transfusion reactions, it must be considered clinically significant.

16. (a) The M and N antigens
    (b) are glycoproteins.
    (c) They appear to be dependent on sialic acid in appropriate linkages for their integrity, and they are well developed at birth.

17. (a)   I antigens show a great
    (b)   range of strength from
    (d)   one individual to another,
          and are possessed by most
          healthy adults. The
          strength of the I antigen
          in any one individual,
          however, appears to be
          a constant property of
          the red cells.

18. (d)   The expression of HLA
          antigens is controlled
          by a region on chromo-
          some number 6.

19. (b)   The first HLA antigen
          to be described was
          called Mac. Under
          current nomenclature,
          this antigen is known
          as HLA-A2.

20. (b)   The antibodies most
          often implicated as
          the cause of hemolytic
          disease of the newborn
          are ABO and Rh antibodies.
          Other blood group anti-
          bodies seldom cause hemo-
          lytic disease of the new-
          born - although any anti-
          body which can occur as
          IgG can be causative.

21. (a)   If a baby has had repeated
    (b)   intrauterine transfusions,
    (c)   erroneous results may be
          obtained in ABO grouping,
          Rh typing and in the
          direct antiglobulin test.

22. (c)   The take-up of antibody
          by the red cells is known
          as adsorption. Absorp-
          tion (choice a) is the
          removal of antibody from
          the serum (usually by
          adsorption) and elution
          (choice b) is the removal
          of antibody from the red

cells.

23. (a)   The causative antibodies
    (c)   in 'cold' antibody auto-
          immune hemolytic anemia
          react best at room tem-
          perature or below and
          may have a wide thermal
          range.

24. (a)   In most cases of drug-
          induced hemolytic anemia,
          the immunoglobulin on
          the red cells is solely
          IgG1.

25. (c)   15 ml of ACD-A is re-
          quired to prevent the
          clotting of 100 ml of
          blood.

26. (b)   The specific gravity of
          the copper sulphate
          solution used for the
          determination of hemo-
          globin levels in male
          donors is 1.055.

27. (b)   The hemoglobin require-
          ment for female donors
          is 12.5 mg/dl.

28. (d)   Blood collected into
          heparin can only be
          stored for 48 hours,
          since the anticoagu-
          lant does not contain
          a preservative.

29. (c)   If the hermatic seal
          has been broken during
          the preparation of red
          blood cells (red cell
          concentrates), the red
          cells must be trans-
          fused within 24 hours.

30. (a)   Washed red blood cells
    (c)   may be used in cases
    (d)   of paroxysmal nocturnal
          hemoglobinuria. They

are prepared by manual washing or with the use of special cell-washing instruments, and they should not be stored, but rather should be prepared for a proposed transfusion.

31. (b) Factor IX concentrate
    (c) may be useful in cases
    (d) of congenital Factor VII deficiency, congenital Factor X deficiency and congenital Factor IX deficiency. Factor IX concentrate is *not* indicated for the treatment of patients with liver disease because of the risk of thrombosis or disseminated intravascular coagulation.

32. (d) When low ionic strength solution is used as a suspending medium in the antiglobulin test, the usual recommended incubation time is ten minutes.

33. (b) The antigen Ch^a is weakened or inactivated by proteolytic enzymes. The antigen Jk^a, C^w and i are generally enhanced in their activity by proteolytic enzymes.

34. (d) The specificity of the lectin derived from the plant *Ulex europaeus* is anti-H.

35. (b) The spontaneous agglutination of all red cells (irrespective of blood group) by a given serum is known as panagglutination.

36. (a) The latent receptor T
    (c) is contained in all
    (d) human red cells. It can be activated by various strains of bacteria, or by the enzymes derived from certain strains of bacteria.

37. (a) Rouleaux formation is
    (b) encountered if red cells
    (c) are allowed to sediment
    (d) in their own plasma, especially in individuals with a high sedimentation rate; in certain disease states involving high levels of immunoglobulin; in patients with serum protein abnormalities and in patients who are on fibrinogen therapy.

38. (a) Febrile transfusion
    (b) reactions may be due to
    (c) leukocyte antibodies, platelet antibodies or pyrogens.

39. (a) The antigens and anti-
    (b) bodies known or suspected of being associated with *anaphylactoid* transfusion reactions include IgG-anti-IgG and IgM-anti-IgM. This type of reaction can also be associated with human albumin transfusion hypersensitivity to passively acquired antibodies, hypersensitivity to passively acquired penicillin antibody or sensitivity to nickel. The severe *anaphylactic* transfusion reaction is usually the result of interaction between the transfused IgA and class-

specific anti-IgA in the
recipient's plasma.

40. (b) The probability of stimu-
         lating one or more anti-
         bodies to red cell anti-
         gens after one blood trans-
         fusion has been estimated
         to be about 1 per cent.

41. (d) 4.5 grams of sodium chlor-
         ide would be required to
         prepare half ($\frac{1}{2}$) a liter
         of physiological saline.

42. (a) The direct antiglobulin
         test is not generally
         performed on donor blood.

43. (c) The Betke-Kleihauer test
    (d) is an acid elution test
         which is used primarily
         to detect fetal red cells
         in the maternal circula-
         tion.

44. (c) The father's genotype is
         R^2r.

45. (b) A full complement of
    (c) chromosomes consists of
         46 single chromosomes
         (23 pairs); twenty-two
         pairs of chromosomes
         being autosomes and the
         remaining pair being
         the sex chromosomes.

46. (b) A 'zygote' is a ferti-
         lized ovum, formed after
         the gametes unite in the
         process of *fertilization*.
         The zygote obtains half
         of its chromosomes from
         the sperm and half from
         the ovum, making a full
         complement of 46 single
         chromosomes (23 pairs).

47. (b) The antigens K and k are
         antithetical. The term

'alleles' (choice a)
refers to genes, there-
fore the genes K and k
would be referred to
as alleles. The term
'amorphs' (choice c)
refers to genes which
produce no detectable
product; since the K
and k genes produce
the K and k antigens
respectively, these
genes are not amorphic.
Since the K and k
genes produce their
respective products
(antigens) regardless
of whether they occur
in the homozygous or
heterozygous state,
they are dominant and
not recessive. The
term 'recessive' refers
to genes and not antigens.

48. (d) According to the numer-
         ical nomenclature in
         the Kell system, Js^a
         is K6. The antigen K
         is K1 (choice a), the
         antigen k is K2 (choice
         b) and the antigen Kp^a
         is K3 (choice c).

49. (b) The majority of bloods
         from black donors
         (about 70 per cent) are
         of phenotype Fy(a-b-).

50. (c) The term 'genotype'
         refers to the total
         sum of genes present
         on a chromosome (with
         respect to one or more
         than one characteristic)
         regardless of whether
         or not they produce
         detectable products.
         By contrast, the term
         'phenotype'; refers
         to *detectable* products

only.

51. (c) *Mitosis* is the process of cell division by which the body grows and replaces discarded cells. Meiosis, on the other hand, is concerned with the production of sperm or ovum cells (known as 'gametes').

52. (a) If antibodies are transferred from mother to fetus, this is an example of *naturally acquired passive immunity*. Active immunity refers to the production of antibodies by the host, whereas passive immunity refers to the injection of antibody which survives temporarily in the host. Artificial immunity refers to the injection of virus (i.e., not acquired by naturally or 'normal' means).

53. (c) IgM consists of five basic structural units. There is no molecule that consists of ten basic structural units. The IgG molecule consists of one basic structural unit (monomer) and secretory IgA occurs in secretions mostly as a dimer (i.e., two structural units).

54. (a) Secretory IgA is made up of two basic structural units with a J-chain. It is not known to fix complement, is not transported across the human placenta and is not detectable in cord serum.

55. (b) Aggregates of IgA activate the alternative pathway of complement activation. Red cell antibodies and IgG activate the classic pathway of complement activation.

56. (b) With anti-H, the order of reactivity of red cells of various ABO groups (from the strongest reaction to the weakest) is dependent on the amount of unconverted H substance on the red cells. Since no conversion of H occurs in group O individuals, these individuals have the most H, and therefore give the strongest reaction with anti-H. In group A_1B individuals, however, almost all of the substance is converted to A and B substance, and therefore these individuals have the least H and give the weakest reaction with anti-H. The order of reactivity usually follows the pattern $O - A_2 - A_2B - B - A_1 - A_1B$.

57. (c) The secretion of ABH substances is controlled by the gene *Se*. The gene *se*, its allele, is amorphic.

58. (a) Anti-A_1 is present in all group O and group B individuals, along with anti-A (assuming normal immunoglobulin levels). The antibody is often IgM in group B individuals, IgG in group O

individuals. The anti-
body does not *always*
occur in group A_2B in-
dividuals (choice c) and,
when reactive below 25°C
(i.e. most examples) is
clinically insignificant.

59. (d) Anomalous results in ABO
testing are caused by a
great variety of factors,
including disease, irreg-
ular antibodies and un-
washed red cells.

60. (b) The inheritance of Lewis
substances is controlled
by the genes *Le* and *le*
and not Le^a and Le^b.
The Jk^a and Jk genes
(choice c) are involved
in the inheritance of
Kidd antigens and the *Se*
and *se* genes control the
inheritance of the ABH
antigens in secretions.

61. (b) The majority of Lewis
antibodies are IgM.

62. (b) An individual whose serum
possesses potent Lewis
antibodies should be
transfused with blood of
phenotype Le(a-b-).

63. (b) The Rh complex has been
assigned to chromosome
number 1.

64. (a) The antigen K1 is found
in 7 - 9 per cent of
random whites.

65. (a) The Fy^a and Fy^b antigens
are thought to be asso-
ciated with susceptibility
to malaria. The antigens
have low antigenicity and
are inactivated by enzyme
treatment of the red cells.

66. (a) The antibodies in
    (c) the Kidd system are
    (d) clinically significant.
They are usually (prob-
ably always) complement
binding, and are usually
found in conjunction
with other red cell
antibodies.

67. (c) There is evidence of
linkage between the
Lutheran and the
Secretor loci.

68. (c) Anti-Lu^a usually reacts
best at 12°C.

69. (a) The *M* and *N* genes give
    (d) rise to three genotypes
(*MM*, *MN* and *NN*) and
three phenotypes (M, MN
and N).

70. (c) Anti-P_1 may bind complement when reactive at
37°C. The antibody is
found in 90 per cent of
pregnant women who are
P_2, and is usually found
as a non-red-cell-immune
antibody. Anti-P_1 is
usually a cold reacting,
IgM antibody.

71. (b) Most infants appear to
be of phenotype i.

72. (c) Anti-Wr^a is not an HTLA
antibody (i.e., high-
titer-low-avidity).

73. (b) Individuals who are
HLA-B17-positive have
red cells possessing
the Bg^b antigen. In-
dividuals who have the
HLA-B7 antigen have
red cells possessing
the Bg^a antigen (choice
a) and individuals who

have the HLA-A28 antigen
have red cells possess-
ing the Bg^c antigen
(choice c).

74. (a) The complement components
    (c) involved in 'warm' anti-
        body autoimmune hemolytic
        anemia are C3d and C4d.
        C5 and C6 can also be
        demonstrated on the red
        cells in this type of
        autoimmune hemolytic
        anemia.

75. (b) When a fetus is ABO in-
        compatible with the
        mother, immunization due
        to Rh through pregnancy
        is less common. It is
        believed that this is
        because the Rh-positive
        fetal red cells are de-
        stroyed immediately on
        entering the maternal
        circulation by the exist-
        ing ABO antibodies.

76. (d) The procedure whereby a
        unit of blood is with-
        drawn from a donor to
        obtain plasma, followed
        by the reinfusion of the
        donor's red cells is
        known as plasmapheresis.

77. (d) The fact that a concen-
        trated form of the re-
        quired fraction can be
        administered, that the
        risk of circulatory over-
        load is reduced, and that
        many patients can be
        effectively treated from
        a single donation are all
        reasons why selective
        transfusion of specific
        blood components is pre-
        ferable to the routine
        use of whole blood.

78. (a) The enzyme papain is
        prepared from *Chorica
        papaya*.

79. (a) Rouleaux formation is
    (b) inhibited by saline,
    (d) glycine and sodium
        salicylate.

80. (b) The type of red cell
        destruction in which
        the red cells rupture
        within the blood stream
        with consequent libera-
        tion of hemoglobin into
        the plasma is known as
        intravascular destruc-
        tion.

81. (a) If you have a 30 per
        cent solution and you
        require a 5 per cent
        solution of the same
        substance, you could
        prepare 3 ml of a 5
        per cent solution with
        0.5 ml of the 30 per
        cent solution.

82. (b) False positive anti-
        globulin reactions may
        be caused by bacterial
        contamination of the
        red cells. Inadequate
        washing of red cells,
        underincuation of
        the cell-serum mixture
        or use of EDTA blood
        samples may cause false
        negative reactions.

83. (a) In the situation de-
        scribed, the woman
        should receive 1 x
        300 μl vial of Rh
        immune globulin.

84. (a) To minimize the risk
    (b) of bacteriogenic reac-
    (d) tions, blood should

(e) remain at refrigerator temperature at all times during storage; the blood container should not be opened or punctured to obtain a specimen; the recommended storage time must not be exceeded, and the blood should be examined visually before issue and after storage for an unusual color or the presence of hemolysis. Note that components prepared by 'open' procedures must be used within *24 hours* after preparation in order to minimize the risk of bacteriogenic transfusion reactions.

85. (a) Chagas' disease, infec-
    (b) tious mononucleosis and
    (c) leishmaniasis can all be transmitted by transfusion. Hypotension, obviously, can not.

86. (a) An extract from the seeds
    (d) of *Salvia sclaera*, when diluted, reacts strongly with Tn red cells and does not react with T-activated red cells.

87. (a) Panagglutination is fre-
    (b) quently the result of bacterial action, which causes the exposure of the T receptor.

88. (c) When bovine albumin solutions are contaminated, no cloudiness occurs because the refractive indices of bacteria and albumin are very similar. This makes it very difficult to detect bacterial contamination in these solutions.

89. (b) A satisfactory bacteriostatic agent for stored serum is sodium azide with a final concentration of 0.01 per cent.

90. (c) Leukocyte concentrates
    (d) should not be stored but should be infused as soon as possible after collection. The concentrates are only prepared by leukapheresis techniques, since the preparation of these concentrates from single units of blood would involve 30 - 50 units of fresh blood for a single infusion.

91. (b) Frozen red blood cells which are prepared in high concentration glycerol must be stored at -65°C or lower and preferably at -80°C.

92. (d) A full donation (450± 45 ml plus up to 30 ml for processing tubes) may be taken from otherwise eligible donors weighing 50 kg or more.

93. (b) Autologous blood may
    (c) be used to provide blood to patients of extremely rare blood type or to provide blood to patients with unexpected antibodies for whom compatible blood cannot be found.

94. (a) Stillbirth, spontaneous
    (b) miscarriage, amniocen-
    (c) tesis and the manual

(d) removal of the placenta
can all increase the
risk of feto-maternal
hemorrhage.

95. (a) In all cases of hemolytic
(b) disease of the newborn,
(c) exchange transfusion is
(d) performed on the baby to
lower the serum bili-
rubin concentration, to
remove the baby's red
cells which have been
sensitized with anti-
body, to provide sub-
stitute compatible red
cells with adequate
oxygen-carrying capacity
and to reduce the amount
of irregular antibody
in the baby.

96. (b) Antibodies which are
directed against an in-
dividual's own tissues
are known as autoanti-
bodies. Alloantibodies
(choice a), also some-
times known as isoanti-
bodies (choice c), are
those which are produced
in response to stimulation
by antigens from another
of the same species, and
xenoantibodies (choice d)
are antibodies which are
directed against the red
cells of many different
species (also known as
heterophile antibodies).

97. (d) The Donath-Landsteiner
antibody commonly has
the specificity anti-P.

98. (a) The frequency of febrile
reactions to blood trans-
fusion in patients with
leukocyte antibodies is
greater than 50 per cent.

(NOTE: If the leuko-
agglutination and lympho-
cytotoxicity tests are
employed in all cases,
the incidence of febrile
reactions in these pa-
tients would probably
reveal itself to be
much higher than 50 per
cent.)

99. (d) HLA antigen typing has
proven useful in organ
transplantation, as an
aid in the differential
diagnosis of certain
disease states and in
parentage disputes.

100. (d) The genes of the Xg
blood group system
are carried on the X
chromosome.

101. (b) To be categorized as
(c) a 'low-frequency' anti-
(d) gen, the antigen in
question must be a dom-
inant character; it
must be defined by a
specific antibody, and
it must be extant. The
antigen must have a fre-
quency of not more than
1 in 400 in the general
population.

102. (d) That part of the I antigen which is developed
after the first eighteen
months of life is known
as I^D (D = developed).
I^F (F = fetal) refers
to that part of the I
antigen which is pres-
ent in fetal red cells
and in the red cells of
i-adults. I-cord is
the antigen that reacts
very weakly with power-

ful anti-I on cord red cells and I^T (T = transitional) is an antigen which is powerful on cord red cells, weaker on normal adult red cells and weaker still on adult i red cells.

103. (a) Anti-I is contained by most normal sera. The antibody is usually non-red-cell-immune.

104. (a) The P_1 antigen is inherited as a dominant mendelian character.

105. (b) In paroxysmal cold hemoglobinuria, the patient's serum contains an antibody which classically has anti-P specificity.

106. (b) Anti-M is usually IgG (though IgM examples are also frequently found). The antibody occurs more commonly in infants than in adults, and it fails to react with enzyme-treated red cells. Anti-M is not found in an extract of the seeds of *Ulex europaeus* - that lectin has anti-H specificity.

107. (c) The MNSs blood group
(d) system was discovered through the injection of human red cells into rabbits with subsequent absorption of the resulting rabbit serum which was then tested against other human red cells. As a result of this work the M, N and P antigens were discovered.

108. (b) Anti-Lu^a has not been clearly incriminated as a cause of hemolytic disease of the newborn or of hemolytic transfusion reaction.

109. (b) Anti-Lu3 appears to be made by individuals of the recessive type of Lu(a-b-). The antibody is inseparable anti-Lu^a plus anti-Lu^b.

110. (a) The majority of black and white individuals are of phenotype Lu(a-b+).

111. (a) Kidd antibodies react
(b) best in the indirect
(c) antiglobulin test.
(d) They are generally enhanced by first enzyme-treating the red cells (a fact that is particularly useful in dealing with weak Kidd antibodies). They commonly show dosage effect, and they deteriorate rapidly on storage.

112. (c) The Jk^a antigen is found in 77 per cent of whites.

113. (d) The Duffy locus has been assigned to chromosome number 1.

114. (a) Under the numerical nomenclature for the Duffy system, the antigen Fy^b is Fy2.

115. (b) The antibody which reacts with all red cells carrying Kell antigens is known as

anti-Ku. This antibody is generally possessed by all K_o individuals.

116. (c) Anti-K and anti-k are usually IgG.

117. (d) Rh antigens have not been detected in saliva or amniotic fluid or on platelets.

118. (a) The Rh antigens are well developed at birth.

119. (c) The most common Rh antibody formed (from the choices given) is anti-G. Anti-Rh_o(D) is, of course, the most common Rh antibody formed.

120. (a) Treatment of red cells with the enzyme papain produces clustering of the Rh antigen. It does not destroy or enhance the activity of the antigen.

121. (c) Lewis antibodies do not cause hemolytic disease of the newborn for the following reasons:

    i) They are predominantly IgM, and therefore do not cross the placenta.

    ii) Most infants type as Le(a-b-), and therefore the antibody would not attach to the infant's red cells.

122. (c) An individual whose saliva contains H substance but no Lewis

substance would be classified as saliva type nL Sec.

123. (b) The strength of anti-A and anti-B antibodies varies considerably in different individuals. The strength of these antibodies is not dependent on the immunoglobulin class of the antibodies, and while there are differences noted when comparing adult and cord samples, this is not the only source of variation.

124. (c) The difference between A_1 and A_2 is believed to be both qualitative and quantitative. While this point is still controversial, there is evidence to support both theories.

125. (b) Individuals who possess the A antigen on their red cells have anti-B in their serum (or plasma). Individuals who possess the B antigen on their red cells have anti-A in their serum (or plasma). Individuals who possess both the A and the B antigens on their red cells (group AB) have neither anti-A nor anti-B in their serum (or plasma) - and individuals who possess neither the A nor the B antigens on their red cells (group O) have both anti-A and

anti-B in their serum
(or plasma).

126. (d) The antigen-antibody
reaction *in vitro* is
affected by antibody
size, ionic strength
of the surrounding
medium and the number
of antibody molecules
present. Several other
factors also influence
the antigen-antibody
reaction.

127. (d) Heating of serum to 56°C
for 30 minutes, anti-
coagulants and storage
at 37°C for 72 hours all
destroy the action of
complement *in vitro*.

128. (c) The three subcomponents
of C1 are known as C1q,
C1r and C1s.

129. (c) The nucleus of a somatic
cell is primarily con-
cerned with body growth
and cell division.
Functions such as phag-
ocytosis and oxidative
processes are the re-
sponsibility of the cell
cytoplasm.

130. (a) A cell which is not actively dividing is said
to be in interphase.
The four main stages of
active division (both
in meiosis and mitosis)
are known as prophase,
metaphase, anaphase and
telophase.

131. (c) The position occupied
by a gene on a chromo-
some is known as the
'locus.' Genes are

coded for by three-
base sequences which
are known as 'triplets'
(or 'codons').

132. (b) The pentose sugar in
RNA is ribose; the
pentose sugar in DNA
is deoxyribose.

133. (a) After cell division,
the new cell enters
a postmitotic period
known as G_1 (or Gap$_1$)
during which there is
no DNA synthesis.
This is followed by
the 'S' period (DNA
synthesis period),
followed by a pre-
mitotic nonsynthetic
period known as G_2
(or Gap$_2$) - followed
by mitosis. This is
known as the mitotic
cycle (or 'cell cycle').

134. (d) The 'segregation' law
states that two mem-
bers of a single pair
of genes are never
found in the same
gamete, but segregate
and pass to different
gametes. The 'inde-
pendent assortment'
law is concerned with
which of a pair of
chromosomes ends up in
the sex cell - being
a matter of chance -
and the 'dependent
assortment' (unit
inheritance) law con-
cerns itself with genes
on the same chromosome
which are so close to-
gether that they are
inherited as a unit
and are said to be

'linked.'

135. (b) When the centromere of a chromosome is close to but not quite at one end, this is classified as acrocentric. Meta-centric = in the center; telocentric = at the very end; submetacentric = at some distance from the end but not quite central.

136. (d) Plasma, the liquid con-stituent of the blood, constitutes 55 - 60 per cent of the total blood volume.

137. (d) The basic precursor sub-stance of all antigens studied so far consists of two molecules of D-galactose, one molecule N-acetyl glucosamine and one molecule of N-acetyl glucosamine. L-fucose is the sugar that is attached to the terminal sugar of the precursor substance to give the molecule H specificity (among others).

138. (a) The addition of L-fucose to the terminal sugar of the precursor substance gives the molecule H specificity. See ques-tion 137.

139. (b) It is generally accepted that the lowest limit for a substance to be a good antigen is between 40,000 and 50,000 MW - though molecules with a greater molecular weight will, of course, be better antigens.

140. (b) The variable portion of the immunoglobulin molecules is thought to determine antibody specificity. Other biological functions (e.g., complement activation, etc.) are the responsibility of the constant portion of the molecule on the heavy chain. The hinge region of the molecule allows for the flexi-bility of the molecule.

141. (b) The antibody formed in the secondary response is usually IgG.

142. (d) The four ABO alleles, A_1, A_2, B and O, give rise to ten genotypes (A_1A_1, A_1A_2, A_1O, A_2A_2, A_2O, BB, BO, OO, A_1B and A_2B) and six phenotypes (A_1, A_2, B, O, A_1B and A_2B).

143. (d) The serum of individuals of group A_3 usually con-tains anti-A_1. The serum of individuals of group A_2, A_{int} and A_m usually does not con-tain anti-A_1.

144. (a) Individuals with ac-quired B antigen have normal anti-B in their serum. They secrete A and H, but no B sub-stance (if secretors). They are not always non-secretors.

145. (c) The A and B antigens are detectable long before birth - however, they are generally not fully developed at

birth. The strength
of these antigens does
not increase during
fetal life.

146. (c) Pure anti-H is found
in Bombay (O_h) indi-
viduals. It is not
found as a non-red-cell-
immune antibody in all
individuals - and it is
not found in an extract
of seeds of *Dolichos
biflorus*. While it is
true that anti-H is
found in a number of
seed extracts, only
Ulex europaeus is
commonly used in the
routine laboratory.

147. (b) In forward grouping,
anti-A, anti-B and
anti-A,B are commonly
used.

148. (a) The genes *le*, *h* and *se*
are amorphic.

149. (c) Anti-Le^a can be produced by secretors who
are Le(a-b-). Anti-Le^a
is generally not found
in Le(a-b+) individuals,
since these individuals
secrete Le^a and Le^b
substances, and the Le^a
substance therefore
neutralizes any anti-
Le^a antibody.

150. (d) Anti-Le^a has been produced in chickens, rab-
bits and goats.

151. (c) Le(a-) parents can produce Le(a-) or Le(a+)
offspring. This is due
to the interaction of
the genes *Lele*, *Hh* and
Sese. For example,

parents who are Le(a-b+)
are secretors of ABH
and therefore possess
the Se gene. If both
parents are heterozygous
for the Se gene (i.e.,
Sese), the offspring
may inherit the se
gene from both parents
and be a non-secretor
of ABH with the Lewis
phenotype Le(a+b-).

152. (a) Anti-Le^x reacts with
the same proportion
of adult and cord red
cells - a fact which
distinguishes it from
anti-Le^a plus anti-Le^b.

153. (d) The guinea-pig anti-
rhesus antibody is
known as anti-LW (after
its discoverers,
Landsteiner and Wiener).
The human antibody
that at first appeared
to be the same as the
guinea-pig antibody
retained the title anti-
Rh because so many
papers had already been
written about this
antibody that a change
seemed impractical.

154. (c) According to the Wiener
genetic theory of Rh
inheritance, there are
an infinite number of
alleles at a single
complex locus, each
determining its own
agglutinogen, which
comprise multiple fac-
tors. The genetic
theory that states
that there are three
closely linked loci
each with a primary
set of allelic genes

is that of Fisher-Race (choice a). The alleles in the Wiener nomenclature are correctly given in choice (b) with the exception of r^X, which should be r^y. The antigens named in choice (d) are the names given in the Fisher-Race nomenclature.

155. (c) The structure of the Rh antigen is maintained by surrounding lipid, which may be essential for the conformation of the determinants.

156. (a) D^u is a weak form of the D antigen, giving some but not all of the reactions of normal D. While D^u can be genetically determined, this is not always so. D^u is usually detectable in the indirect antiglobulin test only. The antigen is considered to be clinically significant.

157. (d) D^u red cells fail to react with 'genuine' saline anti-D. These cells in a recipient of blood transfusion are classified as $Rh_o(D)$-negative. There is no anti-D^u serum.

158. (c) The Rh_{null} condition may be due to an amorphic gene at the *Rh* complex locus. In the Rh_{null} condition, all Rh antigens are lacking; individuals of Rh_{null} type have abnormal red cells.

159. (d) The red cells of individuals who are Rh_{null} appear as stomatocytes and lack some membrane component. They have a reduced life span.

160. (d) Rh antibodies are capable of causing both hemolytic transfusion reactions and hemolytic disease of the newborn. They are, therefore, clinically significant.

161. (a) False negative reactions in Rh typing may be caused by a reagent antibody which recognizes only a compound antigen. The presence of a contaminating antibody in the test serum, panagglutination and polyagglutination all cause false positive reactions in Rh typing.

162. (d) The K^o gene can be considered to be an allele at the Kell locus. It produces no Kell antigens, and could be a rare allele at a Kell operator site which depresses the activity of its neighboring K, Kp and Js sites.

163. (a) In a person who is K+, Kp(a+), the k antigen is weaker than normal when it is produced by the same gene complex which is producing Kp^a.

164. (a) The antibody anti-Claas (anti-K9) is compatible with McLeod red cells. All other cells (including those of phenotype K_0) are incompatible with anti-Claas.

165. (b) The Fy^a antigen occurs in 66 per cent of whites.

166. (c) The gene Fy^x is independent of the Fy gene. It is not the white (Caucasian) equivalent of the Fy gene. It is an independent, modifying gene which affects the expression of the Fy^b gene.

167. (c) The Fy^a and Fy^b antigenic determinants are inactivated by heating the red cells to 56°C for 10 minutes. The antigens are thermolabile and do not exist naturally in a soluble form. These antigens are denatured by formaldehyde treatment.

168. (a) Anti-Fy^a and anti-Fy^b are usually IgG.

169. (b) The Fy3 antigen is unaffected by enzyme treatment of the red cells. The antigen is the product of an allele Fy^3 at the *Duffy* locus. The antigen does not react with anti-Fy^b or with anti-Fy^a.

170. (a) Anti-Fy^a and anti-Fy^b are clinically significant. Being IgG, they are capable of causing hemolytic disease of the newborn, and both antibodies have been involved in delayed hemolytic transfusion reactions.

171. (a) The phenotype Jk(a+b+)
     (c) is most common among whites - and the phenotype Jk(a+b-) is most common among blacks.

172. (b) Anti-Jk^a and anti-Jk^b
     (c) are usually IgG, but may be IgM.

173. (b) The Jk^a and Jk^b anti-
     (c) gens are well developed
     (d) at birth. They make useful anthropological markers, and, since Jk(a-b-) is a common phenotype in Polynesians, they do occur infrequently in this population group.

174. (a) Anti-Jk3 behaves as 'inseparable' anti-Jk^a plus anti-Jk^b. The antibody is known not to be cross-reacting anti-Jk^a plus anti-Jk^b. Only one example of non-red-cell-immune anti-Jk3 has been described. The antibody is only found in individuals of phenotype Jk(a-b-).

175. (d) The Lu(a-b-) phenotype is sometimes inherited as a 'recessive' character and sometimes as a 'dominant' character. The phenotype is sometimes inherited due to homozygosity for the rare allele, *Lu*.

176. (b) The allele which converts the Lu precursor substance into a form such that it is unable to affect the production of Lu antigens is called *In(Lu)*.

177. (a) Anti-Lu^b is found not uncommonly in Lu(a-b-) individuals following transfusion or pregnancy. The antibody is usually immune. While some examples of anti-Lu^b bind complement, they do not cause *in vitro* lysis.

178. (b) When typing for the Lu^b antigen, red cells of phenotype Lu(a+b+) should be used as a positive control.

179. (a) The Lu^b antigen of Lu(a-b+) cord red cells is weaker than that of adults of the same phenotype, and is also weaker than that of Lu(a+b+) cord red cells.

180. (b) Blood samples which give negative reactions with anti-U also give negative reactions with anti-S and anti-s.

181. (b) The so-called Miltenberger sub-system involves five classes of antigens, each of which give different reaction patterns.

182. (a)
     (b)
     (d) Anti-N will agglutinate M-positive red cells at temperatures of 23°C or lower. The antibody is usually non-red-cell-immune, and is found almost exclusively in S-s- individuals. While anti-N has caused hemolytic disease of the newborn, this is extremely unusual.

183. (a)
     (b)
     (d) Anti-s is usually IgG. The antibody usually reacts more strongly at low temperatures than at high temperatures. The antibody has caused both hemolytic disease of the newborn and hemolytic transfusion reactions, and is therefore clinically significant. Only some examples of the antibody bind complement.

184. (a)
     (b) Anti-M and anti-N antisera may be prepared from human or goat serum. These antisera usually react best in room temperature tests which do not involve centrifugation.

185. (c) In light of the discovery that P-negative individuals share a powerful antigen with P-positive individuals and do not lack an antigen of the P system, as was originally thought, the P-negative phenotype became known as P$_2$. The P-positive phenotype became known as P$_1$.

186. (d) The P$_1$ antigen is inhibited by the gene *In(Lu)*. The antigen occurs in a wide variety of strengths and is more common than the P$_2$ antigen.

187. (d) The immunodominant sugar
           of the P_1 antigen is D-
           galactose.

188. (a) Anti-P_1 can cause severe
           adverse transfusion re-
           actions although the
           destruction of P_1 red
           cells by anti-P_1 is
           usually described as
           'occasional.' Examples
           of anti-P_1 that sensitize
           red cells to anti-comple-
           ment should be regarded
           as clinically significant -
           other examples (the ma-
           jority) can be generally
           considered to be clini-
           cally insignificant.
           Anti-P_1 has never been
           implicated as the cause
           of hemolytic disease of
           the newborn.

189. (c) The differences between
           the I antigen on cord
           and adult red cells are
           both qualitative and
           quantitative.

190. (c) Red cells which have a
           small amount of I anti-
           gen are classified as i_2.

191. (a) I substance has been
      (b) found in saliva, human
      (c) milk, amniotic fluid
      (d) and urine. I substance
           has also been found in
           ovarian cyst fluid, hyda-
           tid cyst fluid and plasma.

192. (a) Anti-I is found as a
      (b) weak cold agglutinin in
      (c) the serum of most 'nor-
      (d) mal' individuals. It
           is usually IgM, commonly
           binds complement and is
           usually clinically in-
           significant.

193. (b) Anti-i has been found
      (d) in individuals suffer-
           ing from infectious
           mononucleosis. The
           antibody is usually a
           cold-reacting IgM
           antibody. It has not
           been described as an
           allo-antibody.

194. (c) Anti-I is clinically
      (d) significant when re-
           active at 30 - 37°C
           in vitro. The anti-
           body produces vary-
           ing degrees of red
           cell destruction *in
           vivo*, which is well
           correlated with the
           in vitro thermal range.
           Anti-I has not been
           implicated as the cause
           of hemolytic disease
           of the newborn.

195. (d) The I antigen occurs
           as a glycoprotein in
           secretions. It has
           been suggested that
           the I antigen could
           be a branched carbohy-
           drate chain attached
           at an early stage in
           the biosynthetic path-
           way of the ABO antigens.
           The I antigen develops
           during the first eight-
           een months of life.

196. (b) The Bg antigen Bg^a
           is known to correspond
           with the white cell
           antigen HLA-B7.

197. (a) Anti-Ch^a (Chido) is
      (c) neutralized by the
           plasma and serum (but
           not the saliva) of
           Ch(a+) individuals,
           and is absorbed by
           the leukocytes of

Ch(a+) individuals.
The antibody does not
reduce the survival
of Ch(a+) red cells
in vivo.

198. (b)   The antigen Rg^a (Rogers)
      (c)   is an antigen of C4
            molecules, and occurs
            in more than 95 per cent
            of whites.

199. (c)   The gene locus originally
            named MLC is now known
            as HLA-D. The loci
            originally known as LA,
            Four and AK are now known
            as HLA-A, HLA-B and HLA-C,
            respectively.

200. (b)   There is a dramatic asso-
            ciation between the white
            cell antigen HLA-B27 and
            the disease, ankylosing
            spondylitis.

201. (a)   HLA antibodies are char-
            acteristically IgG.

202. (d)   Cytotoxic HLA antibodies
            occur in approximately
            55 per cent of women
            after three pregnancies.
            The incidence of HLA
            antibodies increases
            with parity.

203. (a)   Causative antibodies in
      (c)   'warm' antibody autoimmune
      (d)   hemolytic anemia usually
            react well at 37°C and
            react as well, or better
            at 37°C than at lower
            temperatures. They are
            usually IgG.

204. (a)   Anti-K, anti-U, anti-Rh$_o$
      (b)   (D) and anti-Jk^a have
      (c)   all been associated with
      (d)   autoimmune hemolytic

anemia of the warm
antibody type.

205. (a)   When fresh serum is
            used, the complement
            components detected
            in vitro in cold anti-
            body type autoimmune
            hemolytic anemia in-
            clude C4c, C4d, C3c
            and C3d.

206. (b)   The most common anti-
            body found in cold
            type autoimmune hemo-
            lytic anemia has the
            specificity anti-I.

207. (b)   The tests used to
      (c)   detect paroxysmal
            nocturnal hemoglobinuria
            are the Ham test and
            the sucrose hemolysis
            test. The direct and
            indirect antiglobulin
            tests have no value
            in this respect.

208. (b)   The drug penicillin
            can cause a positive
            direct antiglobulin
            test and hemolytic
            anemia by the drug
            adsorption mechanism.

209. (a)   The destruction of
            red cells transfused
            to a patient with
            autoimmune hemolytic
            anemia may be greater
            than the destruction
            of the patient's own
            red cells at first,
            but eventually equalizes.

210. (a)   Immune anti-A and anti-
            B in group B and group
            A subjects, is usually
            IgG. Non-red-cell-
            immune anti-A and anti-

B in these subjects is
usually IgM.

211. (a) Routine laboratory tests
     (b) performed on the mother's
     (c) first prenatal specimen
         should include ABO group-
         ing, Rh typing and anti-
         body screening.

212. (b) While anti-Le^a and anti-
     (c) Le^b do occur relatively
         commonly during pregnancy,
         these antibodies do not
         cause hemolytic disease
         of the newborn.

213. (c) If a mother is $Rh_o(D)$-
         negative with no irreg-
         ular antibodies and tests
         on the father reveal him
         also to be $Rh_o(D)$-negative,
         hemolytic disease of the
         newborn can be discounted.
         The disease, however,
         could still occur due
         to 'other' antibodies.

214. (a) Amniocentesis is in-
     (c) dicated if a mother has
         an antiglobulin titer
         of 32 or higher for a
         significant antibody
         or if a mother has a
         history of producing
         children suffering from
         hemolytic disease of
         the newborn. Amnio-
         centesis is never indi-
         cated in cases of ABO
         hemolytic disease of
         the newborn.

215. (a) Blood used for intra-
     (d) uterine transfusion is
         normally group O $Rh_o(D)$-
         negative, and is given
         as packed red cells.

216. (a) Rh immune globulin is

     (c) given to women who
     (d) have had first tri-
         mester amniocentesis
         (if they do not already
         have anti-$Rh_o(D)$),
         women who have had an
         ectopic pregnancy,
         and women who have
         had abortions. In
         all these cases, the
         women should be $Rh_o(D)$-
         negative and should
         not possess anti-$Rh_o(D)$.

217. (b) Except in special
         circumstances and
         with the written
         consent of a physician,
         the interval between
         blood donations must
         be a minimum of eight
         weeks.

218. (a) Citrate toxicity in
         patients undergoing
         discontinuous leuka-
         pheresis or platelet-
         pheresis can be avoid-
         ed by using half-
         strength ACD-A solu-
         tion or sodium citrate.

219. (b) The procedure whereby
     (d) platelets are separ-
         ated centrifugally
         from whole blood with
         the continuous or in-
         termittent return of
         platelet-poor whole
         blood to the donor is
         known as platelet-
         pheresis (also known
         as thrombapheresis).

220. (a) It is important to
     (b) perform antibody
     (d) screening, syphilis
         testing and hepatitis
         screening on a donor's
         serum. ABO and Rh

typing are performed
using the donor's red
cells (although, of
course, ABO grouping is
confirmed using the
donor's serum).

221. (a) To be issued as whole
           blood, a unit must
           contain between 405 and
           495 ml of blood.

222. (a) In the preparation of
      (b) platelet concentrates,
      (c) the donation time should
           not exceed eight minutes,
           the units to be used must
           be kept at room tempera-
           ture at all times before
           and during platelet sepa-
           ration, and the prepara-
           tion of the concentrates
           must begin no more than
           four hours after donation.
           Note that donations from
           individuals who are tak-
           ing aspirin-containing
           compounds are NOT accept-
           able for the preparation
           of platelet concentrates.

223. (a) Leukocyte-poor red blood
      (c) cells can be stored for
           21 days at 2 - 6°C if a
           'closed' system has been
           used in preparation.
           Leukocyte-poor red blood
           cells can be prepared by
           filtration techniques.

224. (a) Stored plasma may be
      (b) prepared from the super-
      (c) natant plasma after cryo-
           precipitate preparation;
           they may be stored at
           2 - 6°C for 26 days from
           phlebotomy, or at -18°C
           for five years.

225. (b) Human serum albumin is

(c) prepared from normal
(d) human plasma by cold
     ethanol plasma frac-
     tionation. The pre-
     paration can be stored
     at room temperature
     for three years - and
     is not indicated in
     cases of chronic
     nephrosis. Note that
     human serum albumin
     should NOT be stored
     frozen.

226. (d) Cryoprecipitated anti-
           hemophilic factor is
           indicated in cases of
           von Willebrand's disease,
           disseminated intravas-
           cular coagulation, and
           for transfusional dilu-
           tion in massive trans-
           fusion.

227. (b) Isotonic saline is
           prepared by dissolving
           8.5 grams of sodium
           chloride in one liter
           of distilled water.

228. (b) Preparations of bovine
           albumin vary greatly
           in their potentiating
           effect, apparently
           depending on the polymer
           content.

229. (d) Anti-I and anti-P_1
           are enhanced in their
           reactions when enzyme-
           treated red cells are
           used. Anti-M, however,
           is weakened (or fails
           to react) with enzyme-
           treated red cells.

230. (c) The reactions of T-
      (d) activated red cells
           are strongest with
           fresh serum. T-activated

cells react better with serum containing anti-A than with those that do not. They are not agglutinated by the sera of most newborn infants - and the reactions are strongest at room temperature - they may be weak or absent at 37°C.

231. (a) Polyagglutination due
     (d) to Tn-activation is persistent rather than transient and may be found in people described as always healthy. Polyagglutination is not associated with gross infection, but rather with hematological disorders such as acquired hemolytic anemia, leukopenia and thrombocytopenia.

232. (a) Wharton's jelly is usu-
     (c) ally present in cord samples which have been collected by cutting the umbilical cord and allowing the blood to drain into the tube. The presence of Wharton's jelly may cause red cells to agglutinate spontaneously.

233. (b) Prozone phenomenon is
     (c) sometimes observed in
     (d) titration of antibodies in which the antibody apparently reacts more strongly with serum when it is *diluted* than when it is undiluted. It has been attributed to lack of proportions between antigen and antibody and/or it may be due to the use of

fresh serum containing complement. Prozone phenomenon is sometimes seen in the antiglobulin test as a result of partial neutralization of the antiglobulin reagent.

234. (d) The non-specific reactions (agglutination) of red cells caused by colloidal silica may be seen when solutions are stored in glass bottles, when tests are performed on glass slides or when solutions are stirred with a glass rod.

235. (a) Adverse reactions to transfusion have been recorded in 6.6 per cent of recipients.

236. (b) The reaction of anti-A or anti-B with their corresponding antigens *in vivo* would be an example of intravascular destruction.

237. (d) The most common signs of extravascular red cell destruction are fever and chills.

238. (a) Hemolytic transfusion
     (b) reactions can be caused
     (c) by the transfusion of
     (d) incompatible red cells to a patient whose plasma contains an antibody directed against an antigen on the transfused red cells, the injection of water into the circulation, the injection

of blood into the circulation under pressure and/or the transfusion of blood containing antibody.

239. (c) In delayed transfusion reaction, the causative antibody is generally too weak to be detected in routine crossmatching, but becomes detectable 3 - 7 days after transfusion.

240. (d) Pyrogens, contamination at the time of blood collection and/or flaws in the blood container can all cause bacteriogenic transfusion reactions.

241. (d) The reaction to circulatory overload is characterized by coughing, cyanosis and difficulty in breathing, leading to congestive heart failure.

242. (b) The amount of CPD anticoagulant in a unit of blood is 63.0 ml.

243. (c) In the auto-absorption procedure for the removal of cold auto-agglutinins from serum, pretreatment of the patient's red cells with ficin is often helpful.

244. (d) Red cells from a patient with cold hemagglutinin disease may be agglutinated by the anti-complement fraction of broad-spectrum antiglobulin reagent. The antibodies

in this reagent attach to the Fab portion of human antibodies; the reagent is not sensitive enough to detect as few as 10 - 20 antibody molecules per red cell and all batches of the reagent are not identically manufactured to ensure rigid quality control - since different manufacturers have their own manufacturing procedures.

245. (c) In the situation described, a direct antiglobulin test on the donor unit should be done first.

246. (d) In the situation described, group A $Rh_o(D)$-negative red cells should be chosen for transfusion.

247. (a) In the situation described,
     (c) treatment of the serum with 2-mercaptoethanol and the addition of saliva from an Le(a+b-) individual would help to identify any other antibodies which might be present.

248. (a) When testing blood
     (b) samples from individuals
     (c) with weak subgroups of A, the red cells may react with anti-A,B, the red cells may type as group O and the serum may contain anti-A_1. Individuals with weak subgroups of A do not have an increased incidence of immune antibodies.

249. (a) The sugar-water test is

(c) a screening test for paroxysmal nocturnal hemoglobinuria. If the test is performed on the blood of a patient who has recently been transfused, the results may be unreliable. The test does not represent a screening test for paroxysmal cold hemoglobinuria and the principle of this test is not used to prepare complement coated red cells.

250. (d) In a centrifuge, the relative centrifugal force does not depend on the diameter of the sample container.

SECTION B: HEADINGS

(1)
251. (b) Bovine albumin

252. (f) Lectin

253. (d) Proteolytic enzyme

254. (a) Isotonic saline

255. (b) Bovine albumin

256. (c) Low ionic strength solution

257. (e) Complement

258. (f) Lectin

259. (a) Isotonic saline

260. (b) Bovine albumin

261. (d) Proteolytic enzyme

262. (e) Complement

263. (d) Proteolytic enzyme

264. (d) Proteolytic enzyme

265. (b) Bovine albumin

(2)
266. (a) Anti-I

267. (c) Anti-I^T

268. (b) Anti-i

269. (c) Anti-I^T

270. (b) Anti-i

SECTION C: TRUE OR FALSE

271. False A single codon (or 'triplet') codes for one amino acid; a sequence of codons contains the code for one polypeptide.

272. False The action of ribosomes is non-specific; they produce whatever kind of protein they are directed to produce by mRNA.

273. True

274. True

275. False The injection of antibody which survives temporarily in the host is known as 'passive' immunity. Active immunity refers to antibody *produced* by the host.

276. False IgM is not transferred

across the placenta
from mother to fetus.
Only IgG is capable
of crossing the
placenta.

277. False   Treatment of IgA with
              2-mercaptoethanol
              reduces the serologi-
              cal activity of the
              immunoglobulin.

278. False   While it was origi-
              nally thought that
              the antibody formed
              initially in the pri-
              mary response was al-
              ways IgM, this finding
              is now disputed. The
              immunoglobulin that is
              formed may be influ-
              enced by the route of
              administration of the
              offending antigen.

279. True

280. False   The term 'secretor'
              refers to individuals
              who secrete ABH sub-
              stances in their saliva
              (and other body fluids).
              These individuals may
              be homozygous *or* heter-
              ozygous for the *Se*
              gene.

281. False   Anti-A$_1$ reactive be-
              low 25°C is clinically
              insignificant. It
              should be noted, how-
              ever, that if anti-A$_1$
              is reactive *above* 25°C,
              it is often clinically
              significant.

282. False   Controls should be con-
              sidered necessary for
              all tests performed in
              the blood transfusion
              laboratory. In the

case of ABO anti-
sera, controls can
either be run with
each test, or as
part of a daily
quality control pro-
gram.

283. True

284. False   Individuals who
              inherit the *le* gene
              are of phenotype
              Le(a-b-). Indivi-
              duals who are of
              phenotype Le(a-b+)
              or Le(a+b-) must
              have inherited the
              Le gene.

285. False   The *Sese* genes con-
              trol the secretion
              of ABH substances
              in saliva and in
              plasma. These genes
              have no control over
              the secretion of
              Lewis substances.

286. True

287. False   R$_1$ is made up of
              three factors: r',
              Rh$_0$ and hr".

288. False   There is no specific
              anti-D^u serum. D^u
              is a weakened form
              of the D antigen;
              it reacts in the
              antiglobulin tech-
              nique with anti-D.

289. False   The *LW* and *Rh* genes
              are inherited sep-
              arately.

290. False   The majority of Rh
              antibodies do not
              bind complement be-
              cause the antigens

are too far apart on
the membrane to allow
IgG molecules to col-
laborate with one
another.

291. True

292. True

293. False Non-red cell immune
            antibodies in the
            Kell system are ex-
            tremely rare. Most
            Kell antibodies are
            immune in nature.

294. False Anti-K is usually IgG,
            and as such can cause
            hemolytic disease of
            the newborn.

295. True

296. False The Fy^b gene is domi-
            nant, since it will
            produce the Fy^b anti-
            gen regardless of
            whether it occurs in
            the homozygous or
            heterozygous state.

297. False Only one example of
            non-red cell immune
            anti-Fy^a has been
            reported.

298. False Duffy antisera fail
            to react in the two-
            stage papain test.
            Duffy antisera react
            best in the indirect
            antiglobulin test.

299. True

300. True

301. True

302. True

303. True

304. True

305. True

306. False Tests for the pres-
            ence of the Lu^a
            antigen are usually
            performed at 12 -
            15°C.

307. True

308. True

309. True

310. True

311. False While the indicator
            locus $In(Lu)$ does
            inhibit the activity
            of the P_1 antigen,
            it is not linked to
            the P locus.

312. False While it is true
            that anti-P_1 is
            frequently found
            in pregnant women
            who are of pheno-
            type P_2, this could
            not be connected
            with alloimmunization
            in pregnancy, since
            the antibody is
            usually IgM, and
            therefore does not
            cross the placenta.

313. True

314. False Anti-P_1 has not
            been implicated
            as the cause of
            hemolytic disease
            of the newborn.

315. True

316. False I inhibiting substances
have been found in
small amounts in urine.

317. True

318. True

319. True

320. True

321. False Antigens of high frequency are also known
as 'public' antigens.

322. True

323. True

324. False The take-up of antibody by the red cells
is known as *adsorption*.

325. True

326. True

327. True

328. True

329. False Any antibody which can
occur as IgG can cause
hemolytic disease of
the newborn.

330. False While the Rh form of
hemolytic disease of
the newborn does not
occur in the first
pregnancy, the ABO
form of the disease
can and often does
occur in the first
pregnancy, since anti-
A and anti-B are al-
ready present and
therefore readily
stimulated.

331. True

332. True

333. False In general, blood
or blood products
intended for auto-
logous transfusion
should not be re-
assigned for homo-
logous use.

334. False Blood products intended for autolo-
gous transfusion
should be handled
and processed as
similarly as pos-
sible to products
intended for homo-
logous use.

335. True

336. True

337. False Platelet transfusions
are seldom useful for
patients with idio-
pathic thrombocyto-
penic purpura, since
in that condition,
transfused platelets
are rapidly destroyed.

338. True

339. True

340. True

341. False Two-stage enzyme
techniques tend to
be more sensitive
than one-stage tech-
niques.

342. True

343. False When animal serum
is used as a source

of complement it *is* necessary to absorb heteroagglutinins out.

344. False   In panagglutination, all red cells are agglutinated by a given serum, often even the cells of the individual from whom the serum was derived.

345. False   Polyagglutination refers to the agglutination of a sample of red cells by many samples of serum.

346. True

347. True

348. False   The most common type of transfusion reaction is febrile (55 per cent). Shivering without recorded fever occurs in only about 14 per cent of cases.

349. True

350. True

351. False   The causative organism of syphilis survives for only 96 hours in stored blood.

352. False   The most common genotype of individuals with the phenotype DCcEe is R^1R^2.

353. True

354. True

355. False   An individual of phenotype Le(a+b-) could be homozygous or hetero-

zygous for the *Lewis* gene.

356. False   Individuals who possess the Le^a antigen (i.e., Le(a+b-)) are *nonsecretors* of ABH substances.

357. False   If an individual has a positive V.D.R.L. test, his/ her blood may be capable of transmitting syphilis, and therefore the blood from that donor may not be used for transfusion.

358. True

359. True

360. False   The 'Bombay' phenotype refers to individuals who *lack* the *H* gene.

361. False   The frequency of secretors who are of genotype *lele* is 80 per cent.

362. True

363. True

364. True

365. True

366. True

367. True

368. True

369. False   The pH of blood stored in CPD is higher than that

of blood stored in
ACD.

370.   True

SECTION D: QUESTIONS AND ANSWERS

371.   Adenine, guanine, cytocine,
       thymine.

372.   Genome.

373.   Erythrocytes (red cells),
       leukocytes (white cells),
       thrombocytes (platelets).

374.   8 - 10 days.

375.   900,000 daltons.

376.   Extravascular destruction.

377.   70 - 80 per cent.

378.   Le(a-b-).

379.   Anti-Rh$_0$(D).

380.   70 per cent.

381.   IgG.

382.   K^0

383.   Fy2.

384.   Jk^b.

385.   Mixed field.

386.   Formaldehyde-N.

387.   IgG.

388.   The Diego blood group system.

389.   Autoantibodies.

390.   "Warm" antibody type auto-

immune hemolytic anemia.

391.   8 weeks.

392.   13.5 mg/dl.

393.   Fresh frozen plasma.

394.   Factor IX complex.

395.   Rg^a antigen is weakened
       or inactivated by pro-
       teolytic enzymes.

396.   Rouleaux formation.

397.   Prozone phenomenon.

398.   Leukocyte antibodies.

399.   Elution.

400.   Six weeks.

401.   1.055.

402.   Anti-H.

403.   Alleles.

404.   Proposita.

405.   Mitosis.

406.   Nine months.

407.   Chimerism.

408.   C1, C2 and C4.

409.   The Matuhasi-Ogata phenom-
       enon.

410.   Cell-mediated immunity.

411.   Secretor.

412.   H substance.

413.   Amorphic gene.

414. Chromosome number 1.

415. Jk(a+b-).

416. Anti-Lu6.

417. Anti-N.

418. Recessive genes.

419. D-galactose.

420. Adsorption.

SECTION E: SPECIAL QUESTIONS

421.

	WIENER	FISHER-RACE	ROSENFIELD
A)	R^1R^2	CDe/cDE	Rh: 1,2,3,4,5
B)	R^1R^1	CDe/CDe	Rh: 1,2,-3,-4,5
C)	R^2R^2	cDE/cDE	Rh: 1,-2,3,4,-5
D)	rr	cde/cde	Rh: -1,-2,-3,4,5
E)	$r''r$	cdE/cde	Rh: -1,-2,3,4,5
F)	r^yr	CdE/cde	Rh: -1,2,3,4,5,
G)	$r'r$	Cde/cde	Rh: -1,2,-3,4,5,
H)	R^Or	cDe/cde	Rh: 1,-2,-3,4,5,
I)	R^2r	cDE/cde	Rh: 1,-2,3,4,5
J)	R^zR^z	CDE/CDE	Rh: 1,2,3,-4,-5

422. (A), (E), (F), (H).

423. A) Rh   F) MNSs
     B) Kell   G) P
     C) Kidd   H) Cartwright
     D) Kell   I) MNSs
     E) Kell   J) MNSs

424. Saline: Anti-M (dosage)
     Antiglobulin: Anti-Fy^a

425. Saline: Anti-Le^a plus anti-Le^b
     Enzyme: Anti-E
     Antiglobulin: Anti-C plus anti-D

HISTOPATHOLOGY

GEORGE L. MUNROE
F.I.M.L.S
Chief Technologist
Laboratory and Nuclear Medicine
York Finch General Hospital
TORONTO, ONTARIO, CANADA

QUESTIONS

SECTION A: MULTIPLE CHOICE

Select the phrase or sentence which answers the question or completes the statement. More than one answer may be correct in each case.

1. As a fixing agent formalin:
   (a) precipitates protein
   (b) penetrates rapidly
   (c) is a reducing agent
   (d) cannot be neutralized

2. As a fixing reagent ethyl alcohol:
   (a) is an oxidizing agent
   (b) precipitates protein
   (c) preserves mitochondria
   (d) is compatible with chromates

3. As a fixing agent mercuric chloride:
   (a) penetrates rapidly
   (b) does not fix chromatin
   (c) swells tissue cells
   (d) precipitates protein

4. As a fixing agent dilute acetic acid:
   (a) penetrates rapidly
   (b) preserves mitochondria
   (c) enhances nuclei
   (d) shrinks collagen fibers

5. As a fixing agent picric acid:
   (a) penetrates rapidly
   (b) is explosive when dry
   (c) forms water soluble picrates
   (d) does not preserve glycogen

6. As a fixing agent chromic acid:
   (a) is a reducing agent
   (b) should be mixed with formalin
   (c) precipitates protein
   (d) should be mixed with alcohol

7. As a fixing agent potassium dichromate:
   (a) is recommended for

myelinated nerve fibers
   (b) renders protein soluble
in water
   (c) penetrates rapidly
   (d) forms dichromate crystals
in tissues

8. As a fixing agent osmium tetroxide:
   (a) denatures fat
   (b) penetrates rapidly and
evenly
   (c) is a strong oxidizing
agent
   (d) preserves Golgi bodies

9. As a fixing agent acetone:
   (a) preserves glycogen
   (b) preserves phosphatase
and lipase
   (c) preserves fat
   (d) penetrates rapidly

10. As a micro-anatomical fixative
formol-saline:
   (a) is unsuitable for museum
specimens
   (b) is recommended for the
central nervous system
   (c) causes tissue shrinkage
   (d) does not preserve fat

11. Zenker's acetic acid fixative:
   (a) keeps well after the
addition of acetic acid
   (b) rapidly penetrates large
pieces of tissue
   (c) is not recommended for
liver and spleen
   (d) allows good staining by
trichrome methods

12. Carnoy's fluid is recommended
for:
   (a) the preservation of
chromosomes
   (b) the preservation of red
blood cells
   (c) the fixation of whole
organs
   (d) the rapid fixation of

biopsy material

13. As a fixative Bouin's fluid:
   (a) causes excessive
hardening and shrinkage
   (b) is not recommended for
trichrome methods
   (c) is ideal for fixing
kidney
   (d) preserves glycogen

14. Heidenhain's Susa fixative:
   (a) allows good elastic
staining by Weigert's
method
   (b) is intolerant
   (c) removes minute calcium
deposits from tissues
   (d) contains 95 per cent
alcohol

15. As a fixative buffered
formol-sucrose:
   (a) has a pH of 7.0
   (b) is unsuitable for
electronmicroscopy
   (c) gives best results
at 4°C on fresh tissues
   (d) does not preserve phospholipids

16. Flemming's fixative has
the following advantages:
   (a) after fixation, tissues
may be taken directly
to alcohol
   (b) large pieces of tissue
are rapidly penetrated
   (c) prepared solutions
keep well on standing
   (d) relatively small volumes are required

17. Formol-sublimate is a fixative which:
   (a) allows brilliant staining with acid dyes
   (b) swells tissues
   (c) is unsuitable for
silver impregnation
techniques

(d) does not preserve cyto-
     plasm and red blood cells

18. Helly's fluid is a fixative
    which:
    (a) contains acetic acid
    (b) contains a reducing and
         an oxidizing agent
    (c) is unsuitable for bone-
         marrow and spleen
    (d) does not impart mercury
         pigment to tissues

19. Fixation is a process which:
    (a) dehydrates tissues
    (b) is not accelerated by
         heat
    (c) prevents putrefaction
         of cells and their in-
         clusions
    (d) renders cells insensi-
         tive to hyper and
         hypotonic solutions

20. Aqueous mounting media:
    (a) have a refractive index
         higher than resinous
         media
    (b) are used for sections
         stained for fat
    (c) always contain sugars
    (d) are always used after
         metachromatic stain-
         ing
    (e) none of the above

21. Bone has the following
    features:
    (a) it does not have a
         blood supply
    (b) it does not contain
         inter-cellular material
    (c) it is classified as
         connective tissue
    (d) it does not contain
         cells
    (e) none of the above

22. Tendons consist mainly of:
    (a) elastic fibers
    (b) collagen fibers

(c) reticulin fibers
(d) muscle and cartilage
(e) none of the above

23. All of the following are
    suitable for decalcification
    except:
    (a) EDTA
    (b) nitric acid
    (c) hydrochloric acid
    (d) acetic acid
    (e) formic acid

24. All of the following are
    section adhesives except:
    (a) Apathy's gum syrup
    (b) egg albumin
    (c) gelatin
    (d) starch
    (e) Mayer's adhesive

25. The alveolar wall:
    (a) contains a basement
         membrane
    (b) is the site of gaseous exchange
    (c) contains elastic fibers
    (d) contains capillaries
    (e) all of the above

26. Tissue that cannot be immedi-
    ately fixed should be:
    (a) moistened with distilled
         water at 4°C
    (b) moistened with saline at
         4°C
    (c) kept in a freezer
    (d) kept at room temperature
    (e) placed in an air-tight
         container

27. Alcoholic picric acid bleaches:
    (a) carbon
    (b) melanin
    (c) acid formaldehyde
         hematin
    (d) mercury pigment
    (e) all of the above

28. After Zenker-formol (Helly's)
    fixation the endpoint of
    decalcification may best be

determined by:
(a) electrolysis
(b) x-rays
(c) neutralization with ammonia
(d) the chemical test
(e) probing with a needle

29. Quality control in histology includes:
(a) appropriate storage of chemicals and reagents
(b) the use of control slides for testing stains
(c) checking stained sections microscopically
(d) checks for accurate labelling
(e) all of the above

30. Celloidinization of tissue sections:
(a) involves a hardening step in absolute alcohol
(b) is not recommended for silver impregnation techniques
(c) is not recommended for glycogen demonstration
(d) renders tissues impervious to dyes
(e) utilizes cellulose nitrate

31. Xylene should be stored in:
(a) safety cans and in a well-ventilated room
(b) a dark cupboard
(c) dark bottles
(d) a cold room
(e) a refrigerator

32. Metallic impregnation of sections:
(a) is the deposition of metallic ions
(b) stains chromotropes

(c) is a physical theory of staining
(d) is the routine stain
(e) is regressive staining

33. The chemical test for the detection of calcium ions requires:
(a) potassium hydroxide and ammonium oxalate
(b) ammonium hydroxide and ammonium oxalate
(c) aluminum hydroxide and ammonium oxalate
(d) potassium hydroxide and aluminum oxalate
(e) ammonium hydroxide and calcium oxalate

34. Crypts of Lieberkuhn:
(a) are compound in structure
(b) are glands
(c) are villi
(d) produce gastric juices
(e) are found in the stomach

35. Cloudiness of an H and E section prior to cover-slipping:
(a) indicates incomplete hydration
(b) occurs because alcohol and xylol are not miscible
(c) indicates incomplete dehydration
(d) indicates the section should be mounted
(e) none of the above

36. Fixation aims to preserve:
(a) shape of cells and tissues
(b) structure of cells and tissues
(c) relationships of cells and tissues
(d) chemical constituents

of cells and tissues
(e) all of the above

37. Vacuum impregnation requires
a negative pressure of:
(a) 400 - 600 mm mercury
(b) 75 - 200 mm mercury
(c) 100 - 150 mm mercury
(d) 300 - 500 mm mercury
(e) none of the above

38. Which fixative best preserves
neutral lipids?
(a) Zenker's
(b) Buffered formalin
(c) Carnoy's
(d) Bouin's
(e) All are of equal value

39. Putrefaction in tissues causes
the following artefacts except:
(a) spaces caused by gas
bubbles
(b) distortion
(c) diffuse staining
(d) lack of cellular detail
(e) excessive shrinkage

40. Which of the following is used
in conjunction with gelatin as
a section adhesive?
(a) Methanol
(b) 10 per cent formalin
(c) Formaldehyde vapor
(d) Chloroform
(e) Ethanol

41. Ascending grades of alcohol
are used in tissue processing:
(a) to raise the refractive
index of tissues
(b) to ensure rapid dehy-
dration
(c) beginning with 95 per
cent alcohol
(d) all of the above
(e) none of the above

42. Decalcification aims to accom-
plish all of the following
except:

(a) prevent distortion
of tissue cells
(b) preserve nuclear
structures
(c) complete removal of
calcium salts
(d) separation of soft
tissues from bone
(e) prevent harmful effects
on staining reactions

43. Sections stained for fat
should be:
(a) mounted from water
in aqueous mounting
media
(b) mounted dry
(c) dehydrated, cleared
and mounted in synthetic
media
(d) dried in air and examined under oil
(e) none of the above

44. The adenohypophysis is
composed of:
(a) basophil cell groups
(b) chromophobe cell
groups
(c) acidophil cell groups
(d) all of the above
(e) none of the above

45. Lacunae are:
(a) connected to vascular
spaces
(b) small spaces with-
in bone
(c) connected to each
other by canaliculi
(d) all of the above
(e) none of the above

46. Insufficient wax impregnation results in:
(a) a hard and brittle
block
(b) a shrunken block
(c) opaque or cloudy
tissue
(d) a moist crumbling

      block
    (e) none of the above

47. Celloidinized slides are
    hardened in:
    (a) 70 per cent ethyl
        alcohol
    (b) absolute alcohol-ether
        mixture
    (c) methanol
    (d) isopropyl alcohol
    (e) acetone

48. Embedding under reduced pres-
    sure is useful for:
    (a) dense tissue
    (b) lung tissue
    (c) spleen
    (d) urgent material
    (e) all of the above

49. Chloroform is a clearing
    solution which:
    (a) causes minimal shrink-
        age in tissues
    (b) is relatively expensive
    (c) is inflammable
    (d) is recommended for
        nervous tissue
    (e) all of the above

50. The following may be used for
    dehydration except:
    (a) cellosolve
    (b) methyl alcohol
    (c) toluene
    (d) dioxane
    (e) acetone

51. Paraffin wax solvents include:
    (a) carbon tetrachloride
    (b) petroleum ether
    (c) carbon bisulfide
    (d) all of the above
    (e) none of the above

52. Mayer's egg albumin adhesive
    contains the following:
    (a) gelatin
    (b) serum
    (c) egg yolk

    (d) dilute ethanol
    (e) none of the above

53. Islets of Langerhans are
    found in:
    (a) the liver
    (b) the spleen
    (c) the stomach
    (d) the pancreas
    (e) the thyroid

54. Skeletal muscle:
    (a) contains regularly
        arranged myofibrils
    (b) is voluntary
    (c) is striated
    (d) does not branch
    (e) all of the above

55. The following apply to
    tissue cassettes except:
    (a) they must be perfor-
        ated
    (b) they must be insoluble
        in processing solvents
    (c) they must be miscible
        with wax
    (d) they must have tight
        fitting closures
    (e) they may be disposable

56. Calcified tissue may be
    satisfactorily decalcified:
    (a) using x-rays
    (b) by chelating agents
    (c) by hypnotics
    (d) by sulphuric acid
    (e) none of the above

57. A cryostat:
    (a) does not require
        decontamination
    (b) is a refrigerated
        cabinet housing a
        microtome
    (c) may be autoclaved
    (d) sections unfixed
        material only
    (e) all of the above

58. The following agents are

flammable except:
- (a) benzene
- (b) carbon tetrachloride
- (c) liquid paraffin
- (d) toluene
- (e) xylene

59. CH_3COOH is:
- (a) acetic acid
- (b) nitric acid
- (c) picric acid
- (d) ethyl alcohol
- (e) glutaraldehyde

60. Quenching:
- (a) destroys tissue enzymes
- (b) is a substitute for chemical fixation
- (c) is necessary for all cryostat sections
- (d) is required for electron-microscopy
- (e) requires the use of heat

61. The rate of fixation may be increased by:
- (a) negative pressure
- (b) volume of fixative
- (c) agitation
- (d) heat
- (e) all of the above

62. Patchy staining is the result of:
- (a) incomplete hydration
- (b) insufficient exposure to stains
- (c) insufficient washing stages
- (d) slides stuck together
- (e) all of the above

63. Foreign tissue artefacts may be derived from:
- (a) the water bath
- (b) the tissue cassettes
- (c) the embedding forceps
- (d) the fingers
- (e) all of the above

64. CCL_3COOH is:
- (a) formic acid
- (b) methyl alcohol
- (c) trichloracetic acid
- (d) formaldehyde
- (e) chloroform

65. A stained cryostat section for rapid diagnosis should be available:
- (a) within one hour
- (b) the next day
- (c) within four hours
- (d) within thirty minutes
- (e) within fifteen minutes

66. Perfusion fixation of a brain involves:
- (a) fixation in a refrig-erator
- (b) injection of fixative through the basilar and cerebral arteries
- (c) fixation under increased pressure
- (d) complete immersion in fixative
- (e) fixation under reduced pressure

67. Serial sectioning:
- (a) is routine paraffin sectioning
- (b) involves picking-up alternate sections from a ribbon
- (c) aids in assessing malignancy in biopsies
- (d) all of the above
- (e) none of the above

68. Mercuric chloride has the following characteristics except:
- (a) it enhances staining with acid dyes
- (b) it interferes with x-ray detection of calcium
- (c) it preserves lipids
- (d) it precipitates pro-tein
- (e) it corrodes metal

69. Sections stained with hematoxylin may be blued by the following except:
    (a) alkaline tap water
    (b) aqueous phenol
    (c) ammonia water
    (d) Scott's tap water substitute
    (e) aqueous lithium carbonate

70. A good substitute for commercial diastase is:
    (a) saline
    (b) chloroform
    (c) potassium permanganate
    (d) human saliva
    (e) urea

71. The predominant component of a normal thyroid gland is:
    (a) colloid
    (b) mucin
    (c) lipid
    (d) cartilage
    (e) collagen

72. Areas of tissue in a block not present in sections may be the result of:
    (a) insufficient clearance angle
    (b) wax too hard
    (c) incomplete tissue impregnation
    (d) a blunt knife
    (e) faulty microtome mechanism

73. Alcoholic iodine removes:
    (a) formalin pigment
    (b) mercury pigment
    (c) dichromate crystals
    (d) melanin
    (e) bile pigment

74. Which of the following is not used with a compound microscope?
    (a) Revolving nosepiece
    (b) Eyepiece lens
    (c) Iris diaphragm
    (d) Electromagnetic lens
    (e) Oil immersion objective

75. The distance between the outer objective lens and the top of the object is:
    (a) the numerical aperture
    (b) the working distance
    (c) the depth of field
    (d) the focal length
    (e) the object-to-image ratio

76. Oxytocin is a secretion of the:
    (a) thyroid
    (b) neurohypophysis
    (c) kidney
    (d) pancreas
    (e) uterus

77. Which of the following are located in the submucosa of the duodenum?
    (a) Brunner's glands
    (b) Microglia
    (c) Rugae
    (d) Astrocytes
    (e) Bowman's capsule

78. The primary function of adipose connective tissue is:
    (a) storage
    (b) support
    (c) protection
    (d) defence
    (e) absorption

79. All of the following tissue elements exhibit basophilia except:
    (a) collagen
    (b) DNA
    (c) nuclei
    (d) mucin
    (e) cartilage matrix

80. The plasmalemma or cell membrane contains:

(a) phospholipid and carbo-
    hydrate
(b) protein and carbohy-
    drate
(c) phospholipid, protein
    and carbohydrate
(d) protein
(e) phospholipid

81. The following are found in
    the small intestine except:
    (a) paneth cells
    (b) argentaffin cells
    (c) Kupffer cells
    (d) goblet cells
    (e) Peyer's patches

82. The trachea contains all of
    the following except:
    (a) cartilage
    (b) elastic fibers
    (c) fibroconnective tissue
    (d) nerves
    (e) striated muscle fibers

83. A sarcomere is the linear
    unit of a myofibril between:
    (a) the I to I band
    (b) the A band to Z line
    (c) the A to A band
    (d) the Z to Z line
    (e) the H to A band

84. For routine automatic tissue
    processing:
    (a) the first bath is always
        alcohol
    (b) wax baths are never
        completely changed
    (c) all dehydrating baths
        must be changed daily
    (d) the last dehydrating
        bath must be changed
        frequently
    (e) the first clearing bath
        is changed to become
        the last clearing bath
        each day

85. Successful staining of micro-
    organisms is most dependent

on:
    (a) critical timing of
        differentiation
    (b) correct counterstain-
        ing
    (c) intact cell wall
    (d) dye purity
    (e) stain concentration

86. Acid alcohol when used as
    a differentiator for alum
    hematoxylin:
    (a) dissolves the dye
    (b) alters the lake com-
        plex
    (c) dissolves the mordant
    (d) splits the lake from
        the tissue
    (e) splits the dye from
        the lake

87. The component in Zenker's
    fixative which necessitates
    washing tissues in running
    water is:
    (a) formalin
    (b) potassium dichromate
    (c) mercuric chloride
    (d) sodium sulphate
    (e) acetic acid

88. Which part of the rotary
    microtome initiates the
    advance mechanism?
    (a) The clearance setting
    (b) The micrometer screw
    (c) The drive wheel
    (d) The ratchet
    (e) The pawl

89. As a general rule, a clear-
    ing agent must be:
    (a) non-flammable
    (b) chloroform
    (c) miscible with alcohol
        and wax
    (d) non-toxic
    (e) miscible with water
        and wax

90. How many milliliters of

stock solution are required
in order to prepare 60 mls of
4 per cent silver nitrate
from a stock solution of 15
per cent silver nitrate?
- (a) 16 ml
- (b) 30 ml
- (c) 12 ml
- (d) 20 ml
- (e) 24 ml

91. In trimming a block using a
    rotary microtome:
    - (a) the block does not
      advance a specific
      number of microns
    - (b) the main rotary wheel
      is used to raise and
      lower the block
    - (c) the coarse advancement
      wheel is used
    - (d) the pawl does not con-
      nect with the ratchet
      wheel
    - (e) all of the above

92. The lateral lobes of the
    thyroid gland are located:
    - (a) anterior to the
      larynx
    - (b) posterior to the
      larynx
    - (c) posterior to the
      esophagus
    - (d) anterior to the
      esophagus
    - (e) superior to the
      larynx

93. Proper dehydration of a piece
    of tissue 5 mm thick:
    - (a) is complete after 60
      minutes
    - (b) takes at least three
      hours
    - (c) is required for frozen
      sections
    - (d) requires the use of
      heat
    - (e) requires the use of
      chloroform

94. A hormone is:
    - (a) a complex chemical
      substance released
      through epithelial
      cells affecting distant
      tissues and organs
    - (b) a complex chemical
      substance released
      into the blood affect-
      ing distant tissues
      and organs
    - (c) any complex chemical
      substance
    - (d) DNA
    - (e) RNA

95. How much water must be
    added to 200 ml of formal-
    dehyde reagent to make a 10
    per cent formalin solution:
    - (a) 1500 ml
    - (b) 800 ml
    - (c) 1800 ml
    - (d) 2000 ml
    - (e) 5000 ml

96. Iodine is added to dehy-
    drating baths:
    - (a) to remove mercury
      pigment
    - (b) to mordant tissues
    - (c) to give color to
      tissues
    - (d) to remove formalin
      pigment
    - (e) to remove chrome
      pigment

97. The portal vein runs from
    the:
    - (a) stomach to the liver
    - (b) liver to the stomach
    - (c) heart to the liver
    - (d) liver to the heart
    - (e) gut to the liver

98. In polaroid microscopy:
    - (a) the specimen is
      illuminated by linear
      polarized light
    - (b) a polarizing filter

is placed below the
specimen
(c) a polarizing filter is
placed between the
objective and the eye
(d) all of the above
(e) none of the above

99. If the drive wheel on an AO
rotary microtome is rotated
in the wrong direction during
sectioning the part most
severely damaged is likely to
be:
(a) the ratchet wheel
(b) the pawl
(c) the micrometer screw
(d) the advance spring
(e) the drive wheel

100. Glucagon is a secretion of
the:
(a) pancreas
(b) parathyroid
(c) ovary
(d) pituitary
(e) liver

101. Gooding and Stewart's decalcifying fluid contains:
(a) hydrochloric acid
(b) nitric acid
(c) acetic acid
(d) citric acid
(e) formic acid

102. When adjacent CHOH groups in
tissue are oxidized with HlO_4
the end-product is:
(a) alkyl amino groups
(b) glycol groups
(c) carboxyl groups
(d) hydroxyl groups
(e) aldehyde groups

103. Alcohol may be employed as
follows:
(a) to harden cellulose
nitrate
(b) as a fixative

(c) as a dehydrating
agent
(d) as a solvent for
hematoxylin
(e) all of the above

104. The lamina propria of the
small intestine is part
of the:
(a) serosa
(b   adventitia
(c) muscularis mucosa
(d) submucosa
(e) mucous membrane

105. The formation of nitrous
acid in nitric acid decalcifying fluid is prevented
by the addition of:
(a) diastase
(b) sodium bicarbonate
(c) urea
(d) formalin
(e) 10 gm of sodium
chloride

106. In paraffin sectioning the
use of dilute alcohol in
floating-out sections:
(a) allows scores to be
observed
(b) aims to remove creases
(c) completes dehydration
(d) prevents the formation
of bubbles under the
section
(e) aids in assessing
section thickness

107. A dye appears colored because:
(a) it absorbs and transmits light
(b) it refracts light
(c) it transmits light
(d) it emits light
(e) it reflects light

108. You are required to prepare 80 ml of 5 per cent

ferric chloride from a stock solution of 20 per cent ferric chloride; how much stock solution and water would you use?
(a) 20 ml stock and 60 ml water
(b) 25 ml stock and 55 ml water
(c) 10 ml stock and 70 ml water
(d) 5 ml stock and 75 ml water
(e) None of the above

109. A blue substage filter used in light microscopy:
(a) enhances trichrome staining
(b) reduces the intensity of illumination
(c) polarizes light
(d) filters ultraviolet light
(e) increases the intensity of illumination

110. Gross examination of tissue specimens requires the following recorded information:
(a) weight
(b) color
(c) consistency
(d) dimensions
(e) all of the above

111. In sharpening a microtome knife the following are always necessary:
(a) abrasive powder
(b) oil
(c) a glass plate
(d) a strop
(e) none of the above

112. Apochromatic lenses correct for chromatic aberration of:
(a) 7 colors
(b) 4 colors
(c) 6 colors
(d) 3 colors
(e) 2 colors

113. Labels which accompany tissues during processing should be marked with:
(a) a ball point pen
(b) a felt tipped pen
(c) a lead pencil
(d) Lugol's iodine
(e) it does not matter

114. The numerical aperture of an objective:
(a) affects the ability of a microscope to resolve
(b) is n X sin u
(c) affects depth of focus
(d) affects flatness of field
(e) all of the above

115. Routine paraffin sections are cut at a thickness of 5 microns; this is equal to:
(a) 0.05 mm
(b) 0.5 mm
(c) 0.005 cm
(d) 0.005 mm
(e) 0.5 cm

116. Alcoholic iodine may be used to remove:
(a) melanin
(b) hemosiderin
(c) mercury pigment
(d) formalin pigment
(e) none of the above

117. In regressive staining the following may be used:
(a) mordants
(b) oxidizing agents
(c) acids
(d) simple solubility
(e) all of the above

118. The dye component of
aldehyde fuchsin is:
  (a) carbol fuchsin
  (b) acid fuchsin
  (c) basic fuchsin
  (d) hematoxylin
  (e) paraldehyde

119. A chromogen:
  (a) is an azo coupling
  (b) is a dye
  (c) has ionizing pro-
      perties
  (d) facilitates ionic
      bonding
  (e) incorporates chromo-
      phoric groupings

120. Prussian blue is the result
of:
  (a) the reduction of ferric
      to ferrous ions
  (b) the splitting of the
      iron-protein complex
      of hemosiderin
  (c) metachromasia
  (d) the combination of ferric
      ions with potassium
      ferrocyanide
  (e) neutral red combining
      with methylene blue

121. Formalin is used in Gomori's
reticulin method as:
  (a) a sensitizer
  (b) a reducing agent
  (c) a bleaching agent
  (d) an oxidizing agent
  (e) a fixing agent

122. Diastase incubation in the
PAS stain is a control for:
  (a) neutral fats
  (b) glycogen
  (c) phospholipids
  (d) enzymes
  (e) amino acids

123. In the Masson Fontana method:
  (a) the fixing agent is
      formalin
  (b) the reducing agent
      is iodine
  (c) the toning agent is
      sodium thiosulphate
  (d) the oxidizing agent
      is potassium perman-
      ganate
  (e) the oxidizing agent
      is chromic acid

124. Oil Red O staining:
  (a) is carried out at
      37°C
  (b) is successful on
      paraffin wax sections
  (c) achieves metachromasia
  (d) accomplishes salt
      linkage between
      tissue and dye
  (e) all of the above

125. Elastic tissue may be
demonstrated by:
  (a) Weigert's resorcin
      fuchsin
  (b) Orcein
  (c) Verhoeff's stain
  (d) Gomori's aldehyde
      fuchsin
  (e) all of the above

126. The following dyes do not
belong to the triphenyl-
methane group:
  (a) aniline blue
  (b) methyl green
  (c) new fuchsin
  (d) eosin
  (e) crystal violet

127. Grocott's methanamine
silver technique:
  (a) does not require
      oxidation
  (b) is an argyrophil
      method
  (c) requires an extraneous
      reducing agent
  (d) is an induced argen-

taffin method
(e) is an argentaffin
method

128. The following are acid dyes
except:
(a) light green
(b) fast green F.C.F.
(c) eosin
(d) Biebrich scarlet
(e) crystal violet

129. A dye consisting of both
colored cations and anions
is:
(a) amphoteric
(b) basic
(c) leuco
(d) acid
(e) neutral

130. Thymol or formaldehyde added
to eosin acts as:
(a) a post fixing agent
(b) an accelerator
(c) a mordant
(d) a bacteriostatic
agent
(e) an accentuator

131. Dyes are classified according to:
(a) their chromophores
(b) their molecular formulae
(c) their auxochromes
(d) none of the above
(e) all of the above

132. The dye/mordant complex is
called:
(a) alum
(b) a clearing agent
(c) lake
(d) a chromogen
(e) a fixative

133. The following are used for
bluing hematoxylin except:
(a) lithium carbonate
(b) Scott's tap water

(c) normal saline
(d) running tap water
(e) ammonia water

134. In a routine H and E eosin
may be substituted by:
(a) saffron
(b) carmine
(c) erythrosin B
(d) safranin
(e) phenol red

135. Acetic acid added to hematoxylin will:
(a) decrease nuclear
staining
(b) enhance nuclear
staining
(c) enhance cytoplasmic
staining
(d) inactivate the stain
(e) decrease cytoplasmic
staining

136. The following groups are
auxochromes except:
(a) amine
(b) carboxyl
(c) hydroxyl
(d) sulphonic
(e) methyl

137. Indirect staining refers
to:
(a) a natural dye
(b) a dye which does
not require a mordant
(c) impregnation with
metallic salts
(d) histochemical reac-
tions
(e) none of the above

138. Attachment of mordant to
hematein:
(a) is an oxidation
procedure
(b) occurs between the
mordant and the
chromophore

(c) produces an anionic
      lake
(d) occurs at the site of
      adjacent hydroxyl
      groups
(e) none of the above

139. The following are anionic
      dyes except:
      (a) ponceau
      (b) light green
      (c) picric acid
      (d) neutral red
      (e) phloxine

140. The following methods may
      assist in the identification
      of fungi except:
      (a) auramine-rhodamine
      (b) periodic acid-
            Schiff
      (c) Grocott's methenamine
            silver
      (d) Gram's
      (e) Gomori's methenamine
            silver

141. The mordant for connective
      tissue stains in Masson's
      trichrome method
      is:
      (a) aqueous light green
      (b) chromic acid
      (c) phosphomolybdic acid
      (d) potassium permanganate
      (e) dilute acetic acid

142. In a reticulin impregnation
      method sodium thiosulphate
      is used to:
      (a) counteract the reduc-
            ing properties of
            formalin
      (b) remove all excess
            toning reagent
      (c) bleach the section
      (d) remove all unreduced
            silver salt
      (e) mordant reticulin
            fibers

143. To establish the proper
      identity of two similar
      dyes, labels should be
      checked for the following:
      (a) batch number
      (b) color index number
      (c) catalogue number
      (d) commission certi-
            fication number
      (e) none of the above

144. Weigert's Van Gieson
      method is most useful for:
      (a) adipose tissue iden-
            tification
      (b) assessing amounts of
            collagen
      (c) central nervous
            tissue
      (d) identifying fungi
      (e) renal basement
            membrane

145. In preparing Schiff's
      reagent, activated char-
      coal is used to:
      (a) break the chromogen
            of basic fuchsin
      (b) adsorb unreacted
            basic fuchsin
      (c) break the chromo-
            phore of acid
            fuchsin
      (d) adsorb non-oxidized
            acid fuchsin
      (e) absorb non-oxidized
            basic fuchsin

146. The quinoid benzene ring
      in a dye molecule is the:
      (a) auxochrome
      (b) accentuator
      (c) chromophore
      (d) chromogen
      (e) none of the above

147. The accentuator added to
      Harris's hematoxylin is:
      (a) phenol
      (b) alcohol
      (c) mercuric oxide

(d) acetic acid
(e) potassium permanganate

148. In a well differentiated
      H and E stain prior to eosin
      staining, the cell cytoplasm
      should be:
      (a) pink
      (b) blue
      (c) yellow
      (d) bluish-black
      (e) none of the above

149. To which group of dyes does
      picric acid belong?
      (a) Azo
      (b) Xanthene
      (c) Nitro
      (d) Triphenylmethane
      (e) None of the above

150. Verhoeff's elastic stain is
      prepared by adding the re-
      agents in the following se-
      quence:
      (a) hematoxylin, ferric
           chloride, iodine
      (b) iodine, ferric chloride,
           hematoxylin
      (c) hematoxylin, iodine,
           ferric chloride
      (d) ferric chloride, hema-
           toxylin, iodine
      (e) no sequence is required

151. Melanin pigment is:
      (a) bleached by iodine and
           hypo
      (b) bleached by strong
           oxidizing agents
      (c) always black
      (d) unstable
      (e) an exogenous pigment

152. Basophilia exhibited by cal-
      cium after H and E staining
      is dependent on:
      (a) a laking process
      (b) negative charges of
           calcium salts
      (c) negative charges of

      hematoxylin
      (d) simple salt linkage
      (e) none of the above

153. A well decolorized Ziehl-
      Neelsen stain prior to
      counterstaining shows:
      (a) all bacteria red,
           RBC pink
      (b) tubercle bacilli
           pink, all other
           tissue red
      (c) tubercle bacilli
           red, RBC pink, other
           tissue colorless
      (d) all bacteria red, all
           other tissue colorless
      (e) tubercle bacilli and
           RBC red, other tissue
           colorless

154. Van Gieson's solution:
      (a) stains collagen
           yellow
      (b) is used with alum
           hematoxylin
      (c) contains a basic dye
      (d) is used in Masson's
           trichrome method
      (e) none of the above

155. Post mordanting:
      (a) decreases dye binding
           sites in tissue
      (b) involves lake forma-
           tion in tissue
      (c) is used after Bouin's
           fixation
      (d) is post fixation
      (e) involves the use of
           potassium dichromate
           solution

156. The plasmal reaction requires
      the use of:
      (a) Schiff's reagent
      (b) mercuric chloride
      (c) unfixed frozen
           sections
      (d) sulphurous acid
      (e) all of the above

157. Melanin may be identified
     by:
     (a) solubility and bleach-
         ing
     (b) silver reduction
     (c) induced fluorescence
     (d) enzyme methods
     (e) all of the above

158. Weigert's iron hematoxylin
     stain contains all of the
     following except:
     (a) ferric chloride
     (b) an artificial ripening
         agent
     (c) hydrochloric acid
     (d) hematoxylin
     (e) absolute alcohol

159. The color of collagen after
     Mallory's trichrome stain-
     ing is:
     (a) orange
     (b) blue
     (c) green
     (d) red
     (e) yellow

160. Weigert's resorcin fuchsin
     best demonstrates:
     (a) tubercle bacilli
     (b) amyloid
     (c) elastic fibers
     (d) reticulin
     (e) collagen

161. Turnbull's blue is:
     (a) ferric chloride
     (b) potassium ferrocyanide
     (c) ferrous ferricyanide
     (d) ferric ferricyanide
     (e) ferric ferrocyanide

162. In the Grocott-Gomori method
     for fungi the silver solu-
     tion is used at a temperature
     of:
     (a) 60°C
     (b) room temperature
     (c) 4°C
     (d) 45°C

(e) none of the above

163. In the Ziehl-Neelsen method
     carbol fuchsin is decolorized
     by:
     (a) aqueous hydrochloric
         acid
     (b) acetone/HCl
     (c) alcohol/acetone
     (d) HCl/alcohol
     (e) alcohol

164. Dye powders should be stored
     in:
     (a) humid atmosphere
     (b) sealed plastic bags
     (c) warm atmosphere
     (d) well-lit locations
     (e) air-tight containers

165. Gram positive bacteria in
     Gram's stain are colored
     by:
     (a) natural dyes
     (b) amphoteric dyes
     (c) basic dyes
     (d) neutral dyes
     (e) acid dyes

166. Gomori's aldehyde fuchsin
     solution requires all of
     the following except:
     (a) paraldehyde
     (b) isopropyl alcohol
     (c) ripening
     (d) HCl
     (e) basic fuchsin

167. Sudan IV:
     (a) is a lysochrome
     (b) stains by adsorption
     (c) is soluble in water
     (d) stains fat black
     (e) is basic in action

168. Verhoeff's elastic stain
     is differentiated with:
     (a) acetone
     (b) 95 per cent alcohol
     (c) acid/alcohol
     (d) 2 per cent ferric

chloride
(e)   20 per cent ferric
      chloride

169.   In silver impregnation meth-
       ods for reticulin, gold
       chloride is used as:
       (a)   a toning agent
       (b)   a trapping agent
       (c)   a sensitizer
       (d)   an accentuator
       (e)   an accelerator

170.   The following dyes are anionic
       except:
       (a)   phloxine
       (b)   safranin
       (c)   eosin
       (d)   acid fuchsin
       (e)   picric acid

171.   The mordant used in Mallory's
       PTAH method is:
       (a)   potassium alum
       (b)   phosphotungstic acid
       (c)   ferric chloride
       (d)   ferric ammonium sulphate
       (e)   none of the above

172.   Which of the following is used
       to oxidize Harris's hematoxy-
       lin?
       (a)   sodium iodate
       (b)   strong sunlight
       (c)   glycerine
       (d)   potassium permanganate
       (e)   mercuric oxide

173.   The Feulgen reaction for DNA
       requires the following except:
       (a)   Schiff's reagent
       (b)   acid hydrolysis
       (c)   heat
       (d)   sulphite rinse
       (e)   fixation in Bouin's
             solution

174.   Best's carmine stain:
       (a)   demonstrates amyloid
       (b)   contains sodium chlor-
             ide

(c)   contains methyl alcohol
(d)   does not require heat
(e)   is stored at room
      temperature

175.   The following is true of
       Altman's technique for
       mitochondria except:
       (a)   heat is required
       (b)   mitochondria are
             stained yellow
       (c)   picric acid is the
             differentiator
       (d)   aniline oil is used
       (e)   a high concentra-
             tion of acid fuchsin
             is required

176.   The following is true of
       Grocott's technique for
       fungi except:
       (a)   sodium tetraborate
             affects the pH of
             the working solution
       (b)   silver is reduced by
             fungal wall aldehydes
       (c)   the oxidant is potas-
             sium permanganate
       (d)   incubation at 60°C is
             necessary
       (e)   sodium bisulphite is
             used

177.   Which of the following is
       stained most strongly with
       eosin in an H and E?
       (a)   muscle
       (b)   cartilage
       (c)   collagen
       (d)   elastic fibers
       (e)   nuclei

178.   Saffron used in Masson's
       HPS technique:
       (a)   is red
       (b)   precedes staining
             with phloxine
       (c)   is an alcoholic
             solution
       (d)   is basic in action
       (e)   stains muscle

179. An acid dye:
    (a) stains metachromatically
    (b) has a cationic dye ion
    (c) stains nuclei
    (d) has an anionic dye ion
    (e) stains only in an acid medium

180. Which structure is not demonstrated by Weigert's van Gieson method?
    (a) collagen
    (b) muscle
    (c) fibrin
    (d) red blood cells
    (e) elastin

181. An acid dye:
    (a) when dissolved has a pH below 7.0
    (b) when dissolved has a pH above 7.0
    (c) has a colored acidic molecular component
    (d) stains acid tissue components
    (e) is none of the above

182. Lipids may be demonstrated in ultra-thin sections using:
    (a) sudan black
    (b) osmium tetroxide fixation
    (c) oil red O
    (d) sudan IV
    (e) glutaraldehyde

183. The dye used in Ziehl-Neelsen's staining solution is:
    (a) basic fuchsin
    (b) methylene blue
    (c) phenolic acid fuchsin
    (d) neutral red
    (e) safranin

184. Von Kossa's technique is used to demonstrate:
    (a) calcium in tissue
    (b) hemosiderin
    (c) aldehyde groups
    (d) keratin
    (e) reticulin

185. Verhoeff's elastic tissue stain:
    (a) is regressive
    (b) is unstable
    (c) contains iodine
    (d) all of the above
    (e) none of the above

186. In Masson's trichrome technique, differentiation of collagen is accomplished by:
    (a) acetic acid
    (b) phosphomolybdic acid
    (c) hydrochloric acid
    (d) phosphotungstic acid
    (e) none of the above

187. Reticulin is demonstrated by the theory of:
    (a) leuco staining
    (b) celloidinization
    (c) metallic impregnation
    (d) toning
    (e) simple solubility

188. Ferrous iron is demonstrated by:
    (a) potassium ferrocyanide
    (b) polaroid microscopy
    (c) Turnbull's blue reaction
    (d) silver reduction
    (e) Perl's Prussian blue reaction

189. Production of a colored chemical substance in tissues using a colorless solution:
    (a) is a histochemical reaction
    (b) is metachromasia
    (c) relies on the use of a mordant
    (d) is a physical theory of staining
    (e) is vital staining

190. A quinoid benzene ring:
     (a) is found in hematein
     (b) is a chromophore
     (c) is an auxochrome
     (d) always has a positive charge
     (e) none of the above

191. The approximate solubility of picric acid in water:
     (a) is 10 per cent
     (b) is 5.5 per cent
     (c) is 1.2 per cent
     (d) is 8 per cent
     (e) is insoluble in water

192. When using oil soluble dyes it is important that:
     (a) tissues are fixed in alcohol
     (b) only cryostat sections are used
     (c) sections are mounted in resinous mountants
     (d) the working solution is filtered
     (e) sections are blotted before mounting

193. Van Gieson's solution:
     (a) contains trinitro-phenol
     (b) is a compound stain
     (c) is anionic
     (d) all of the above
     (e) none of the above

194. Ringing media are used:
     (a) in floating-out water baths
     (b) to seal the space between coverslip and slide
     (c) to assist the cutting of frozen sections
     (d) to dilute aqueous media
     (e) none of the above

195. The solvent used in the preparation of Papanicolaou's cytoplasmic stains is:
     (a) ethyl alcohol
     (b) methyl alcohol
     (c) distilled water
     (d) isopropyl alcohol
     (e) none of the above

196. With regard to enzyme histochemistry the following is true except:
     (a) oxidative enzymes hydrolyze various substrates
     (b) histochemical reactions can occur by simultaneous capture
     (c) fixation destroys most oxidative enzymes
     (d) the phosphatases are hydrolyzing enzymes
     (e) the dehydrogenases are oxidative enzymes

197. The following is true of Lendrum's phloxine tartrazine method except:
     (a) tartrazine is dissolved in 2-ethoxyethanol
     (b) the phloxine solution includes calcium chloride
     (c) Paneth cell granules are stained yellow
     (d) viral inclusions are stained red
     (e) the tartrazine solution differentiates the phloxine

198. The Golgi apparatus may be demonstrated by:
     (a) silver impregnation
     (b) osmium tetroxide
     (c) electron microscopy
     (d) all of the above
     (e) none of the above

199. True colorless leucobases:
     (a) stain by a physical theory
     (b) include Schiff's reagent

(c)   become colored by the reconstitution of their chromophores
(d)   include silver salts
(e)   none of the above

200.   Unna-Pappenheim's methyl green-pyronin technique requires:
(a)   an acetate buffer of pH 4.1
(b)   a staining temperature of 37°C
(c)   methyl green washed in chloroform
(d)   all of the above
(e)   none of the above

201.   The identification of tubercle bacilli by fluorescence requires all of the following except:
(a)   a dust-free atmosphere
(b)   heat
(c)   fluorochrome dyes
(d)   acid alcohol differentiation
(e)   polaroid discs

202.   Lipofuscins may be successfully demonstrated by the following methods except:
(a)   PAS reaction
(b)   Ziehl-Neelsen technique
(c)   leuco-patent blue method
(d)   Schmorl's ferric ferricyanide method
(e)   sudan black B method

203.   In enzyme histochemistry the following produce a colored reaction product with tissues:
(a)   diazonium salts
(b)   dyes, e.g., pararosanilin
(c)   tetrazonium salts
(d)   all of the above
(e)   none of the above

204.   Nissl granules may be success-

fully demonstrated using the following except:
(a)   pyronin
(b)   picric acid
(c)   cresyl fast violet
(d)   neutral red
(e)   gallocyanin chrome alum

205.   The results of silver techniques in neurohistology can be affected by:
(a)   concentration of reduction solutions
(b)   length of washing
(c)   variations in time
(d)   pH
(e)   all of the above

206.   Which statement does not apply to the Marchi method for degenerate myelin?
(a)   strong sunlight is a prerequisite for impregnation
(b)   impregnation takes 7 - 12 days
(c)   small blocks of tissue are recommended
(d)   the reduction product is osmium dioxide
(e)   after impregnation frozen sections give the best results

207.   Holzer's modified method for glial fibers is applicable to:
(a)   frozen sections
(b)   paraffin sections
(c)   nitrocellulose sections
(d)   all of the above
(e)   none of the above

208.   Which statement is not true of Holmes' method for axons?
(a)   silver protargol

is employed
(b) the working solution
    contains pyridine
(c) boric acid-buffered
    silver is the impreg-
    nating solution
(d) paraffin sections may
    be used
(e) hydroquinone/sodium
    sulphite is the reducer

209. Which of the following best
     demonstrates myelin?
     (a) P A S
     (b) sudan IV
     (c) luxol fast blue
     (d) Gomori's aldehyde
         fuchsin
     (e) oil red O

210. The following require the
     mandatory use of positive
     controls except:
     (a) Masson's Fontana method
     (b) Masson's trichrome method
     (c) Ziehl-Neelsen's method
     (d) Gram's stain
     (e) Grocott's methenamine
         silver technique

211. Which method does not require
     the use of picric acid?
     (a) Schmorl's method for
         bone matrix
     (b) Van Gieson's stain
     (c) Verhoeff's elastic
         stain
     (d) Altman's method for
         mitochondria
     (e) Masson's trichrome

SECTION B: TRUE OR FALSE

*Mark the following statements
either TRUE (T) or FALSE (F).*

212. Ground cytoplasm is a homo-
     geneous watery substance
     containing albumins and

globulins in colloid solution.

213. Mitochondria are minute
     spherical or rod-shaped
     bodies which lie within
     the structure of the nucleus.

214. Neutral red vacuoles are
     minute structures situated
     in the cytoplasm of live
     cells and are capable of
     absorbing neutral red prior
     to fixation.

215. Chromatin is a nucleo-
     protein which has a basic
     reaction and stains intensely
     with acid dyes.

216. Chromosomes are formed by
     the aggregation of chroma-
     tin during the process of
     mitotic cell division.

217. The normal human cell
     contains 46 chromosomes.

218. The achromatic spindle
     consists of crystallized
     protoplasm capable of
     polarization.

219. Plasmosomes and karyosomes
     are nucleoli which may be
     identified by their morpho-
     logical appearance as well
     as by histochemical stain-
     ing reactions.

220. The four successive stages
     of mitotic cell division
     are prophase, anaphase,
     telophase and metaphase.

221. Yolk is a metaplasmic
     inclusion present only in
     embryonic tissues or in ova.

222. Goblet cells have a charac-
     teristic shape, they contain

mucin and occur in bronchial epithelium.

223. Histiocytes are free cells capable of ingesting secretory granules such as microorganisms within their cytoplasm.

224. The cell membrane is impervious to pressure exerted by surrounding fluids or by the ground cytoplasm.

225. Centrioles may be found in nerve cells.

226. Lysosomes have a finely granular structure said to contain enzymes responsible for autolysis.

227. A single karyosome is found in each nucleus.

228. Because of the colloidal nature of cell protoplasm, it can revert from sol to gel and vice versa.

229. Deoxyribonucleic acid (D.N.A.) is found in the nucleoli and in the cytoplasm of cells.

230. Ribonucleic acid (R.N.A.) is also found in the nuclei of cells.

231. In mitotic cell division each daughter cell contains the same number of chromosomes as the parent cell.

232. Certain fats can be demonstrated in paraffin sections when special fixatives are used.

233. Argentaffin granules may be found in the terminal ileum (small intestine).

234. Chromaffin granules are found in the adrenal cortex.

235. Axons, dendrites, myelin, Nissl substance and nerve fibers are found in the cerebellum.

236. Basement membranes are found in the kidney and skin.

237. Collagen is found in abundance in normal lung, kidney and skin.

238. A dye is a chemical in a wet pure state used as a colorant in industry.

239. A stain is a purified chemical in solution used in the biological field.

240. Melanin can reduce ferricyanide to ferrocyanide to give a positive Schmorl's reaction.

241. Glycogen is a simple polysaccharide consisting of glucose chains and is found in liver and muscle.

242. Cytological stains demonstrate minute structures in nuclei and cytoplasm without necessarily aiding in the differentiation of the various tissue types.

243. Direct staining is facilitated by the use of a mordant.

244. To prevent formalin pigment formation in tissues, the fixing solution should be filtered before use.

245. Histopathology may be

appropriately defined as that branch of biology concerned primarily with the microscopic examination of tissues.

246. Nissl granules or substance are found in astrocytes and fibrocytes.

247. Shrinking and hardening of stored paraffin blocks is likely due to incomplete dehydration.

248. Osmium tetroxide is a fixing agent which can be used to demonstrate fat.

249. The bevel angle of a microtome knife is the same as the wedge angle.

250. The resolving power of a microscope is the highest attainable magnification.

251. Transitional epithelium is found in the bladder, ureter and renal pelvis.

252. Calcified tissues are processed in the following sequence: fixation, dehydration, decalcification, clearing, embedding, sectioning.

253. Solutions A and B of the Weigert's iron hematoxylin stain are mixed immediately before use because the mixture deteriorates after 10 minutes.

254. Dilute ferric chloride may be used as a differentiating solution in hematoxylin staining.

255. The following groups are all auxochromes: amine, hydroxyl, carboxyl, sulphonic.

256. Rays of white light passing through a lens being dispersed into their component colors is the principal cause of spherical aberration.

257. If the clearance angle of a microtome knife is too great there would be insufficient support of the bevel by the body of the knife.

258. The principal function of a clearing agent in processing tissue is to remove alcohol from tissue because alcohol is not miscible with paraffin wax.

259. Formaldehyde is a gas soluble in water to approximately 40 per cent by weight.

260. As a clearing agent chloroform is more intolerant than benzene, toluene, carbon tetrachloride and xylene.

261. Chattering in a tissue section may be the result of a nick in the knife edge.

262. Fixation of a whole organ in 10 per cent buffered formalin is best accomplished by immersing the entire organ in fixative at 4°C.

263. The cutting quality of a microtome knife can best be assessed by splitting a hair or by slicing through a piece of paper.

264. The fixative of choice for bone marrow where cytological detail is important is Zenker-acetic acid fixative.

265. The main purpose of infiltrating tissue with paraffin wax is to remove the clearing agent and to give support to the tissue during sectioning.

266. An H and E stained section may contain the following brown to black granular pigments: dichromate, carbon, mercury and acid formaldehyde hematin.

267. During sectioning the temperature of the floating-out water bath should be approximately that of the melting point of the wax being used.

268. When performing the chemical test to determine the endpoint of decalcification the addition of ammonium hydroxide is essential mainly because calcium oxalate is soluble in ammonium hydroxide.

269. Tissues prepared for examination by electronmicroscopy require fixation, dehydration, clearing and embedding.

270. Insufficient time in absolute alcohol at the beginning of the hydration procedure results in white opaque spots when the tissue section is immersed in a weaker strength alcohol.

271. Fluorochromes are quinoid dyes which have the capacity of altering ultraviolet light into visible light when combined with tissues.

272. Normal myelin is birefringent and in fresh or formalin fixed frozen sections mounted in aqueous media it will polarize with a maltese cross effect.

273. Simple lipids are esters of fatty acids and alcohols which are readily soluble in water but insoluble in acetone and ether.

274. Propylene glycol, isopropyl alcohol, 70 per cent alcohol in acetone and triethyl phosphate are solvents commonly used for dissolving oil soluble dyes.

275. Saponification is a process by which the staining reaction of simple acid mucopolysaccharides is restored by the treatment of tissue sections with N/10 potassium hydroxide.

276. Commercially supplied Nile blue has a blue and a red component. The presence of the latter may be confirmed by treating a small amount of the powder with dilute alcohol, the red component becoming immediately visible.

277. Mitochondria may be demonstrated successfully by histological methods, enzyme histochemistry and by electron microscopy.

278. In electronmicroscopy, sections of methacrylate - embedded tissue are unstable in the electron beam and are subject to sublimation.

279. Double embedding employs the use of two waxes of different melting points and aims to give support to large blocks of tissue during sectioning.

280. Osteoclasts, osteoblasts and osteocytes are marrow cells belonging to the hemopoietic system.

281. Astrocytes may be identified by protoplasmic processes arising from their cell bodies called axons and dendrites.

282. A combination of paraldehyde and basic fuchsin in a strongly acid solution has an affinity for elastic fibers, mast cell granules and certain mucins.

283. Schmorl's method stains lipofuscins dark-blue. Other reducing substances which will stain blue include intestinal argentaffin granules, melanin and tissue components with active sulphydryl groups.

284. Solochrome cyanine R.S. and eriochrome cyanine R. are synonomous dyes used to demonstrate myelin sheaths in peripheral nerves.

285. Paraffin wax sections are preferable to frozen sections for the impregnation of nerve fibers in peripheral nervous system material because it is easier to cut thicker sections, thus enabling greater lengths of fibers to be seen in each preparation.

286. Phenolic compounds such as argentaffin granules have the capacity of reducing silver solutions to metallic silver. This direct reduction can only be achieved after alcoholic fixation.

287. The Ziehl-Neelsen technique for acid-fast bacilli depends upon the resistance of certain bacilli, after staining with carbol fuchsin, to decolorization with alcohol or acids.

288. Staining with sudan black B in triethyl phosphate is of value in the rapid demonstration of normal myelin in frozen sections or teased preparations.

289. Evaporation of clearing agents, impregnation with paraffin wax and removal of trapped air in specimens occur more quickly and completely if carried out at reduced pressure.

290. A substance in tissue which carries basic groups and is incapable of altering the color of a metachromatic dye is a chromotrope.

291. Toning is a procedure used in silver impregnation techniques to remove nonspecific background precipitate.

292. Secondary fluorescence is induced in specific tissue components by interaction with flourescent dyes known as fluorochromes, e.g., acridine orange

293. All synthetic dyes are derived from coal tar.

294. Allochromasia is a selective color change shown by tissue components in a method employing two staining reactions in sequence.

295. Elastic fibers are soluble in 2 per cent acetic acid.

296. The potentially explosive nature of stored ammoniacal silver solutions is well documented. Two recommendations for avoiding explosions are (a) prepare solutions in well-silvered glassware and (b) inactivate unused solutions by adding an excess of sodium thiosulphate solution or of dilute sulphuric acid.

297. Acetone and ethanol are preferable to propylene and ethylene glycol as solvents for fat stains.

298. All natural or synthetic mounting media in routine use are soluble in xylene.

299. As a general guideline, the volume of the impregnating medium, e.g., paraffin wax, should be at least 5 times the volume of tissues.

300. Dioxane is miscible with water, alcohol, mounting media, xylol and paraffin wax.

301. The presence of glycerol in Ehrlich's acid alum hematoxylin has the effect of rapidly oxidizing the solution and of counterbalancing the destabilizing action of acetic acid.

302. Ideally, a mounting medium should have a refractive index approaching 1.518, which is the refractive index of glass.

303. In decalcification, formic acid is almost twice as fast as nitric acid; however, nitric acid provides better tissue preservation and staining.

304. Bouin's fixative is useful for bone marrow aspirations because the marrow tends to form a yellow coagulum which is easily seen in the paraffin wax block.

305. With the exception of enzyme preparations, frozen sections of fixed tissue are easier to handle and give better results than frozen sections of fresh tissue.

306. The optimum working temperature of a cryostat is -18°C - -20°C.

307. Chromate fixatives oxidize phospholipids, rendering them nonextractable by alcohols, xylene, toluene or chloroform in paraffin wax processing.

308. Alkaline fixatives precipitate and preserve mucins.

309. Glycogen is insoluble in water but soluble in absolute ethanol.

310. Alcian blue is an alcohol-soluble amphoteric dye related to water-soluble luxol fast blue.

311. The principal constituent of colloidal iron stock solution is ferric sulphate.

312. When heat is used to expedite decalcification, subsequent nuclear staining as well as staining by trichrome methods is considerably enhanced.

313. Paraffin wax sections are ideal for fluorescent antigen-antibody techniques.

314. The ideal method by which amyloid may be identified involves the use of the electron microscope.

315. Paneth cells are known to manufacture heparin and to store it in their granules.

316. Hematoidin, carbon, hemosiderin and silica are all endogenous pigments.

317. After formalin fixation enterochromaffin cells show yellow autofluorescence on exposure to ultraviolet light.

318. Ceroids are believed to be comprised of complex unsaturated fatty acids which are insoluble in fat solvents and may be demonstrated by fat stains on paraffin wax sections.

319. Asbestos bodies are beaded, yellow structures with bulbous ends which give a positive Prussian blue reaction.

320. Neurons are the specialized connective tissue of the central nervous system (C.N.S.).

321. The Feulgen reaction involves acid hydrolysis; the optimum time required is dependent on the fixative used.

322. The presence of an abundance of neurons (nerve cells) gives parts of the brain a white appearance (white matter) whereas an abundance of myelin gives the brain a grayish appearance (gray matter).

323. Nissl substance or tigroid is present in abundance in the cytoplasm of injured neurons.

324. Because of their cytoplasmic basophilia, nerve cells are well stained by such dyes as methylene blue, toluidine blue and thionine.

325. Protargol is a silver proteinate used in conjunction with copper for the demonstration of axis cylinders and neurofibrils.

326. Holzer's stain for neuroglial fibers gives enhanced results after mercury fixation.

327. Dilute ammonia water is recommended for neutralizing formaldehyde in sections of formalin-fixed nervous tissue, prior to impregnation with silver solutions.

328. Myelin is a lipoprotein as it consists of cholesterol, phospholipids and cerebroside, bound to proteins.

329. In the central nervous system the white matter is

surrounded by the gray matter.

330. The periodic acid, Schiff (PAS) method on paraffin sections as well as the Gordon and Sweet's silver impregnation method is recommended for the demonstration of brain capillaries.

331. Gitter cells or compound granular corpuscles are microglia, which act as scavenger or macrophage cells when injured brain tissue undergoes degeneration.

SECTION C: MISSING WORDS

Insert the appropriate missing word(s).

332. Soon after death, tissues begin to undergo _____ changes, which may be either putrefactive or autolytic.

333. The animal cell consists largely of _____ which may be precipitated and preserved by the action of simple fixatives.

334. _____ cell division occurs in four stages the first being prophase.

335. Ethyl alcohol is a _____ agent which should not be mixed with osmium tetroxide, chromic acid or potassium dichromate.

336. Picric acid is potentially _____ when dry.

337. The incorporation of an ion exchange resin into formic acid decalcifying solution speeds up the process of decalcification by increasing the rate of _____ of the calcium from the tissue.

338. Proof spirit is legally defined as that which at a temperature of 51°F weighs exactly twelve-thirteenth parts as an equal volume of _____ .

339. The period necessary for dehydration may be _____ by processing at 37°C instead of room temperature.

340. Clearing agents must be _____ with both alcohol and paraffin wax.

341. Clearing often causes tissue to acquire a transparent appearance. This transparency is due to the raising of the _____ .

342. Inadequate wax impregnation will result in crumbling of the _____ during sectioning.

343. During microtomy, continued movement of the operating handle causes a _____ to engage in the ratchet wheel of the feed mechanism, turning it according to a pre-set thickness.

344. A plano-concave knife is one with an upper surface which is _____ and the lower surface plane.

345. If the face of the block and the upper and lower edges are _____ to the knife edge, sections are likely to form a ribbon.

346. Carmine is a _____ dye produced by the treatment of cochineal with alum.

347. Synthetic dyes are a large group of organic compounds derived from _____ .

348. Basic stains color ___(a)___ tissue components such as nuclei. Acid stains color ___(b)___ tissue components such as cytoplasm.

349. Stained sections of cartilage, epithelial mucins, amyloid and mast cell granules are capable of exhibiting _____ .

350. Potassium hydroxide in Loeffler's methylene blue and phenol in carbol fuchsin act as _____ , increasing the intensity and selectivity of staining.

351. Certain bacteria stained with gentian violet followed by iodine resist alcohol decolorization. Iodine used in this way acts as a _____ agent.

352. Because of the potentially explosive properties of ammoniacal silver solutions they should never be exposed to strong _____ .

353. Acid mucopolysaccharides are the only large group of _____ compounds that are not strongly PAS positive.

354. Lipofuscin, melanin and hemoglobin derivatives are _____ pigments.

355. Malaria pigment is ___(a)___

and this may be sufficient to distinguish it from formalin pigment which is ___(b)___ .

356. Formalin pigment may be removed from tissue sections with a saturated alcoholic solution of _____ .

357. The classic methods for hemosiderin and inorganic iron are the ___(a)___ reaction for ferric iron and the ___(b)___ reaction for ferrous iron.

358. A brown/black pigment normally found in the skin, eye and brain which is insoluble in normal solvents except normal sodium hydroxide solution but can be bleached is _____ .

359. A fresh solution of Ehrlich's hematoxylin may be partially oxidized and used immediately by the addition of _____ .

360. Tissues from the central nervous system are particularly prone to _____ changes; therefore, prompt fixation is desirable.

361. _____ is a complex mixture of lipids combined with protein and forms a sheath around nerve fibers in the central and peripheral nervous system.

SECTION D: QUESTIONS AND ANSWERS

Give a brief answer to each question.

362. State the principle of the periodic acid, Schiff (PAS) reaction for the demonstration of glycogen.
ANSWER: _____

363. Describe reticulin.
ANSWER: _____

364. What is the objective of bleaching in the identification of melanin? How is it achieved?
ANSWER: _____

365. What is a metachromatic dye? How does it act on tissue? Give four examples of metachromatic dyes.
ANSWER: _____

366. Differentiate between progressive and regressive staining.
ANSWER: _____

367. What do you understand by the phenomenon of adsorption?
ANSWER: _____

368. What is the color index?
ANSWER: _____

369. Describe an amphoteric dye.
ANSWER: _____

370. Differentiate between hematein and hematin.
ANSWER: _____

371. Describe polychromasia in histological staining.
ANSWER: _____

372. Briefly explain selective (simple) solubility.
ANSWER: _____

373. What is endothelium?
ANSWER: _____

374. Describe pseudo-stratified columar epithelium. Where is it found?
ANSWER: _____

375. Describe transitional epithelium.
ANSWER: _____

376. Name the common sites where mucous, serous and synovial membranes are found.
ANSWER: _____

377. Describe fibrin.
ANSWER: _____

378. Describe methylation. How is it achieved?
ANSWER: _____

379. Quenching is the first stage of the freeze drying process producing three specific effects on tissue. List these effects.
ANSWER: _____

380. Give a simple definition of a micron.
ANSWER: _____

381. Describe the function of the anti-roll plate used in a cryostat.
ANSWER: _____

ANSWERS

SECTION A: MULTIPLE CHOICE

1. (c) Formalin is a reducing
         agent.

2. (b) Ethyl alcohol precipi-
         tates protein.

3. (a) Mercuric chloride pene-
         trates rapidly.

4. (a) Acetic acid penetrates
    (c) rapidly. Acetic acid
         enhances nuclei.

5. (b) Picric acid is explosive
    (c) when dry. Picric acid
         forms water soluble pic-
         rates.

6. (c) Chromic acid precipitates
         protein.

7. (a) Potassium dichromate is
    (d) recommended for myeli-
         nated nerve fibers.
         Potassium dichromate
         forms dichromate crystals

in tissues.

8. (c) Osmium tetroxide is a
    (d) strong oxidizing agent.
         Osmium tetroxide pre-
         serves Golgi bodies.

9. (b) Acetone preserves phos-
         phatase and lipase.

10. (b) Formol-saline is recom-
         mended for the central
         nervous system.

11. (d) Zenker's acetic acid
         fixative allows good
         staining by trichrome
         methods.

12. (a) Carnoy's fluid is recom-
    (d) mended for the preserva-
         tion of chromosomes.
         Carnoy's fluid is recom-
         mended for the rapid
         fixation of biopsy mate-
         rial.

13. (d) Bouin's fluid preserves

glycogen.

14. (b) Heidenhain's Susa fixa-
    (c) tive is intolerant.
        Heidenhain's Susa fixa-
        tive removes minute cal-
        cium deposits from tis-
        sues.

15. (c) Buffered formol-sucrose
        gives best results at
        4°C on fresh tissues.

16. (d) Relatively small volumes
        of Flemming's fixative
        are required.

17. (a) Formol-sublimate is a
        fixative which allows
        brilliant staining with
        acid dyes.

18. (b) Helly's fluid is a fixa-
        tive which contains a
        reducing and an oxidizing
        agent.

19. (c) Fixation prevents putre-
    (d) faction of cells and their
        inclusions. Fixation
        renders cells insensitive
        to hyper and hypotonic
        solutions.

20. (b) Aqueous mounting media
        are used for sections
        stained for fat.

21. (c) Bone is classified as
        connective tissue.

22. (b) Tendons consist mainly
        of collagen fibers.

23. (d) Acetic acid is considered
        unsuitable for decalcifi-
        cation.

24. (a) Apathy's gum syrup is
        not a section adhesive.

25. (e) The alveolar wall
        contains a basement
        membrane, elastic
        fibers and capillaries
        and is the site of
        gaseous exchange.

26. (b) It is desirable to
        fix tissue immediately.
        If it is impossible to
        do this, the tissue may
        be moistened with saline
        at 4°C for a short per-
        iod, followed by fixa-
        tion.

27. (c) Alcoholic picric acid
        bleaches acid formal-
        dehyde hematin.

28. (d) After Zenker-formol
        fixation the endpoint
        of decalcification
        may best be determined
        by the chemical test.

29. (e) All of the above.

30. (e) Celloidinization util-
        izes cellulose nitrate.

31. (a) Flammable liquids such
        as xylene should be
        stored in safety cans
        in a well-ventilated
        room.

32. (c) Metallic impregnation
        of tissues is a phys-
        ical theory of stain-
        ing.

33. (b) The chemical test for
        the detection of cal-
        cium ions requires
        the use of ammonium
        hydroxide and ammonium
        oxalate.

34. (b) Crypts of Lieberkuhn
        are glands found in

the large and small in-
testine.

35. (c) Cloudiness of an H & E
          section prior to cover-
          slipping indicates incom-
          plete dehydration.

36. (e) All of the above.

37. (d) Vacuum impregnation re-
          quires a reduced (negative)
          pressure of 300 - 500 mm
          mercury.

38. (b) Of the four fixatives
          listed, buffered formalin
          best preserves neutral
          lipids.

39. (a) Putrefaction in tissues
          does not result in spaces
          caused by gas bubbles.

40. (c) When gelatin is being used
          as a section adhesive, a
          further precaution to pre-
          vent section detachment is
          to use formaldehyde vapor.

41. (e) None of the above.

42. (d) Separation of soft tissues
          from bone.

43. (a) Sections stained for fat
          should be mounted from water
          in aqueous mounting media.

44. (d) The adenohypophysis is
          composed of all of the
          above.

45. (d) Lacunae are all of the
          above.

46. (d) Insufficient wax impreg-
          nation results in a moist
          block which tends to crum-
          ble.

47. (a) Celloidinized slides
          are hardened in 70
          per cent ethyl alcohol.

48. (e) Vacuum embedding or
          embedding under re-
          duced pressure is use-
          ful for all of the a-
          bove.

49. (e) All of the above.

50. (c) Toluene is a clearing
          agent.

51. (d) All of the above.

52. (e) None of the above.

53. (d) Islets of Langerhans
          are found in normal
          pancreas.

54. (e) All of the above.

55. (c) They must be miscible
          with wax.

56. (b) Calcified tissue may
          be satisfactorily de-
          calcified by chelating
          agents.

57. (b) A cryostat is a re-
          frigerated cabinet
          housing a microtome.

58. (b) Carbon tetrachloride is
          inflammable.

59. (a) CH_3COOH is acetic acid.

60. (b) Quenching is a substi-
          tute for chemical fix-
          ation.

61. (e) All of the above.

62. (e) All of the above.

63. (e) All of the above.

64. (c) CCL_3COOH is trichloracetic acid.

65. (e) A stained cryostat section for rapid diagnosis should be available within fifteen minutes.

66. (b) Perfusion fixation of a brain involves injection of a fixative through the basilar and cerebral arteries at their base.

67. (c) Serial sectioning aids in assessing malignancy in biopsies.

68. (c) Mercuric chloride does not preserve lipids.

69. (b) Aqueous phenol or carbolic acid is unsuitable for blueing hematoxylin.

70. (d) A good substitute for commercial diastase (as a glycogen control) is human saliva.

71. (a) The predominant component of a normal thyroid gland is colloid.

72. (c) Areas of tissue in a block not present in sections may be the result of incomplete tissue impregnation.

73. (b) Alcoholic iodine removes mercury pigment.

74. (d) Electromagnetic lens.

75. (b) The distance between the outer objective lens and the top of the object is the working distance.

76. (b) Oxytocin is a secretion of the neurohypophysis.

77. (a) Brunner's glands are submucosal glands situated in the duodenum.

78. (a) The primary function of adipose connective tissue is storage.

79. (a) Collagen.

80. (c) The plasmalemma or cell membrane contains phospholipid, protein and a small amount of carbohydrate.

81. (c) Kupffer cells line the sinusoids of the liver.

82. (e) The trachea contains smooth muscle fibers.

83. (d) A sarcomere is the linear unit of a myofibril between the Z to Z line.

84. (d) For routine automatic tissue processing the last dehydrating bath must be changed frequently.

85. (a) Successful staining of microorganisms is most dependent on critical timing of differentiation.

86. (d) Acid alcohol when used as a differentiator for alum hematoxylin splits the lake from the tissue.

87. (b) The component in Zenker's fixative which necessitates washing tissues in running water is potassium dichromate.

88. (c) The drive wheel initiates the advance mechanism of the rotary microtome.

89. (c) As a general rule, a clearing agent must be miscible with alcohol and wax.

90. (a) Calculation:

$$\frac{60 \times 4}{15} = 16 \text{ ml}$$

91. (e) All of the above.

92. (a) The lateral lobes of the thyroid gland are located anterior to the larynx.

93. (b) Proper dehydration of a piece of tissue 5 mm thick takes at least three hours.

94. (b) A hormone is a complex chemical substance released into the blood effecting distant tissues and organs.

95. (c) 200 ml of formaldehyde reagent plus 1800 ml of water is 10 per cent formalin.

96. (a) Iodine is added to dehydrating baths to remove mercury pigment.

97. (e) The portal vein runs from the gut to the liver.

98. (d) All of the above.

99. (a) If the drive wheel on an AO rotary microtome is rotated in the wrong direction during sectioning the part most severely damaged is likely to be the ratchet wheel.

100. (a) Glucagon is a secretion of the pancreas.

101. (e) Gooding and Stewart's decalcifying fluid contains formic acid.

102. (e) When adjacent CHOH groups in tissue are oxidized with $H10_4$ the end-product is aldehyde groups.

103. (e) All of the above.

104. (d) The lamina propria of the small intestine is part of the submucosa.

105. (c) The formation of nitrous acid in nitric acid decalcifying fluid is prevented by the addition of urea.

106. (b) In paraffin sectioning the use of dilute alcohol in floating-out sections aims to remove creases.

107. (a) A dye appears colored because it absorbs and transmits light.

108. (a) 20 ml stock and 60 ml water.

109. (b) A blue substage filter used in light microscopy reduces the intensity of illumination.

110. (e) All of the above.

111. (e) None of the above is always necessary.

112. (d) Apochromatic lenses correct for chromatic aberration of three colors.

113. (c) Labels which accompany tissues during processing should be marked with a lead pencil.

114. (e) All of the above.

115. (d) 5 microns = 0.005 mm.

116. (c) Alcoholic iodine may be used to remove mercury pigment.

117. (e) Mordants, oxidants, acids or simple solubility may be used in a regressive staining technique.

118. (c) Basic fuchsin is the dye component of aldehyde fuchsin.

119. (e) A chromogen incorporates chromophoric groupings.

120. (d) Prussian blue is produced by the combination of ferric ions with potassium ferrocyanide.

121. (a) Formalin acts as a sensitizer in Gomori's reticulin method.

122. (b) Diastase controls glycogen in the PAS technique.

123. (e) In the Masson Fontana method the oxidizing agent is chromic acid.

124. (a) Oil Red O staining is carried out at 37°C.

125. (e) Elastic tissue may be demonstrated by each listed method but more specifically by orcein.

126. (d) Eosin does not belong to the triphenylmethane group but to the xanthene group.

127. (d) Grocott's methenamine silver technique is an induced argentaffin method.

128. (e) Crystal violet is a basic dye.

129. (e) A dye consisting of both colored cations and anions is neutral.

130. (d) Thymol or formaldehyde added to eosin acts as a bacteriostatic agent.

131. (a) Dyes are primarily classified according to their chromophores.

132. (c) The dye/mordant complex is called lake.

133. (c) Normal saline is unsuitable for bluing hematoxylin.

134. (c) In a routine H & E eosin may be substituted by erythrosin B.

135. (b) Acetic acid added to

hematoxylin will enhance nuclear staining.

136. (e) Methyl groups are not auxochromes.

137. (e) Indirect staining requires the use of a mordant.

138. (d) Attachment of mordant to hematein occurs at the site of adjacent hydroxyl groups.

139. (d) Neutral red is not an anionic dye.

140. (a) Auramine-rhodamine is not helpful in the identification of fungi.

141. (e) In the Masson trichrome method, phosphomolybdic acid mordants connective tissue stains.

142. (d) In a reticulin impregnation method sodium thiosulphate is used to remove all unreduced silver salt.

143. (b) The color index numbers are the only reliable checks for the proper identity of dyes.

144. (b) Weigert's Van Gieson method is most useful for assessing amounts of collagen.

145. (e) In preparing Schiff's reagent, activated charcoal is used to absorb non-oxidized basic fuchsin.

146. (c) The quinoid benzene ring in a dye molecule is the chromophore.

147. (d) The accentuator added to Harris's hematoxylin is acetic acid.

148. (e) In routine H & E staining after differentiation and bluing, the cytoplasm of cells should be unstained.

149. (c) Picric acid belongs to the nitro group of dyes.

150. (a) Hematoxylin, ferric chloride, iodine.

151. (b) Melanin pigment is bleached by strong oxidizing agents.

152. (a) Basophilia of calcium deposits stained with hematoxylin and eosin is dependent on a laking process.

153. (c) A well decolorized Ziehl-Neelsen stain prior to counterstaining shows tubercle bacilli red, RBC pink, other tissue colorless.

154. (e) None of the above.

155. (e) Post mordanting involves the use of potassium dichromate solution.

156. (e) All of the above.

157. (e) All of the above.

158. (b) Weigert's iron hematoxylin is ripened naturally.

159. (b) The color of collagen after Mallory's tri-chrome staining is blue.

160. (c) Weigert's resorcin fuchsin best demonstrates elastic fibers.

161. (c) Turnbull's blue is ferrous ferricyanide.

162. (a) In the Grocott-Gomori method for fungi the silver solution is used at a temperature of 60°C.

163. (d) In the Ziehl-Neelsen method carbol-fuchsin is decolorized by HCl/alcohol.

164. (e) Dye powders should be stored in air-tight containers.

165. (c) Gram positive bacteria in Gram's stain are colored by basic dyes.

166. (b) Gomori's aldehyde fuchsin does not require isopropyl alcohol.

167. (a) Sudan IV is a lysochrome (oil soluble dye).

168. (d) Verhoeff's elastic stain is differentiated with 2 per cent ferric chloride.

169. (a) In silver impregnation methods for reticulin, gold chloride is used as a toning agent.

170. (b) Safranin.

171. (b) The mordant used in Mallory's PTAH is phosphotungstic acid.

172. (e) Mercuric oxide is used to oxidize Harris's hematoxylin.

173. (e) Fixation in Bouin's fluid is not recommended.

174. (c) Best's carmine solution contains methyl alcohol.

175. (b) In Altman's technique mitochondria are stained red.

176. (c) In Grocott's technique for fungi the oxidant is chromic acid.

177. (a) Muscle.

178. (c) Saffron used in Masson's HPS technique is an alcoholic solution.

179. (d) An acid dye has an anionic dye ion.

180. (e) Elastin.

181. (c) An acid dye has a colored acidic molecular component.

182. (b) Lipids may be demonstrated in ultra-thin sections (for electron-microscopy) using osmium tetroxide fixation.

183. (a) The dye used in Ziehl-Neelsen's staining solution is basic fuchsin.

184. (a) Von Kossa's technique is used to demonstrate calcium in tissues.

185. (d) All of the above.

186. (a) In Masson's trichrome technique, differentiation of collagen is accomplished by acetic acid.

187. (c) Reticulin is demonstrated by the theory of metallic impregnation.

188. (c) Ferrous iron is demonstrated by Turnbull's blue reaction.

189. (a) Production of a colored chemical substance in tissues using a colorless solution is a histochemical reaction, e.g., Schiff's reagent and Perl's Prussian blue reaction.

190. (a) A quinoid benzene ring is found in hematein.

191. (c) The approximate solubility of picric acid in water is 1.2 per cent.

192. (d) When using oil soluble dyes it is important that the working solution is filtered.

193. (d) All of the above.

194. (b) Ringing media are used to seal the space between coverslip and slide.

195. (a) The solvent used in the preparation of Papanicolaou's cytoplasmic stains is ethyl alcohol.

196. (a) Oxidative enzymes oxidize substrates.

197. (c) Paneth cell granules are stained red.

198. (d) All of the above.

199. (c) True colorless leucobases become colored by the reconstitution of their chromophores.

200. (d) All of the above.

201. (e) Polaroid discs are not required.

202. (c) Leuco-patent blue method demonstrates hemoglobin.

203. (d) All of the above.

204. (b) Picric acid.

205. (e) All of the above.

206. (a) Impregnation should be carried out in the dark and at room temperature.

207. (d) All of the above.

208. (a) Silver protargol is not employed in Holmes' method for axons.

209. (c) Luxol fast blue.

210. (b) Masson's trichrome method.

211. (e) Masson's trichrome.

SECTION B: TRUE OR FALSE

212. True

213. False   Mitochondria are found in cell cytoplasm.

214. True

215. False   Chromatin has an acid reaction and stains intensely with basic dyes.

216. True

217. True

218. True

219. True

220. False   The four successive stages of mitotic cell division are prophase, metaphase, anaphase and telophase.

221. True

222. True

223. True

224. False   The cell membrane is semi-permeable and is subject to the osmotic pressure of surrounding fluids and ground cytoplasm.

225. False   Centrioles are said to be absent from nerve cells. Nerve cells have lost the power of division.

226. True

227. False   There may be several karyosomes present in a single nucleus.

228. True

229. False   D.N.A. is located in the chromosomes of cell nuclei.

230. True

231. True

232. True

233. True

234. False   Chromaffin granules are found in the adrenal medulla.

235. False   These elements are found in the cerebrum.

236. True

237. True

238. False   A dye is dry and usually impure.

239. True

240. True

241. True

242. True

243. False   In direct staining a mordant is not required.

244. False   To prevent formalin pigment the fixing solution should be buffered.

245. True

246. False   Nissl granules are found in neurons.

247. True

248. True

249. False   The bevel angle is greater than the wedge angle.

250. False   Its ability to distinguish minute particles as separate entities is the resolving power of a microscope.

251. True

252. False   Calcified tissues are processed in the following sequence: fixation, decalcification, dehydration, clearing, wax infiltration, embedding, sectioning.

253. False   Solution B acts as the mordant without which solution A will fail to stain.

254. True

255. True

256. False   Spherical aberration results when rays of light entering the periphery of a lens fail to come to the same focus as those passing through the center of the lens.

257. False   The sides of the blade would interfere with sectioning.

258. True

259. True

260. False   Of the five listed clearing agents chloroform is the most tolerant.

261. False   Factors contributing to chattering may include a loose block, a loose knife, a hard tissue or a soft tissue which is cut too cold.

262. True

263. False   Sectioning a chilled block of wax and noting the absence of compression is a reliable assessment of the cutting quality of a microtome knife.

264. False   Helly's is the fixative of choice.

265. True

266. True

267. False   The temperature of the water bath should be maintained at 8 - 10°C below the melting point of the wax in use.

268. False   Ammonium hydroxide is essential because calcium salts do not precipitate in an acid medium.

269. True

270. True

271. True

272. True

273. False Simple lipids are es-
            ters of fatty acids
            and alcohols which
            are insoluble in water
            and are readily solu-
            ble in fat solvents
            such as acetone and
            ether.

274. True

275. True

276. False The presence of the
            latter may be con-
            firmed by treating
            a small amount of
            the powder with xylene,
            the red component
            becoming immediately
            visible.

277. True

278. True

279. False Double embedding is
            a procedure which
            combines the advan-
            tages of paraffin wax
            and nitrocellulose as
            embedding media and
            is designed to facil-
            itate the sectioning
            of tissues of mixed
            consistency such as
            cortical bone and
            soft tissue.

280. False These are types of
            active bone cells.

281. False Axons and dendrites
            are protoplasmic pro-
            cesses arising from
            neurons or nerve cells.

282. True

283. True

284. True

285. False The reverse is true.

286. False Alcoholic fixation
            inhibits the direct
            reduction of silver
            solutions by phenolic
            compounds except where
            an additional reducing
            substance is used in
            the silver impregnation
            technique.

287. True

288. True

289. True

290. False A chromotrope carries
            acidic groups and can
            alter the color of a
            metachromatic dye.
            Amyloid and cartilage
            are chromotropes.

291. True

292. True

293. True

294. True

295. False Elastic fibers are
            insoluble in most
            organic and inorganic
            solvents. Collagen
            is soluble in 2 per
            cent acetic acid.

296. False (a) Well-silvered
                 glassware should
                 never be used.
            (b) Inactivate unused
                 solutions by add-
                 ing an excess of
                 sodium chloride
                 solution or of
                 dilute hydro-

chloric acid.

297. False Acetone and ethanol are solvents which remove from tissues a significant portion of lipids; for this reason, propylene or ethylene glycol is the preferred solvent for fat stains.

298. True

299. False The volume of the impregnating medium should be at least 25 times the volume of tissues.

300. True

301. False Glycerol prevents overoxidation and together with acetic acid stabilizes Ehrlich's hematoxylin. It also slows the staining action and allows a gentler and more even staining.

302. True

303. False Nitric acid is almost twice as fast as formic acid, but formic acid provides better tissue preservation and staining.

304. True

305. True

306. True

307. True

308. False Mucins are readily dissolved by dilute

alkalis.

309. False Glycogen is soluble in all aqueous media and is insoluble in concentrations of alcohol greater than 70 per cent.

310. False Alcian blue is water-soluble. Luxol fast blue is alcohol-soluble. Alcian blue is amphoteric and is related to luxol fast blue.

311. False Ferric chloride is the principal constituent of colloidal iron stock solution.

312. False Heat during decalcification considerably reduces nuclear staining of tissues and impairs the effectiveness of trichrome staining.

313. False Cryostat sections of unfixed tissues give the best and most consistent results with fluorescent antigen-antibody techniques.

314. True

315. False Mast cells manufacture and store heparin.

316. False Hematoidin and hemosiderin are endogenous pigments. Carbon and silica are exogenous pigments.

317. True

318. True

319. True

320. False   Neurons are nerve cells which are supported by specialized cells and fibers known as neuroglia. The latter comprise the connective tissue of the C.N.S.

321. True

322. False   Areas of the brain where nerve cells abound have a grayish appearance (gray matter); the presence of an abundance of myelin gives to the brain a white appearance (white matter).

323. False   Nissl substance or tigroid disappears rapidly from a neuron whose cell body or axon is injured.

324. True

325. True

326. False   Mercury fixation inhibits (if not prevents) staining in the Holzer technique. Formalin fixation gives the best results.

327. True

328. True

329. False   The reverse is true.

330. True

331. True

SECTION C: MISSING WORDS

332. Post-mortem

333. Protein

334. Mitotic

335. Reducing

336. Explosive

337. Solubility

338. Distilled water

339. Reduced

340. Miscible

341. Refractive index

342. Tissue

343. Pawl

344. Hollow-ground (Concave)

345. Parallel

346. Natural

347. Benzene

348. (a) Acid
     (b) Basic

349. Metachromasia

350. Accentuators

351. Trapping

352. Sunlight

353. Carbohydrate

354. Endogenous

355. (a) Intra-cellular
     (b) Extra-cellular

356. Picric acid

357. (a) Prussian blue
      (b) Turnbull blue

358. Melanin

359. Sodium iodate

360. Autolytic

361. Myelin

SECTION D: QUESTIONS AND ANSWERS

362. The principle of the PAS
      reaction for glycogen is
      that periodic acid will
      effect an oxidative cleavage
      of the carbon to carbon bond
      in 1:2 glycols to form di-
      aldehydes. The aldehydes
      will react with fuchsin-
      sulphurous acid, which com-
      bines with the basic para-
      rosanilene to form a magenta-
      colored compound.

363. Reticulin is comprised of
      fine delicate fibers nor-
      mally found connected to
      stronger coarser fibers
      of collagen and forms the
      supporting framework of
      tissues such as liver,
      spleen and lymph nodes.
      They are practically un-
      stained by routine meth-
      ods but are PAS positive
      on frozen sections and are
      birefrigent and argyro-
      philic in metallic im-
      pregnation methods.

364. The technique of bleaching
      melanin aims to produce a
      negative result. Duplicate
      slides are prepared, one

bleached and the other
not treated. They are
both subsequently impreg-
nated with a silver solu-
tion and compared. The
bleached slide should be
negative for melanin and
the untreated slide posi-
tive. Melanin may be
bleached by using strong
oxidizing agents such as
potassium permanganate,
performic acid or hydrogen
peroxide.

365. A metachromatic dye is a
      basic stain belonging to
      the coal tar or aniline
      group. It exhibits meta-
      chromasia in its ability
      to differentiate certain
      substances by staining
      them a different color
      from that of the original
      dye. Certain tissue sub-
      stances known as chromo-
      tropes carry acidic groups
      which react with the dye.
      The negative charges on
      these chromotropes attract
      the positive polar groups
      of the dye to form dye
      polymers. These dye poly-
      mers then exhibit a shift
      of absorption towards the
      shorter wavelengths.

      Examples of metachromatic
      dyes are thionin, azur A,
      methylene blue and methyl
      violet.

366. Progressive staining attempts
      to color varying tissue ele-
      ments differentially, in a
      particular sequence, for a
      given period of time.

      In regressive staining, all
      cellular elements are simul-

taneously overstained followed by careful differentiation or decolorization to remove the stain from unwanted tissue elements.

367. Adsorption is a physical theory of staining although Bayliss (1906) used the term 'electrical theory of staining' to describe this phenomenon. Dyes have the capacity to combine with tissues by a surface phenomenon of adsorption. While the mechanism by which this combination occurs is not fully understood, one theory recently advanced suggests that a loose combination occurs between tissue components and dye molecules by means of latent valences of atoms in the surface layers. It is an established fact that dyes attached to tissue by adsorption are readily differentiated in water or in alcohol.

368. The color index is an internationally accepted nomenclature of dyes. It consists of a five digit coding system developed by a joint committee representing the Society of Dyers and Colorists in England and the American Association of Textile Chemists and Colorists.

369. Histology utilizes acid, basic, neutral or amphoteric dyes. An amphoteric dye has a point in its pH range where there is an equilibrium of positive and negative charges. This is known as the isoelectric point. A dye with amphoteric properties will be basic in action below this point and acid in action

above this point.

370. Hematein is a reddish-brown compound with a metallic luster produced by the oxidation of the natural dye hematoxylin. Hematein contains a quinoid chromophore.

Hematin is a substance resembling hemosiderin and is produced by the action of strong acids and alkalis on hemoglobin.

371. When polychrome methylene blue is applied to sections of fresh frozen tissue a variety of colors are produced. This phenomenon is known as polychromasia. Polychrome methylene blue is not a metachromatic dye but is the result of the treatment of methylene blue with an alkali with the production of a variety of colored breakdown products.

372. Selective or simple solubility is a physical process by which lipids are stained. When applied to the tissue, the dye is more soluble in the lipid than in its solvent.

373. Endothelium is a lining of simple squamous cells covering an internal surface such as the internal lining of blood vessels and lymph channels, with no access to the outside.

374. Pseudo-stratified columnar epithelium is comprised of cells whose nuclei appear at varying levels in relation to the lumen, creating

the impression that several basement membranes are present. In fact there is a single basement membrane. This type of epithelium is found lining the respiratory passages and the excretory ducts of the male reproductive system.

375. Transitional epithelium consists of a basal, intermediate and superficial layer of cells all lying on a common basement membrane. Since transitional epithelium lines the urinary system (renal pelvis to the urethra) it is subject to variations in internal pressure; therefore, its cells tend to vary in shape according to the degree of distention.

376. Mucous membranes line the alimentary, respiratory and urinogenital tracts. Serous membranes are found in the pleura, pericardium and the peritoneum. Synovial membranes line the joint cavity of bones.

377. Fibrin is an acidiophilic substance found in hemorrhagic and inflammatory areas in tissue. It can occur as a fine network, as coarser fibers or as an amorphous mass. It is derived through the blood-clotting process where fibrinogen in the presence of calcium ions is converted by thrombokinase to fibrin. It often exhibits variation in staining reaction due to the presence of a mixture of new as well as old fibrin. It is believed that during infection, the bacteriolytic effect on fibrin causes it to stain similarly to collagen.

378. Methylation is a blocking procedure used to prevent the staining reactions of simple acid and complex sulphated mucopolysaccharides. In this procedure, two serial sections are prepared. After hydration, one is treated with preheated 1 per cent hydrochloric acid in absolute methyl alcohol and the other is untreated. Both are subsequently stained with alcian blue or alcian green. The loss of positive staining in the blocked section and positive staining of the untreated section confirms the presence of simple acid and complex sulphated mucopolysaccharides.

379. Quenching has the following effects on tissue:
    (a) It arrests chemical reactions within the tissue.
    (b) It stops the diffusion of tissue constituents by bringing the tissue to a solid state.
    (c) It produces ice crystals formed by the freezing of unbound water in the tissue.

380. A micron is the standard unit of measurement in microscopy, it is equal to 0.001 mm and is expressed as u.

381. The anti-roll plate used in a cryostat prevents the natural tendency of

frozen sections to curl. By
aligning the plate parallel
to and fractionally above the
edge of the microtome knife,
suitably flat sections are
obtained. Additional pre-
requisites for successfully
sectioning frozen tissue
include the absence of damage
to the plate's upper edge and
its appropriate angle in relation to the body of the
knife.

BIBLIOGRAPHY

CHEMISTRY

1. CAMPBELL, J.B. and CAMPBELL, J.B. *Laboratory Mathematics*, 2nd Ed., The C.V. Mosby Company, Toronto, 1980

2. DAVIDSOHN, I. and HENRY, J.B. *Todd-Sanford-Davidsohn Clinical Diagnosis by Laboratory Methods*, 16th Ed., W.B. Saunders Company, Philadelphia, 1979

3. FREE, A.H. and FREE, H. *Urodynamics*, Ames Company, Elkhart, 1974

4. GORNALL, A.G. *Applied Biochemistry of Clinical Disorders*, Harper & Row, New York, 1980

5. GUYTON, A.C. *Textbook of Medical Physiology*, 5th Ed., W.B. Saunders Company, Philadelphia, 1976

6. MONTGOMERY, R., DYER, R.L., CONWAY, T.W. and SPECTOR, A.A. *Biochemistry: A Case-oriented Approach*, The C.V. Mosby Company, Toronto, 1974

7. PADMORE, G.R.A. *Elementary Calculations in Clinical Chemistry*, Churchill Livingstone, London, 1972

8. SCHWARZ, V. *A Clinical Companion to Biochemical Studies*, W.H. Freeman & Company, San Francisco, 1978

9. TIETZ, N.W. *Fundamentals of Clinical Chemistry*, 2nd Ed., W.B. Saunders Company, Philadelphia, 1976

10. WALLACH, J. *Interpretation of Diagnostic Tests*, 3rd Ed., Little, Brown & Company, Boston, 1978

11. ZILVA, J.F. and PANNELL, P.R. *Clinical Chemistry in Diagnosis and Treatment*, 3rd Ed., Lloyd-Luke Ltd., London, 1979

MICROBIOLOGY

1. BALOWS, A.(Ed.) *Diagnostic Procedures for Bacterial, Mycotic and Parasitic Infections*, 6th Ed., American Public Health Association, 1981

2. BENEKE, E.S. and ROGERS, A.L. *Medical Mycology Manual*, 4th Ed., Burgess Publishing Company, 1980

3. COWAN, S.T. (Revised by) *Cowan and Steel's Manual for the Identification of Medical Bacteria*, 2nd Ed., Cambridge University Press, 1974

4. CUMITECH PUBLICATIONS published by American Society for Microbiology

5. EDWARDS, P.R. and EWING, W.H. *Identification of Enterobacteriaceae*, 3rd Ed., Burgess Publishing Company, 1972

6. FINEGOLD, S.M. and MARTIN, W.J. *Diagnostic Microbiology*, 6th Ed., The C.V. Mosby Company, 1982

7. GILARDI, G.L. (Ed.) *Glucose Nonfermenting Gram-Negative Bacteria in Clinical Microbiology*, CRC Press Inc., 1978

8. *Laboratory Safety Manual*, 2nd Ed., Toronto Institute of Medical Technology, 1981

9. LENNETTE, E.H. (Editor in Chief) *Manual of Clinical Microbiology*, 3rd Ed., American Society for Microbiology, 1980

10. LORIAN, V. (Ed.) *Antibiotics in Laboratory Medicine*, Williams and Wilkins, 1980

11. *Manual of Methods for General Bacteriology*, 1st Ed., American Society for Microbiology, 1981

HEMATOLOGY

1. BAKER, F.T., SILVERTON, R.E. and LUCKOCK, E.D. *Introduction to Medical Laboratory Technology*, 2nd Ed., Butterworth and Company, Toronto, 1957

2. BARNETT, R.N. *Clinical Laboratory Statistics*, Little, Brown and Company, Boston, 1971

3. DACIE, J.V. and LEWIS, S.M. *Practical Haematology*, 5th Ed., Churchill and Livingstone, New York, 1975

4.   GOLDBERG, et al. *Recent Advances in Haematology*, Churchill and
     Livingstone, London, 1971

5.   HIRSH, J. BRAIN, E.A. and SKOV, K.C. *Concepts in Hemostasis and
     Thrombosis*, McMaster University, Hamilton, Canada, 1976

6.   HUTCHINSON, H.E. *An Introduction to the Haemoglobinopathies and
     the Methods used for Their Recognition*, E. Arnold Ltd., London,
     1967

7.   PLATT, W.R. *Color Atlas and Textbook of Hematology*, Lippincott,
     Philadelphia and Toronto, 1969

8.   THOMSON, J.M. *Blood Coagulation and Haemostasis*, 2nd Edition,
     Churchill and Livingstone, New York, 1980

9.   WILLIAMS, W.J., BEUTLER, E., EROLEV, A.J. and RUNDLES, R.W.
     Hematology, McGraw-Hill Company, New York and Toronto, 1972

10. WINTROBE, M.M. *Clinical Hematology*, 8th Edition, Lea and
     Febiger, Philadelphia, 1981

IMMUNOHEMATOLOGY

1.   BRYANT, N.J. *An Introduction to Immunohematology*, 2nd Ed.,
     W.B.Saunders Company, Philadelphia, 1982

2.   ERSKINE, A.G. and SOCHA, W.W. *The Principles and Practice
     of Blood Grouping*, 2nd Ed., The C.V. Mosby Company, Saint
     Louis, 1978

3.   HENRY, J.B. *Clinical Diagnosis and Management by Laboratory
     Methods*, 16th Ed., W.B.Saunders Company, Philadelphia, 1979

4.   ISSITT, P.D and ISSITT, C.H. *Applied Blood Group Serology*,
     2nd Ed., Spectra Biologicals, 1975

5.   MOLLISON, P.L. *Blood Transfusion in Clinical Medicine*, 6th Ed.,
     Blackwell Scientific Publications, Oxford, 1979

6.   RACE, R.R. and SANGER, R. *Blood Groups in Man*, 6th Ed.,
     Blackwell Scientific Publications, Oxford, 1975

7.   RAPHAEL, S.S. (Senior Author) *Lynch's Medical Laboratory
     Technology*, 4th Ed., W.B.Saunders Company, Philadelphia, 1983

8. *Technical Manual of the American Association of Blood Banks*,
    8th Ed., American Association of Blood Banks, Washington, D.C.,
    1981

9. THOMPSON, J.S. and THOMPSON, M.W. *Genetics in Medicine*, 3rd Ed.,
    W.B.Saunders Company, Philadelphia, 1980

10. ZMIJEWSKI, C.M. *Immunohematology*, 3rd Ed., Appleton-Century-
    Crofts, New York, 1978

HISTOPATHOLOGY

1. BANCROFT, J.D. and STEVENS, A. *Theory and Practice of Histological
    Techniques*, Churchill Livingstone, 1977

2. DRURY, R.A.B. and WALLINGTON, E.A. *Carleton's Histological
    Technique*, 4th Ed., Oxford University Press, 1967

3. LEESON, R.C. and LEESON, T.S. *Histology*, 4th Ed., W.B. Saunders
    Company, 1981

4. LILLIE, R.S. and FULLMER, H.M. *Histopathologic Technique and
    Practical Histochemistry*, 4th Ed., McGraw-Hill Book Company

5. RAPHAEL, S.S., *Lynch's Medical Laboratory Technology*, Vol II,
    4th Ed., W.B. Saunders Company, 1983

NOTES

335

NOTES